Global Health, Global Health Education, and Infectious Disease: The New Millennium, Part II

Guest Editor

ANVAR VELJI, MD

INFECTIOUS DISEASE CLINICS OF NORTH AMERICA

www.id.theclinics.com

Consulting Editor
ROBERT C. MOELLERING Jr, MD

September 2011 • Volume 25 • Number 3

SAUNDERS an imprint of ELSEVIER, Inc.

W.B. SAUNDERS COMPANY
A Division of Elsevier Inc.
1600 John F. Kennedy Blvd., Suite 1800, Philadelphia, PA 19103-2899.
http://www.theclinics.com
INFECTIOUS DISEASE CLINICS OF NORTH AMERICA Volume 25, Number 3
September 2011 ISSN 0891–5520, ISBN-13: 978-1-4557-1106-2

Editor: Stephanie Donley
Developmental Editor: Teia Stone

Infectious Disease Clinics of North America (ISSN 0891–5520) is published in March, June, September, and December by Elsevier Inc., 360 Park Avenue South, New York, NY 10010-1710. Periodicals postage paid at New York, NY and additional mailing offices. Subscription prices are $251.00 per year for US individuals, $435.00 per year for US institutions, $124.00 per year for US students, $297.00 per year for Canadian individuals, $538.00 per year for Canadian institutions, $355.00 per year for international individuals, $538.00 per year for international institutions, and $171.00 per year for Canadian and international students. To receive student rate, orders must be accompanied by name of affiliated institution, date of term, and the *signature* of program/residency coordinator on institution letterhead. Orders will be billed at individual rate until proof of status is received. Foreign air speed delivery is included in all *Clinics* subscription prices. All prices are subject to change without notice. **POSTMASTER:** Send address changes to *Infectious Disease Clinics of North America*, Elsevier Health Sciences Division, Subcription Customer Service, 3251 Riverport Lane, Maryland Heights, MO 63043. **Customer Service: 1-800-654-2452 (US). From outside of the US and Canada, call 1-314-447-8871. Fax: 1-314-447-8029. E-mail: JournalsCustomerService-usa@elsevier.com (print support) or JournalsOnlineSupport-usa@elsevier.com (online support).**

Infectious Disease Clinics of North America is also published in Spanish by Editorial Inter-MÅdica, Junin 917, 1er A 1113, Buenos Aires, Argentina.

Reprints. For copies of 100 or more, of articles in this publication, please contact the Commercial Reprints Department, Elsevier Inc., 360 Park Avenue South, New York, New York 10010-1710. Tel. (212) 633-3812, Fax: (212) 462-1935, E-mail: reprints@elsevier.com.

Infectious Disease Clinics of North America is covered in *MEDLINE/PubMed (Index Medicus), Current Contents/ Clinical Medicine, Science Citation Alert, SCISEARCH,* and *Research Alert.*

Printed and bound by CPI Group (UK) Ltd, Croydon, CR0 4YY

Transferred to Digital Print 2011

Contributors

CONSULTING EDITOR

ROBERT C. MOELLERING Jr, MD
Shields Warren-Mallinckrodt Professor of Medical Research, Harvard Medical School; Department of Medicine, Beth Israel Deaconess Medical Center, Boston, Massachusetts

GUEST EDITOR

ANVAR VELJI, MD, FRCP(C), FACP, FIDSA
Chief of Infectious Disease, Department of Infectious Disease, Kaiser Permanente, South Sacramento, Sacramento, California; Co-Founder, Global Health Education Consortium (GHEC); Clinical Professor, School of Medicine, University of California, Davis, California

AUTHORS

MARCELLA M. ALSAN, MD, MPH
PhD Candidate in Economics, Fellow in Infectious Diseases, Division of Infectious Diseases, Department of Economics, Brigham and Women's Hospital, Harvard University, Boston, Massachusetts; Partners In Health

SHAHELA ANWAR, MPH
Professor, Health & Family Planning Systems Programme, International Centre for Diarrhoeal Disease Research, Bangladesh (ICDDR,B), Mohakhali, Dhaka, Bangladesh

SCOTT BARNHART, MD, MPH
Professor, Director, Division of Health Systems, Department of Global Health and Medicine, International Training and Education Center for Health, University of Washington, Seattle, Washington

MARY E. BLACK, MPH, FRCP, DTM&H
International Office, Royal College of Physicians, London, United Kingdom

JOEL G. BREMAN, MD, DTPH, FIDSA
Fogarty International Center, National Institutes of Health, Bethesda, Maryland

KENNETH BRIDBORD, MD, MPH
Fogarty International Center, National Institutes of Health, Bethesda, Maryland

PIERRE BUEKENS, MD, PhD
Chair, Association of Schools of Public Health Global Health Core Competency Development Project; Dean, School of Public Health and Tropical Medicine, W.H. Watkins Professor, Epidemiology, Tulane University, New Orleans, Louisiana

PAULO BUSS, MD, MPH
Oswaldo Cruz Foundation (FIOCRUZ), Brazil; Professor, FIOCRUZ National School of Public Health; Director, FIOCRUZ Center for Global Health, Manguinhos, Rio de Janeiro, Brazil

ALEXANDER BUTCHART, MA, PhD
Department of Violence and Injury Prevention and Disability, World Health Organization, Geneva, Switzerland

JUDITH G. CALHOUN, PhD, MBA
Faculty Consultant, Association of Schools of Public Health; Senior Research Investigator, Office of the Dean, Medical School, University of Michigan, Ann Arbor, Michigan

THOMAS J. COATES, PhD
Michael and Sue Steinberg Professor of Global AIDS Research, Co-Director, University of California Global Health Institute, San Francisco, California; University of California, Los Angeles David Geffen School of Medicine, Los Angeles, California

CORDELIA E.M. COLTART, MPH, MRCP, DTM&H
International Office, Royal College of Physicians, London, United Kingdom

ALEJANDRO CRAVIOTO, PhD, MD
Executive Director, International Centre for Diarrhoeal Disease Research, Bangladesh (ICDDR,B), Mohakhali, Dhaka, Bangladesh

HAILE T. DEBAS, MD
Senior Global Health Advisor; Maurice Galante Distinguished Professor of Surgery, Director, University of California Global Health Institute, University of California, San Francisco, California

RICHARD J. DECKELBAUM, MD
Institute of Human Nutrition, College of Physicians and Surgeons, Columbia University; Department of Pediatrics, Columbia University Medical Center, New York, New York

PHILIPPA J. EASTERBROOK, MPH, FRCP, DTM&H
International Office, Royal College of Physicians, London, United Kingdom

PAUL E. FARMER, MD, PhD
Co-Founder, Partners In Health; Chair, Chief, Division of Global Health Equity, Department of Global Health and Social Medicine, Brigham and Women's Hospital, Harvard Medical School, Boston, Massachusetts

JULIO FRENK, MD, PhD
Dean, Harvard School of Public Health, Boston, Massachusetts

NISHA JAIN GARG, PhD
Professor of Microbiology and Immunology and Pathology, Associate Director of Center for Tropical Diseases, Sealy Center for Vaccine Development, Faculty of the Institute for Human Infections and Immunity, The University of Texas Medical Branch, Galveston, Texas

ROGER I. GLASS, MD, PhD
Fogarty International Center, National Institutes of Health, Bethesda, Maryland

OCTAVIO GÓMEZ-DANTÉS, MD, MPH
Researcher, Center for Health Systems Research, National Institute of Public Health, Cuernavaca, Morelos, México

HADLEY K. HERBERT, MD
International Injury Research Unit, Department of International Health, Bloomberg School of Public, Johns Hopkins University, Baltimore, Maryland

MICHAEL HERCE, MD, MPH
Abwenzi Pa Za Umoyo, Partners In Health, Malawi; Division of Global Health Equity, Department of Global Health and Social Medicine, Brigham and Women's Hospital, Harvard Medical School, Boston, Massachusetts

ADNAN A. HYDER, MD, MPH, PhD
International Injury Research Unit, Department of International Health, Bloomberg School of Public, Johns Hopkins University, Baltimore, Maryland

ILONA KICKBUSCH, PhD
Professor, Director, Global Health Programme, Graduate Institute of International and Development Studies, Geneva, Switzerland

FELICIA M. KNAUL, PhD
Director, Harvard Global Equity Initiative; Associate Professor, Department of Global Health and Social Medicine, Harvard School of Public Health, Boston, Massachusetts

TRACEY PÉREZ KOEHLMOOS, PhD, MHA
Programme Head, Centre for Control of Chronic Diseases, Health and Family Planning Systems Programme, International Centre for Diarrhoeal Disease Research, Bangladesh (ICDDR,B), Mohakhali, Dhaka, Bangladesh

LINDA E. KUPFER, PhD
Fogarty International Center, National Institutes of Health, Bethesda, Maryland

ROBERT MARTIN, MPH, DrPH
Professor, Director, Laboratory Systems Development, Department of Global Health, International Training and Education Center for Health, University of Washington, Seattle, Washington

KOJI NAKASHIMA, MD, MHS
Zanmi Lasante, Partners In Health, Haiti; Instructor in Medicine, Division of Global Health Equity, Brigham and Women's Hospital, Harvard Medical School, Boston, Massachusetts

ROBYN NORTON, MPH, PhD
The George Institute for Global Health, The University of Sydney, Sydney, New South Wales, Australia

JAMES M. NTAMBI, PhD
Departments of Biochemistry and Nutritional Sciences, Madison, Wisconsin

SOLOMON NWAKA, PhD
Unit Leader, Innovation Networks, Stewardship, UNICEF/UNDP/World Bank/World Health Organization Special Programme for Research and Training in Tropical Diseases, Geneva, Switzerland

WALTER K. PATRICK, MD, MPH, PhD
Professor, Global Health and Medicine, John A. Burns School of Medicine, University of Hawaii; Secretary General, Asia Pacific Academic Consortium for Public Health (APACPH), Department of Public Health Science, John A. Burns School of Medicine, University of Hawaii at Manoa, Honolulu, Hawaii

ROSANNA W. PEELING, PhD
Professor and Chair of Diagnostics Research, London School of Hygiene and Tropical Medicine, London, United Kingdom

HARRISON C. SPENCER, MD, MPH, DTMH, CPH
President and CEO, Association of Schools of Public Health, Washington, District of Columbia

ANVAR VELJI, MD, FRCP(C), FACP, FIDSA
Chief of Infectious Disease, Department of Infectious Disease, Kaiser Permanente, South Sacramento, Sacramento, California; Co-Founder, Global Health Education Consortium (GHEC); Clinical Professor, School of Medicine, University of California, Davis, California

MICHAEL WESTERHAUS, MD, MA
Partners In Health; Division of Global Health Equity, Department of Global Health and Social Medicine, Brigham and Women's Hospital, Harvard Medical School, Boston, Massachusetts

DEBRA J. WOLGEMUTH, PhD
Institute of Human Nutrition, College of Physicians and Surgeons, Columbia University; Departments of Genetics and Development and Obstetrics and Gynecology, New York, New York

Contents

> Chronic and infectious diseases, including health care-associated infections and tropical diseases, represent a large portion of the global health burden. Solutions need to be found while addressing other health priorities identified by the Millennium Development Goals. A number of organizations and initiatives have been created to meet this need. Developing countries in Latin America and several African countries are taking a larger role in the development of robust health systems, capacity building, and education. Integrated, efficient, and equitable health systems that incorporate primary, secondary, and tertiary care models with a research focus are critically needed to fill this void.

> The creation of the University of California Global Health Institute represents a paradigm shift in structure and function. Its 3 centers of expertise (Migration and Health, One Health, and Women's Health and Empowerment) not only involve all 10 of the University of California campuses but also bring together a wide range of disciplines from both the health and nonhealth sciences. They have created truly interdisciplinary and transdisciplinary programs that are addressing complex global health challenges of the twenty-first century, training future global health leaders, and forging international academic partnerships.

> The Fogarty International Center (FIC) of the US National Institutes of Health has supported long-term training and research for more than 3600 future leaders in science and public health from low-income and middle-income countries; tens of thousands more persons have received short-term training. More than 23 extramural training and research programs plus an intramural program are now operating. Newer FIC training programs are addressing chronic, noncommunicable diseases and strengthening the quality of medical schools and health care provider training. Most FIC trainees return to their countries of origin, where they mentor and train thousands of individuals in their home countries.

Developmental strategies over the last 4 decades have generally tended to transfer knowledge and technology along north–south axes as trickle-down theories in development, especially in health knowledge transfers, prevailed. Limited efforts in development assistance for health (DAH) were made to promote south-south cooperation for basic health needs. Globalization with increased educational networks and development health assistance has enhanced the potential for more effective south-south partnerships for health. The stages of development in a consortium and key catalysts in the metamorphosis to a south-south partnership are identified: leadership, resources, expertise, visibility participation, and dynamism of a critical mass of young professionals.

In this article, the authors review recent global health activities in the United Kingdom in several defined areas: UK government and international aid, role of UK academic and other institutions in international partnerships, and undergraduate and postgraduate training opportunities.

Competency specification and competency-based education (CBE) are increasingly being viewed as essential for optimizing educational outcomes for the next generation of global health workers. An overview is provided of this movement in graduate health professions education in the United States, the Association of Schools of Public Health (ASPH) contributions to advancing and researching related CBE processes and best practices, and the evolving ASPH competency model for graduate global health education.

This article discusses the nature of the health challenges created by globalization and proposes new forms of international cooperation to confront them. The discussion of global health challenges includes both the transfer of health risks, with an emphasis on infectious diseases, and the international dissemination of health opportunities, including the transfer of knowledge and technology. The authors argue that the health-related challenges and opportunities of an increasingly interdependent world demand new forms of international cooperation. The authors suggest the promotion of 3 elements that, in their essence, contain the idea of collaboration: exchange, evidence, and empathy.

Diplomacy and health are in a period of rapid transition, so this article elaborates on the complex multilevel, multiactor negotiation processes that shape and manage the global policy environment for health. It explores the dynamic relationship between health and foreign policy and provides examples from the national, regional, and global levels. Reflecting on the deliberations in different international bodies, it discusses key questions and opportunities that could contribute to moving forward both health and peace agendas. The concluding remarks draw attention to the importance of bridging the capacity gap.

Poverty and infectious diseases interact in complex ways. Casting destitution as intractable, or epidemics that afflict the poor as accidental, erroneously exonerates us from responsibility for caring for those most in need. Adequately addressing communicable diseases requires a biosocial appreciation of the structural forces that shape disease patterns. Most health interventions in resource-poor settings could garner support based on cost/benefit ratios with appropriately lengthy time horizons to capture the return on health investments and an adequate accounting of externalities; however, such a calculus masks the suffering of inaction and risks eroding the most powerful incentive to act: redressing inequality.

Infectious diseases have had a decisive and rapid impact on shaping and changing health policy. Noncommunicable diseases, while not garnering as much interest or importance over the past 20 years, have been affecting public health around the world in a steady and critical way, becoming the leading cause of death in developed and developing countries. This article discusses emergent issues in global health related to noncommunicable diseases and conditions, with focus on defining the unique epidemiologic features and relevant programmatic, health systems, and policy responses concerning noncommunicable chronic diseases, mental health, accidents and injuries, urbanization, climate change, and disaster preparedness.

The World Health Organization has developed a comprehensive plan to deal with neglected tropical diseases (NTDs). Compared with a decade ago, more resources are being spent to address the problem of neglected diseases, and considerable progress has been made. However, NTDs remain neglected, deepening the global inequities in health. The current efforts do not implement a multiprong strategy and are effective in the short term, but do not generate long-term, sustainable solutions. This article discusses the current successes in providing access to medicine for treatment of a multitude of neglected diseases, and the opportunities to achieve global equality in health.

new drugs and diagnostics is too slow to keep up with the emergence and spread of infectious diseases around the world. Innovative collaborative research and development involving disease endemic countries and developed countries are urgently needed to accelerate progress along the path from discovery to product adoption. These emerging approaches and the need for increased investment in human and financial resources to support them are discussed.

VISIT THE CLINICS ONLINE!
Access your subscription at:
www.theclinics.com

Preface

Global Health, Global Health Education, and Infectious Disease: The New Millennium, Part II

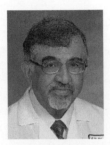

Anvar Velji, MD, FRCP(C), FIDSA
Guest Editor

In this second volume of *Global Health, Global Health Education, and Infectious Disease: The New Millennium*, thought leaders and opinion makers in global health continue the dialogue and discuss their experiences and visions for global health, global health education, research service, development, policy, and diplomacy to achieve Health for All in an equitable manner.

I continue to be inspired by the exceptional membership of the Global Health Education Consortium (GHEC)—students, faculty and administrators, and institutions—who for 20 years have been deeply committed to changing the landscape of global health and global health education through networking between academic institutions, nongovernmental organizations, civil society, and other global partners. At the various global health conferences, student activism and leadership for global health continue to be very visible. For example, see the student perspective on the 17th Annual GHEC Sacramento Conference, held in Sacramento, California, in 2008.[1]

The role of universities and other health institutions in global health and the impending merger of GHEC and the Consortium of Universities for Global Health (CUGH) are

---

This work was supported by funding from Kaiser Permanente. The author wishes to thank Naomi L. Ruff, PhD, ELS, for copyediting assistance.

The author currently serves on the Global Health Education Consortium (GHEC), the Transition Board of GHEC-Consortium of Universities for Global Health (CUGH), the Kaiser Permanente Global Health Program Advisory Committee, and the U.S. Center for Citizen Diplomacy Global Health Task Force.

Infect Dis Clin N Am 25 (2011) xiii–xxii
doi:10.1016/j.idc.2011.07.013
0891-5520/11/$ – see front matter

well summarized by Dr Haile Debas, Chair of the Transition Board of the new CUGH (personal communication, June 30, 2001):

Global health problems have been growing increasingly complex, and to address them successfully many disciplines and sectors have to work together like never before. This statement is especially true of the academic community, whose contribution to education, training, and research is pivotal. Until now, two consortia of universities have been attempting to ensure that the role of universities is coordinated and significant. GHEC has for 20 years dedicated itself to global education and service, and its contribution has been significant. CUGH, on the other hand, was established only 3 years ago to promote further extensive collaboration of universities in education, research, and service, as well as to advocate for funding for global health in general, and funding of university-based global health programs in particular. It is evident that not only are GHEC and CUGH complementary in their goals but they also serve the same constituencies. The expected merger of these two consortia in November 2011 is, therefore, historical and most welcome. The new Consortium of Universities for Global Health, strengthened by expanded membership and united in its efforts, will ensure that the university will play a transformational role in global health. No other organization is as able as this new Consortium of Universities to play an effective and sustained role in capacity building through long-term partnership with universities in low- and middle-income countries in education, research, and service.

An important recent development in Europe was the creation of the European Academic Global Health Alliance, which brings together several academic institutions and is hosted by the Association of Schools of Public Health.[2] Their ideals and actions resonate with those of the Asia Pacific Academic Consortium for Public Health, GHEC-CUGH,[3] and efforts by academic institutions in Great Britain and by the new Latin American and Caribbean Consortium for Global Health.[4] Strong links must be established with like-minded academic organizations worldwide in order to have nonduplicative close collaboration for undertaking important global health and global health education projects to benefit the populations of the geographic south. Health advocacy, policy development, research, service, and diplomacy are clearly priorities and mandates for all of these organizations.

The road map for comprehensive health policies in the 21st century was laid out in the statement in 2007 of the Ministers of Foreign Affairs of Brazil, France, Indonesia, Norway, Senegal, South Africa, and Thailand. In their Oslo Ministerial Declaration, they emphasized that *global health is a pressing foreign policy issue of our time* and pointed to the truism that *our most precious assets, no matter where we live on this planet, are life and health.* Furthermore, they emphasized that *health today is deeply inter-connected with environment, trade, economic growth, social development, national security, human rights, and dignity.* I firmly believe that the articles in the two volumes of the *Infectious Disease Clinics of North America* on global health have addressed all these major issues and more and set the foundations for further discussions and actions.

In my editorial in the current issue of the *Infectious Disease Clinics of North America*, I address ways that global health, global health education, infectious disease, and chronic conditions are being transformed in the 21st century, a perspective gained by having spent a third of my life in Kenya; been for 20 years the "guardian angel/godfather of GHEC," a very honorific and weighty responsibility placed on me by the founding president of the International Health Medical Consortium, a predecessor of GHEC[5]; and having practiced within a very exceptional and exciting health system—Kaiser Permanente—over the last 31 years. Today the breaking down of barriers to global health development gives us an unprecedented opportunity not only for a new intergenerational dialogue but also for sustained focus and action on the evolving paradigm of global health, global health education, and emerging health systems and on the relevant research agendas. How we view health and education will be changed by the renewed focus on and action around the Millennium Development Goals, health system strengthening, and reinvention of primary care with its *moral-ethical backbone* and *framework*; by action on chronic and infectious diseases and neglected tropical diseases; and by increased attention to poverty, education, climate change, and long-neglected mental health, trauma, and surgical and anesthesia needs. We must continue to advocate for a comprehensive definition and compass of "*global health with a face,*" a concept that goes beyond being a discipline or goal, but which has a moral underpinning and is accepted worldwide. The hard lessons we have learned teach us that all of these activities in the field and vision of global health must be integrated and intersectoral for sustained human development and the social good of all humankind.

The article by Haile Debas and Thomas Coates shares their valuable experiences, challenges, and opportunities in setting up the unique University of California Global Health Institute (UCGHI), a collaborative effort of the 10 University of California (UC) campuses that represents a paradigm shift in both structure and function of universities. By bringing together a wide range of disciplines from both the health and the non-health sciences, they have created truly inter- and transdisciplinary programs that are addressing the complex global health challenges of the 21st century, training future global health leaders, and forging international academic partnerships. This pioneering effort of a university-wide initiative will focus on producing leaders and practitioners of global health, conducting innovative and important research, and developing international collaborations to improve the health of vulnerable people and communities in California and worldwide. *The programs of UCGHI are action-oriented and go beyond those of traditional academic programs, which focus on education, research, publication, and dissemination.* The first three programs, the Center of Expertise on Migration and Health; Center of Expertise on One Health: Water, Animals, Food and Society; and Center of Expertise on Women's Health and Empowerment, are setting high standards and demonstrating a new form of interdepartmental and interdisciplinary collaborations. As Debas and Coates state, "the metrics by which UCGHI will judge itself will include not only the usual metrics for academic success, *but just as importantly, the actual impact its programs make to the health and welfare of poor people on the ground everywhere* [emphasis added]."

Joel G. Breman, Kenneth Bridbord, Linda E. Kupfer, and Roger I. Glass articulate in great detail the vision, mission, programs, and accomplishments of the Fogarty International Center (FIC) of the US National Institutes of Health (NIH). In 1988, FIC started the flagship HIV/AIDS International Training and Research Program in response to the global pandemic. Since then, more than 23 extramural training and research programs and an intramural program have begun operating, all in collaboration with other Institutes and Centers at NIH, US government agencies, foundations, and partner institutions in the low- and middle-income countries (LMICs) and the US. Today, FIC training programs are addressing chronic, noncommunicable diseases and are strengthening the quality of medical schools and health care provider training, in addition to expanding expertise in infectious diseases. The FIC model for successful training is based on long-term commitments, institutional strengthening, "twinning" of research centers, focus on local problems, and active mentoring. Because the FIC programs are institution-strengthening partnerships and candidates are carefully selected and mentored, close to 90% of FIC trainees return to their countries of origin and in turn help develop the next generation of leaders and global health workers in LMICs. FIC has an enviable record of supporting long-term (>6 months) basic, clinical, and applied research training for over 3600 future leaders in science and public health from LMICs; tens of thousands more have also received short-term training. The wide variety of programs, projects, and initiatives supported by FIC reflects FIC's goals of providing comprehensive training and tools to investigators to ultimately—and sustainably—build capacity in global health research and lessen the burden of global disease and illness worldwide. FIC thus sets a very high bar for existing and future institutions involved in global health.

Walter Patrick shares the long and valuable experiences of the Asia Pacific Academic Consortium for Public Health's (APACPH) in strengthening South-South and South-North Collaborations in global health education, development policy, and networking for the public good. To date, limited efforts and investment have been made to promote South-South cooperation between and within LMICs for basic health needs. As a result, there are very few stable South-South cooperative networks. However, the evolution of APACPH demonstrates how an academic organization that originated as a North-South collaboration with strong interest in fostering developments in the South has since emerged as South-North-South organization with South-South academic networks established nationally and regionally. Patrick also points to the newer shift in global cooperation and collaboration involving the African–South American collaboration. Although these collaborations initially focused primarily on energy and trade, their focus now includes issues of peace, security, health needs, and poverty reduction. Patrick identifies the strengths and weaknesses of sustaining such partnerships and key catalysts in the stages of development for such a metamorphosis. He further focuses on how universities, nongovernmental organizations, and international agencies involved in population health improvement have expanded the social responsibility of medical and public health schools to the marginalized populations and have promoted South-South regional and national academic networks through access to knowledge on the Internet as well as cultural compatibilities.

Cordelia Coltart, Mary Black, and Philippa J. Easterbrook trace the rich roots of global health activities in the UK, going back a little over a century to their origins in "Tropical Medicine and Hygiene," and describe how these activities have now broadly evolved to encompass multiple arenas, especially the government and university sectors. These efforts are built on the central idea, launched as a UK government-wide strategy in 2008, *that health is global*. The authors address the role of government and international aid, the role of UK academic and other institutions in international partnerships, and undergraduate and postgraduate training opportunities. Global health enables the harmonization of international and domestic health concerns and the adoption of a more global outlook than that afforded by a development or foreign-assistance perspective alone. The development of the UK global health strategy is built around the UK Department of Health's five key areas for the promotion of global health: global security and health protection, sustainable development, trade by promoting health as a commodity, maximization of global public good, and encouragement of the human rights approach to health. The strategy was based on five key areas for action, with key goals remaining the elimination of poverty and the delivery of clean water, sanitation, basic health care, and education to the world's poorest people. The authors point out that there has been limited discussion and debate in the UK as to the optimal role of UK universities in global health and to the type of institutional partnerships that will meet the needs and priorities of southern institutions, as well as building and sustaining the capacity of these institutions for the future. Finally, the authors provide examples of academic courses and degrees in global health in the UK.

Judith Calhoun, Harrison C. Spencer, and Pierre Buekens address competencies for Global Health Graduate Education to drive global health education initiatives. There is an urgent need to focus on competencies, uniform standards, and interprofessional education beyond silos. The authors provide an overview of competency-based education (CBE) and its impact in the US today. Of great significance, the Association of Schools of Public Health (ASPH) Initiative focuses on CBE processes and best practices and the development of a standardized ASPH global health competency model. The authors also provide recommendations addressing potential future trends and barriers to acceptance of CBE to help the many educators and trainers who are just embarking on the competency journey. Acceptance by professional organizations, accrediting bodies, and school-wide leadership is critical for the wider diffusion and success of the program and for the development of an adaptable and productive workforce for global health and well-being.

Julio Frenk, the recipient of the GHEC Distinguished Service Award [2008], Octavio Gomez-Dantes, and Felicia Knaul address globalization and infectious diseases through the lenses of human security and interdependence. International transfer of risks, especially in the realms of infectious disease and noncommunicable/chronic conditions, has also generated interdependence, new opportunities for collaborating across boundaries, joint learning, and international collective action to ensure the public good. The authors have contributed significantly to our understanding of global health. Aside from knowledge translation and its foundational support to build policies for the public good, the important concept of "global health with a human face" gives us another window on global health.

Ilona Kickbusch and Paulo Buss (recipient of the GHEC Distinguished Service Award 2010) have enriched us considerably over the past many years in the exciting field of Global Health Diplomacy and Peace. The authors elaborate on the complex multilevel multi-actor negotiation processes that shape and manage the global policy environment for health. They further explore the dynamic relationship between health and foreign policy and provide examples from the national, regional, and global levels. Reflecting on the deliberations in different international bodies, they discuss key questions and opportunities that could contribute to moving health and peace agendas forward in today's rapidly evolving global health and development landscape. In the geopolitical marketplace, "soft power" and "smart power" in reference to global health initiatives have increasingly replaced the "hard power" of the last century. In the negotiations on global health policy, the other side of the coin—the interests and desires of the LMICs—is mostly neglected. However, the authors point out that these interests were amply represented at the recent deliberations of the 128th Executive Board in 2011 and echoed in the UN General Assembly Resolutions. The authors stress that it is critical to empower the LMICs through capacity building to take the initiative in managing their own development and growth.

Marcella M. Alsan, Michael Westerhaus, Michael Herce, Koji Nakashima, and Paul E. Farmer discuss how to apply a biosocial framework to the design of health systems based on their valuable experience and long involvement in Haiti and Rwanda. They review ways in which poverty, structural violence, and infectious disease and chronic conditions confine poor populations to vicious cycles of suffering and despair and then examine the implications of these understandings on the design of health interventions. As they forcefully argue, it is the failure to employ a biosocial lens that often gives rise to charity and development models of health intervention that replicate preexisting unequal structures. Such models localize blame for disease with the poor themselves.

In contrast, a biosocial lens makes clear that disease among the poor results from the embodiment of structural violence and requires that any serious attempt to address disease in resource-poor settings incorporate efforts for social change. Through commitment to models built upon the principles of social justice, Partners In Health (PIH) has found that advocacy and long-term partnerships between the public sector and the communities in which they work are indispensable for creating sustainable transformations in health that reduce suffering caused by infectious and chronic disease. Thus, the authors challenge the prevalent model of just providing diagnostic tools, pharmaceuticals, and trained clinicians without addressing the consequences of deep poverty: limited transportation, poor housing, and food scarcity, among others. In essence, PIH and local partners provide care that integrates social and economic programs. Such solutions, which privilege a biosocial approach to identifying and breaking down barriers to care, have resulted in remarkable successes in addressing epidemics of HIV/AIDS, TB, malaria, and other communicable and chronic diseases in some of the most challenging domestic and global settings.

Tracey Koehlmoos, Shahela Anwar, and Alejandro Cravioto bring their unique experience from Bangladesh to address noncommunicable diseases (NCDs), mental health, accidents, occupational injuries, urbanization, climate change, and disaster preparedness. This perspective is important because clearly the largest burden of NCDs occurs in LMICS. Of the deaths due to NCDs, 80% occur in developing countries, and only 2.3% of international development assistance for health is directed to NCDs. The economic impact and burden of NCDs are therefore likely to be dramatic and overwhelming. These challenges, together with ongoing classical challenges of infectious disease and emerging infectious disease, will place significant strains on these fragile economies. The authors define the unique epidemiological features and relevant programmatic health systems and policy responses that are necessary to successfully negotiate the current and impending challenges.

Nisha Garg focuses on neglected diseases and access to medicines. The essential thesis is that there are not only neglected diseases but also neglected populations who are resource poor, lack fundamental amenities, and are overlooked even in the presence of available resources. Garg outlines several key challenges and opportunities for promoting local ownership of problems and responsibility for solutions, strengthening health systems, sustained donor commitments, logistics, and poverty reduction. She outlines successful programs and reasons for failure. Empowering the local populations to fully partake in their health decisions, preventive efforts, and education can significantly change the dynamics and help improve productivity, as was the case with the control of Guinea worm disease. Policies to control and in certain cases eliminate neglected tropical diseases must be multipronged and involve decision-makers and resources from both the donor and the recipient countries.

Hadley Herbert, Adnan Hyder, Alexander Butchart, and Robyn Norton discuss in a very comprehensive and succinct manner one of the most neglected areas of global health: that of injury and violence, which rank among the top ten leading causes of death worldwide. They further examine how injury and violence relate to global health using recent global burden of disease data and selected key studies and databases, and they explore risk factors and intervention initiatives that address unintentional and intentional injuries. This article serves as a call to action to enhance our understanding of the growing burden of injury and violence, especially in LMICs, where over 90% of injuries occur. The article by Koehlmoos, Anwar, and Cravioto also adds to this rich perspective.

Richard J. Deckelbaum, James M. Ntambi, and Debra J. Wolgemuth provide evidence that basic science research and education should be a priority for training and capacity building in developing countries. They pose several important questions, such as: Is there a need?, What is the current status of basic science training in global health?, How can the problems of lack of financial and human resources, physical infrastructure, and poor recognition of the need for local basic science related to indigenous health issues be addressed?, and how will strengthening basic science research in developing countries be achieved? Currently, there are tremendous gaps between strong science education and research in developed countries (the North) as compared to developing countries (the South). In addition, science research and education appear to be low priority in many developing countries. The authors point out the acute need to stress basic science research beyond the typical investment in infectious disease. Basic service and research laboratories in developing areas contribute meaningfully to society in terms of the benefits not only to education, but also to economic strengthening and development of human resources. There are some indications that appreciation of basic science research education and training is increasing, but this still needs to be applied more rigorously and strengthened systematically in developing countries. They further point out that what is required is the will and the financial, physical, and human resources to implement basic science programs. A recent special issue of *Nature* has also focused on this need of building science in Africa.[6–14]

Robert Martin and Scott Barnhart address the long-neglected topic of global laboratory systems development, with a particular focus on sub-Saharan Africa. Laboratory systems are an integral part of any robust, efficient, integrated health system and are necessary for country capacity building. The new directions outlined by the authors call for development of leadership, education of laboratory scientists, quality assurance, resource management, and country ownership and responsibility. Furthermore, networking within the country and between countries for setting and maintaining quality and standards is critical for the accreditation process and patient safety. A particular statement from Easterly[15] quoted by the authors is worth restating here, as it has a broad applicability in global health: "It would be worth testing and exploring the hypothesis that most successful development is homegrown. And if so, research should concentrate more on homegrown determinants of development rather than spend so much time on outsider's actions… Perhaps then we might find that the ones most likely to 'save Africa' are Africans themselves."

Rosanna W. Peeling and Solomon Nwaka discuss new business models for research and development to accelerate progress along the path from discovery of drugs and diagnostics to product adoption and implementation. While funding for research and development is critical, an accompanying increase in investment to build capacity for drug and diagnostic research and development, as well as development of robust health care infrastructure, is critical if the full impact of these innovative approaches is to be realized. A new paradigm is emerging from a convergence of several key insights and developments that includes proof-of-concept funds, networks linking scientists and entrepreneurs, and physical centers providing shared research infrastructure. The involvement of developing-country scientists and institutions as key partners continues to be an urgent challenge. This is in keeping with the WHO's Global Strategy and Plan of Action developed by the Inter-governmental Working Group on Innovation, Intellectual Property, and Public Health that promotes innovation as a way to improve the range and affordability of medical interventions for diseases that disproportionately affect developing countries. As the authors emphasize, the commitment of public-private partnerships to share resources, share risks (crossing the valley of death), and share rewards is a critical element of the new paradigm and most urgently needed.

These two volumes of the *of North America of North America* have focused mostly on universities and consortia, but I would be remiss if I did not acknowledge the excellent work in global health and global health education being carried out by the Bill and Melinda Gates Foundation, The Aga Khan Development Network, the Rockefeller Foundation, the William J. Clinton Foundation, the Carter Center, and many other nongovernmental organizations, religious organizations, and other leading health systems both abroad and in North America.

In the US, the recently passed Affordable Care Act focuses on reducing disparities, improving quality, and reducing costs and waste. President Obama pointed out four institutions as health care models for the future: Kaiser Permanente, the Mayo Clinic, the Cleveland Clinic, and the Geisinger Health System.[16] It is important to highlight some unique features that make these models so successful, since there is a rush globally to create new markets for health care delivery without consideration of equity cost, quality, or safety. Due to lack of space, I will discuss only the largest and most successful model, Kaiser Permanente (KP), below.

Over the last 60 years, KP has transformed how medicine is practiced in the US, and its pervasive influence has been felt around the world. KP is a nonprofit, integrated, managed care system. Physicians and hospitals collaborate effectively to mitigate health care cost increases and improve the quality, safety, and accountability of care. This process requires input from other arenas of health care, and at KP this expertise is provided by three Institutes: Health Policy, Research, and Culturally Competent Care. The cornerstone of the KP Health Systems is the integration of the principles of population management, evidence-based medicine, team-based chronic care management, multicultural health, diversity and inclusion, community outreach, and cost effectiveness, with recent emphasis on same-day access. KP today has the most comprehensive electronic health record system in the world, which securely connects all members' medical records across both ambulatory and inpatient settings; integrates billing, scheduling, and registration; and provides members access to personal health records on the organization's Web-based member portal and through member–physician secure e-mail communication. These tools and technologies of the 21st century simultaneously make health and health care more personalized and convenient, safer, and more cost effective. KP's ubiquitous motto "Live well, be well, and thrive" focuses on preventive care and promotes healthy living. KP also offers a unique training opportunity for residents from university- and community-based programs throughout the Northern California Region, including Stanford, UC Davis, and UC San Francisco. Approximately 900 affiliated residents rotate through the KP Northern California facilities each year for 1 to 6 months at a time. "Our increasing involvement in global health is a natural outgrowth of our mission, of improving the health of the communities we serve, and for the past two years, approximately one third of the incoming class of new residents and fellows at Kaiser Permanente Northern California have reported participating in some type of global health rotation during medical school" (Bruce Blumberg, KP Northern California Director of Graduate Medical Education, personal communication, July 12, 2011). Recently, KP global health residency training sites have been established in Ugenya, Kenya (the TIBA/Mati Babu Foundation); University Teaching Hospital at Lusaka, Zambia; and the Sihanouk Hospital in Phnom Penh, Cambodia, and many others are currently being evaluated.[17]

The Kaiser Permanente Medical Group (TPMG) in the Northern California Region is the largest medical group in the US, comprising over 7000 physicians and 25,000 staff members. It operates 19 medical centers in Northern California and is responsible for 3.3 million members. Similar sister groups exist in seven other regions: Southern

California, Oregon, Georgia, Hawaii, Colorado, Ohio, and the Mid-Atlantic.[18] Many of the physicians, nurses, and other health workers are in academia and contribute significantly to the global health programs in the US and many parts of the world and will continue to be a significant force after retirement as they continue to train the global health workforce. These tremendous resources are generally overlooked outside the academic centers, but the new millennium has ushered in a new spirit of cooperation among universities and organizations such as KP to train the new global health workforce in a manner that is culturally competent and sensitive and socially accountable.

Another generally overlooked and underappreciated aspect of global health is the significant contributions of US volunteers who are involved in global health and citizen diplomacy. A Global Health Task Force (of which I am a member) was created in 2010, with goals of increasing the impact of US health volunteers worldwide and improving their monitoring and evaluation, as well as strengthening and leveraging the contributions of US citizens to meet the goals of the Global Health Initiative and the goal of doubling the number of American citizen diplomats in the next 10 years. Mary Flake Flores, the Former First Lady of Honduras (a GHEC Distinguished Service Award recipient for 2008 for her remarkable work and dedication to the people of Honduras following Hurricane Mitch), was a guest speaker at the first meeting of the US Citizen Diplomacy Summit in Washington DC. The First Lady very movingly recollected the very real contributions that the US and other volunteers made to alleviate the tremendous loss and destruction of life, property, and environment in Honduras. A monograph is available that lists organizations and members of the Task Force and its initiatives.[19]

In conclusion, I wish to extend my sincerest appreciation to all the experts who have contributed to this second volume and to the enlightened leadership at TPMG, including Dr Robert Pearl, the Executive Director of TPMG; Dr Richard Isaacs, Physician In Chief of Kaiser Permanente; and Dr Boone Seto, Chief of Medicine at KP South Sacramento, for their robust support of my efforts in global health over the last several years. Finally, I wish to extend my sincere thanks to Dr Robert Mollering, Consulting Editor of the *Infectious Disease Clinics of North America* for giving me another opportunity to focus on global health issues. I also wish to express my sincere thanks to the wonderful staff at Elsevier, in particular, the editor for this edition, Stephanie Donley; journal manager, Diana Schaeffer; and Teia Stone, who were so helpful to me and to the authors who contributed to this edition of the *Clinics*.

Anvar Velji, MD, FRCP(C), FIDSA
Department of Infectious Disease, Kaiser Permanente
South Sacramento
6600 Bruceville Road
Sacramento, CA 95823, USA

E-mail address:
Anvarali.Velji@kp.org

REFERENCES

1. Hafiz S. Global Health Activism Among Medical Students. Sierra Sacramento Valley Medicine 2008;59. Available at: http://www.ssvms.org/ssv_medicine/archives/2008/03/articles/0803-hafiz.pdf. Accessed March 2, 2011.
2. Haines A, Flahault A, Horton R. European academic institutions for global health. Lancet 2011;377(9763):363–5.

3. Velji AM. Global Health Education Consortium (GHEC): 20 years of leadership in Global Health and Global Health Education. Infect Dis Clin North Am 2011;25(2): 323–35.
4. Ministers of Foreign Affairs of Brazil F, Indonesia, Norway, Senegal, South Africa, and Thailand. The Oslo Ministerial Declaration. Lancet 2007;369(9570):1373–8.
5. Global Health Education Consortium. Minutes of the International Health Medical Education (IHMEC) Governing Council. June 14, 1992, Arlington, VA; reiterated at the GHEC Board Meeting. Salt Lake City (UT), April 15, 2011.
6. A helping hand. Nature 2011;474(7353):542.
7. Murenzi R. Give the new generation a chance. Nature 2011;474(7353):543.
8. Irikefe V, Vaidyanathan G, Nordling L, et al. Science in Africa: The view from the front line. Nature 2011;474(7353):556–9.
9. Science in Africa: Lands of promise. Nature 2011;474(7353):555.
10. Nordling L. Science in Africa: Enter the dragon. Nature 2011;474(7353):560–2.
11. Vaidyanathan G. Agriculture: The wheat stalker. Nature 2011;474(7353):563–5.
12. Turok N. Africa AIMS high. Nature 2011;474(7353):567–9.
13. Bonfoh B, Raso G, Inza Koné I, et al. Research in a war zone. Nature 2011; 474(7353):569–71.
14. Ruxin J, Habinshuti A. Crowd control in Rwanda. Nature 2011;474(7353):572–3.
15. Easterly W. Can the West save Africa? J Econ Lit 2009;47(2):373–447.
16. Obama B. Remarks by the President at Town Hall, Broughton High School, Raleigh (NC); July 29, 2009. Available at: http://www.whitehouse.gov/the_press_office/ Remarks-by-the-President-at-Town-Hall-in-Raleigh-North-Carolina/. Accessed July 19, 2011.
17. Kaiser Permanente. Global Health Program. Available at: http://residency.kp.org/ ncal/about_us/global_health.html. Accessed July 19, 2011.
18. Kaiser Permanente. Fast Facts about Kaiser Permanente. Available at: http://xnet. kp.org/newscenter/aboutkp/fastfacts.html. Accessed July 20, 2011.
19. Global Health Task Force: Contributions of U.S. Volunteers Towards the Improvement of Global Health and U.S. Diplomacy. Washington, DC: U.S. Center for Citizen Diplomacy; November 16–19, 2010. Available at: http://uscenterforcitizendiplomacy.org/ images/pdfs/summit-reports/Task-Force/TF_Global-health.pdf. Accessed March 30, 2011.

Editorial: Transforming Global Health, Global Health Education, Infectious Disease, and Chronic Conditions in the 21st Century

Anvar Velji, MD, FRCP(C), FIDSA[a,b,*]

KEYWORDS

- Global health • Global health education
- Global health diplomacy • Global health policy
- Global health law • Poverty • Infectious disease
- New world order

GLOBAL HEALTH, GLOBAL HEALTH EDUCATION, INFECTIOUS DISEASE, AND CHRONIC CONDITIONS: THE UNACCEPTABLE AND OBSCENE SITUATION

Billions of humans are currently neglected, marginalized, and deprived. Four seminal volumes on global health in the *Infectious Disease Clinics of North America* Series— International Health, International Health Beyond the Year 2000, and the two current volumes on Global Health, Global Health Education, and Infectious Disease[1-4]— have taken on the challenge of focusing on *this unacceptable situation,* reminding us that we should all continue to share the plight of these people and that we should advocate on their behalf at every opportunity through transformational changes in global health education, research, service, advocacy, policy, or diplomacy. Infectious

Conflict of interest disclosure: The author serves on the Board of Global Health Education (GHEC) and the Transition Board of the GHEC- Consortium of Universities for Global Health (CUGH).

[a] Department of Infectious Disease, Kaiser Permanente, 6600 Bruceville Road, South Sacramento, CA 95823, USA
[b] School of Medicine, University of California, Davis, CA, USA
* Department of Infectious Disease, Kaiser Permanente, 6600 Bruceville Road, South Sacramento, CA 95823.
E-mail address: Anvarali.Velji@kp.org

Infect Dis Clin N Am 25 (2011) 485–498
doi:10.1016/j.idc.2011.05.002
0891-5520/11/$ – see front matter © 2011 Elsevier Inc. All rights reserved.

id.theclinics.com

diseases such as HIV-AIDS, neglected diseases of tropical medicine, chronic diseases, trauma, violence, and mental health problems disproportionately affect the poor. In the 1930s, James Grant, who served as the Director of UNICEF, felt that addressing poverty should be the priority of societies because it was clearly immoral not to act when 40,000 children a day were dying, two-thirds from preventable causes. He called this an "obscene situation." He reasoned that if one lived in a world in which not much could be done about poverty, then doing little or nothing about it would not be a crime. However, when it was possible to do something about poverty, or about its worst manifestations, than it was clearly immoral not to act.[5] Even today, poverty continues to be a major determinant and driver of ill health and non-productivity.[6]

A SAFER AND MORE SECURE FUTURE

A more secure and safer future is achievable by bridging the gaps between ideas, ideals or values, and transformational actions for global health, global health education, infectious disease, and chronic conditions. Goals continue to shift, but the deep values that we espouse as humans are eternal within the context of specific cultures. The hallmarks of universal shared values are expressed as equity, rights, fairness, justice, and solidarity. These values underpin the universal processes of interdependence, independence, collaboration, and interdisciplinary approaches to solving global health problems and the challenges of rich and poor alike by focusing on the social determinants of health across economic and geopolitical boundaries, including in one's own backyard. Aside from the recognition of shared vulnerability, we now understand that we have shared responsibility, which calls for shared security. Shared vulnerabilities arise from chronic conditions, infectious diseases, climate change, natural and human-made disasters, adverse effects of globalization, wars, and individual and group violence. The response to addressing shared vulnerability must consist of shared responsibility, mutual trust, accountability, transparency, and mutual respect. The building blocks of these efforts include shared knowledge; generation and application of new knowledge; a shared global workforce; resources, including natural resources; peace; and effective, fair, representative governance. Shared safety and security have many components, such as basic rights to food, clean water, shelter, jobs, education, and freedom of worship.[7–10] The recent events in Haiti, including an earthquake, political chaos, and outbreak of cholera, and the transformation of the political scene in the Middle East with much destruction of human life and displacement, provide great lessons and an opportunity to get involved seriously in root-cause analysis, joint learning, and realization of social justice, rights, and participatory governance.

THE 21ST CENTURY AND THE NEW WORLD ORDER: TRANSFORMATIONAL STRATEGIES AND POLICIES

In the early 1990s, in a brief editorial and response to Alfred Sommer's insightful commentary,[11] I indicated that the search for President Bush's "new world order" and the World Health Organization (WHO) agenda "Health for All by the Year 2000" were neither theoretical nor rhetorical. The major challenges and some solutions to global health problems were reviewed in two issues of *Infectious Diseases Clinics of North America*[1,2] and I suggested that, if the United States adopted global leadership in efforts to improve the health of people everywhere, then health for the "global person" could translate into "the new diplomacy" and better health could be the new *lingua franca*, replacing the arms race and the cold war.[12] In contrast, aside from the creation of the President's Emergency Plan for AIDS Relief (PEPFAR), which was a significant event, no clear indication was delivered from the US Presidency until the recent President's Global Health Initiative, which will be transformative in scope if performed as planned. President Obama, recalling the centrality of the United Nations Charter and the Universal Declaration of Human Rights, pledged to work to promote the economic and social advancement of all people and to recognize the inherent dignity and rights of every individual, including the right to a decent standard of living. Furthermore, President Obama pointed out that, in addition to freeing men, women, and children from the injustice of extreme poverty, the new initiative would focus on several issues: (1) moving nations from poverty to prosperity, by harnessing all the tools from diplomacy to trade and investment policies, and addressing how aid is structured, (2) offering people a path out of poverty by breaking the cycle of dependency, (3) unleashing transformational change through broad-based economic growth; combating corruption; promoting good governance and democracy, the rule of law, and equal administration of justice; and creating transparent institutions with strong civil societies and respect for human rights, and (4) mutual accountability from all parties. Additionally, investments in health, education, and the rights of women, entrepreneurs, and leaders will be a critical part of development and global health policy. The core principles, implementation components, and program areas have been summarized elsewhere.[13] Other transformative and innovative thinking on global health comes from planning and action by the rising economic powers. The acronyms BRIC (Brazil, Russia, India, and China), IBSA (India, Brazil, and South Africa), and BASIC (Brazil, South Africa, India, and China) point to the new reality that these countries have growing influence within the global health policy status quo previously dominated by European and American interests.[14] The increased influence of these countries and creation of solidarity in the global south–south partnership and alliance configuration brings creative thinking to the fields of economics, politics, health issues, and global health diplomacy. For instance, Brazil has emerged as a dominant global health player in the 21st century. The core of its unique understanding of global health is rooted in the nation's constitution (1988), which stresses health as a human right. "Brazil's global health outreach is premised on the idea of 'health in all policies,' and themes of solidarity, human rights, and the priority of health over patent protections inform the perspective Brazilian program implementers and policymakers...."[14] Brazil's new model of international development calls for structural cooperation in health with capacity building in education, research, human resource training, health service, use of local skills and expertise, knowledge generation, involvement of civil societies, and the strengthening of health systems. However, there is also a need to structure institutions such as health ministries, schools of public health, national health institutes, and faculties of higher education to work cooperatively in developing efficient and integrated health systems.[15,16]

INFECTIOUS DISEASE AND GLOBAL HEALTH: THE MILLENNIUM DEVELOPMENT GOALS

The recent interest in the emerging vision, variously described as the field, discipline, enterprise, or goal of global health, has drawn many North American and European academic institutions and philanthropic organizations to seriously engage in the problems of the middle- and lower-income countries (MLCs) that have been devastated by infectious and chronic disease, droughts, wars, natural disasters, forced migration, and global climate change. The specialties of infectious disease and public health are keystones of global health. Those who pursue research and practice in these specialties have played a critical role in elucidating the epidemiology of the HIV-AIDS pandemic, neglected diseases prevalent in the tropics, and travel-associated diseases; in developing vaccines and antimicrobics; and in making a panoply of other contributions to tackling emerging and remerging diseases and population health, population displacement, and health care-associated infections (HAIs). Many universities are now also engaged in creating centers of "Global Health Excellence" to coordinate the multidisciplinary activities and interests in transuniversity and intrauniversity research, teaching, and service; as well as advocacy, policy, and diplomacy.[17,18] Infectious disease specialists direct a number of these centers. Infectious disease physicians also take active roles in the Society of Tropical Medicine & Hygiene, Public Health, and Travel Medicine.

In 1987, the UNICEF Report Adjustment with a Human Face dealt with the negative impact of the poorly thought out Structural Adjustment Programs on societies, especially with reference to education and health.[19] Today, as we become more enlightened and bridge the schism between medicine and public health we need to craft global health with a human face[9] and, by extension, global health education, global health policies, global health diplomacy, and global health law with a human face. With this new mindset, we can clearly overcome the schisms between public health and medicine and the ephemeral schisms present within universities and between universities locally and globally.[20]

We in medicine, public health, and the diverse fields and disciplines involved in global health owe a deep debt of gratitude to WHO and UNICEF, which together launched the greatest public health enterprise of the last three centuries, Health for All, at Alma Ata in the former Soviet Union in 1978. This was a clarion call, a simple slogan to mobilize the world's values and commitment to aid billions in desperate need, from those in our backyards to the globally marginalized. A host of other collaborative initiatives followed, such as the Convention on the Rights of the Child (1990), the World Summit for Children (1990), the African Program for Onchocerciasis (1995), UNAIDS (1996), Stop-TB Initiative (1998), Roll Back Malaria Partnership (1998), and Global Alliance for Vaccines and Immunizations (1999). The Millennium Development Goals, another major milestone in global health, were unanimously adopted by the leaders at the United Nations (UN) in September 2000. Eight development goals were established, starting with the elimination of extreme poverty and hunger. The sixth goal was to combat HIV-AIDS, malaria, and other infectious diseases, but neglected conditions such as chronic diseases and tropical diseases that contribute to the massive morbidity and mortality globally were not included. In all, infectious disease accounts for 29 of the 96 major causes of human morbidity and mortality,[21] causes 25% of global deaths (over 14 million deaths annually), and continues to be a major challenge worldwide.[22] For instance a comprehensive literature review identified 1415 species of infectious organism known to be pathogenic to humans, including 217 viruses and prions, 538 bacteria and rickettsia, 307 fungi, 66 protozoa, and 287 helminthes; of these, 868 (61%) are zoonotic, and 175 pathogenic species are associated with a disease considered to be "emerging."[23] Every year brings a new emerging infection and multiple issues of antimicrobic resistance. The Infectious Disease Society of America (IDSA) has presented several dire scenarios to the US Congress of the ongoing crises in antimicrobic availability, increasing resistance, and dwindling production of new antimicrobics and antihelminthes,[24] but without much response. In the MLCs, the epidemic of HAIs has the potential to deplete scarce global resources.

HAIs: PATIENT AND POPULATION SAFETY

In 2005, the state of California mandated the creation of the HAIs Advisory Committee. The committee, of which I was a member, was charged with making recommendations to the California Department of Public Health on the prevention of HAIs.[25] Based on estimates from 2004, approximately 240,000 HAIs likely occurred in California among 4 million patient discharges, with a cost of approximately $3.1 billion. This excludes the economic cost to individuals and society from lost wages, productivity, and medico-legal costs.[25] As a committee, we felt that aside from our core missions of the prevention of antimicrobial resistance through antibiotic stewardship programs, surgical-site infections, ventilator-associated pneumonia, central-line-related bloodstream infections, and influenza transmission in health care facilities, it was critical to develop and implement public health infrastructure for surveillance and effective interventions, including the development of an effective HAI surveillance and prevention program and an electronic database for public reporting, and to strengthen lab capacity.[25] In contrast, the MLCs in most instances lack both a national surveillance system and the capacity within the health systems to address the mounting burden of HAIs.[26] Over the last 8 years, significant progress has been made in benchmarking regional and international data from the MLCs and identifying the relative economic and social burdens of HAI.[27] A major step 8 years ago was the founding of the International Nosocomial Infection Control Consortium (INICC) to standardize surveillance and control HAIs in hospitals in developing countries. In the INICC report of March 2010, there were no surprises. As expected, the rate of infections was several-fold higher in MLCs than in developed countries in all categories of HAIs, and most of the bacteria were resistant to multiple antimicrobics.[28]

THE NEGLECTED AND SEVERELY NEGLECTED TROPICAL DISEASES

Emerging infectious diseases such as Ebola virus, West Nile virus, avian influenza (H5N1), severe acute respiratory syndrome (SARS), and the so-called swine flu (H1N1) represent the tip of the iceberg but capture a lot of attention and emergency funding. In contrast, the rest of the iceberg contains neglected and severely neglected tropical diseases that cause approximately 534,000 deaths annually.[29] The 13 neglected tropical diseases are among the most disabling chronic conditions. They target the world's bottom billion in terms of poverty and perpetuate the intergenerational cycle of poverty. The seven most prevalent neglected tropical diseases within this group (ascariasis, trichuriasis, hookworm infection, schistosomiasis, lymphatic filariasis, trachoma, and onchocerciasis) have been targeted for control and elimination by the Global Network for Neglected Tropical Diseases and their partners.[29,30] A hopeful sign is the inclusion of the neglected tropical diseases in the new Presidential Global Health Initiative.

CHRONIC AND NONCOMMUNICABLE DISEASES

By one estimate, chronic diseases such as cardiovascular disease, diabetes, respiratory disease, and cancers will account for 69% of all global deaths by 2030, with 80% of these deaths in the MLCs.[31] They are already surpassing infectious diseases as the major burden in the new century. A number of chronic diseases have a microbial cause or are driven by an infectious disease. This is in addition to other negative social determinants of health, such as poverty and lack of education, access to clean water, food, and human security. A whole complex of interactive social determinants and environmental factors such as poverty, discrimination, access to health care, availability of employment, adverse marketing of tobacco and products containing high salt and sugar, climate change, natural and human-made disasters, exposure to microbial threats, environmental toxins, and breakdown of public health play a significant role in both well-to-do nations and fragile states. These factors, which are usually beyond individual control, are now well recognized and form the basis of the historic WHO resolution on noncommunicable diseases and the high-level UN meeting scheduled for September 2011: "[T]he Resolution and the High Level meeting will place chronic diseases at the center of other development and health initiatives, including the need to strengthen health systems, the focus on prevention and control of disease, and the importance of whole-government approaches" to global health.[32] Both infectious diseases and chronic conditions (including mental health and cancers) require a robust and functioning health system to provide continuity of care through all stages of life, and primary health care within an integrated health system has been determined to be an indispensable point of entry for coordination of preventive, promotive, equity-based, quality affordable care.

TRANSFORMING HEALTH SYSTEMS, PRIMARY HEALTH CARE, AND UNIVERSAL HEALTH CARE

Health systems are "all organizations, people, and actions whose main intent is to promote, restore, or maintain health."[33] This definition includes efforts to address the determinants of health and to direct activities to improve health. The WHO has also identified six "building blocks" for an efficient health system: (1) service delivery, (2) health workforce, (3) health information systems, (4) access to essential medicines, (5) financing, and (6) leadership or governance. A health system is therefore "more than a pyramid of publicly owned facilities that deliver personal health services."[33] A critical element of efficient and equitable health systems rests on health policy and systems research (HPSR), which is very often divorced from health systems, especially in the MLCs. HPSR is "the production of new knowledge to improve how societies organize themselves to achieve health goals," and HPSR can address any or all of the six "building blocks."[10] The achievement of health goals rests on an integrated system of primary care within a comprehensive health system. The primary care movement has been driven by the global values of equity, social justice, and solidarity and aims to create universal health care for all.[34] Increasingly, it is realized that effective primary care, regardless of its location, is best situated within a dynamic integrated health system that in turn reaches out and interacts with other sectors of the economy and civil societies. It is critical that these integrated primary care models include anesthesia, obstetric care, acute surgical care, ongoing surgical needs, and trauma care.[35] Excellent supportive laboratory and imaging systems are critical to all integrated health systems. Quality assurance and safety processes guide developing health systems to excellence.

TRANSFORMING GLOBAL HEALTH EDUCATION, RESEARCH, SERVICE, ADVOCACY, AND POLICY

In 1997, there were two sets of organizations involved in global health. One group derived their legitimacy from their mission and global constitutional basis; this group includes the WHO, UNICEF, and the United Nations Population Fund. The other group included organizations in North America that derived their legitimacy from their constituency, such as the National Council for International Health (now Global Health Council), whose main mission was to improve global health by providing vigorous leadership and advocacy to increase private and public sector commitment to international health issues; the Canadian Society for International Health, a professional organization also advocating for international health issues; and, importantly, the academic institutions represented by the International Health Medical Education Consortium (now the Global Health Education Consortium [GHEC]).[36] These three organizations shared the same challenge of how to attract and maintain interest in problems that often seemed distant. As Alleyne[36] stated, "The prize for most of these institutions and associations lay in development of new knowledge that had a value in and of itself as well as success in seeding in those who participated a new appreciation of the reality of health in other settings." He further said, "It is interesting to note that these entities in *international public health have been virtually ignored in the debate on how international or global public health problems might be addressed* [emphasis added]. As far as I am aware, little systematic attention has been given to the possibility of having this kind of institution become international or multinational in the sense of being replicated in several countries of the world."[36] Except for these organizations, a state of disinterest and noncollaboration in global health prevailed. A prominent member of the Institute of Medicine (IOM) Committee on International Health stated, "The last time I was on the committee, everybody was saying we might as well shut down this committee because nobody cares anymore and there is no interest in the US in international health. Some of us argued that we should produce a white paper that would try to find a reason people should care. So we did. We ended up doing the report that focused on what is America's self-interest in having our country remain active in global health."[37] Much has been achieved at IOM in global health since then including several groundbreaking reports such as the one on global health, chronic conditions, HIV-AIDS, and other topics, as can be seen on their Web site: http://www.iom.edu/Global/Topics/Global-Health.aspx.

Today, we would also say that GHEC has had considerable success in cultivating interest and involvement in global health in North American universities, and the launching of The Network for Equity represents a unique international model of education of health care professionals, based on the principles of global equity.[38,39]

TRANSFORMATIVE MODELS OF EDUCATION: LESSONS FROM AFRICA

Pliny the Elder, a Roman scholar and scientist (23 to 79 AD) famously stated, "There is always something new out of Africa."[40] Having lived the first third of my life in Africa, I agree with this statement and recently participated in several major initiatives, in differing capacities, in reforming and transforming medical education. These initiatives included The Afiya Bora ("good health" in Swahili) in Nairobi, Kenya[41]; Developing Health Care Leadership, sponsored by the Institute of Infectious Disease at Makerere University, Kampala[42]; the sub-Saharan Africa Medical School Study (SAMSS)[43,44]; Celebrating Accountable Medical Education in Africa at the Walter Sisulu University in Mthatha, South Africa; and the Global Consensus for Social Accountability of Medical Schools (GCSA).[45] These efforts have given me another valuable perspective on the rapid pace of development and transformation of educational leadership emanating from Africa. Some of these remarkable achievements and ongoing efforts are highlighted in the following sections, including the formation of the African Science Academy.

SAMSS

This pathbreaking study examined the challenges, innovations, and emerging trends in medical education in sub-Saharan Africa. This study made 10 recommendations (**Box 1**)[43,44] relevant to universities in Africa and their current and prospective partners, including donors, policy makers, and governments (especially the ministries of health, education, and finance, which often do not work cohesively in ensuring the needs of their populations). The study resulted in funding to transform African medical education. It is important to mention the leadership role of Francis Omaswa, the Director of

---

Box 1
Recommendations of the SAMSS

1. Launch campaigns to develop medical school faculty capacity, including recruitment, training, and retention

2. Ramp up investment in medical education infrastructure

3. Institute structures to promote interministerial collaboration for medical education

4. Fund research and research training at medical schools

5. Promote community-oriented education based on principles of primary health care

6. Establish national and regional postgraduate medical education programs to promote excellence and retention

7. Establish national or regional bodies responsible for accreditation and quality assurance of medical education

8. Increase donor investment in medical education aligned with national health needs

9. Recognize and review the growing role of private institutions in medical education

10. Revitalize the association of medical schools in Africa

The African Center of Global Health and Social Transformation, who has also been a significant force in the global health workforce development.

GCSA: A New Paradigm of Medical Education

An International Reference Group of 130 organizations and individuals was formed to create a consensus document on the social accountability of medical schools. Sixty-five delegates from medical educational and accrediting bodies around the world, including GHEC and the Training for Health Equity Network, recently met in East London, South Africa, to finalize the document. A clear consensus was achieved on the direction of action on 10 interlinked areas (**Box 2**), in order that medical schools will have a greater impact on health system performance and on health status globally.[45]

Box 2
Areas of action from the GCSA of medical schools

Area 1. Anticipating society's health needs

Area 2. Partnering with the health system and other stakeholders

Area 3. Adapting to the evolving roles of doctors and other health professionals

Area 4. Fostering outcome-based education

Area 5. Creating responsive and responsible governance of the medical school

Area 6. Refining the scope of standards for education, research, and service delivery

Area 7. Supporting continuous quality improvement in education, research, and service delivery

Area 8. Establishing mandated mechanisms for accreditation

Area 9. Balancing global principles with context specificity

Area 10. Defining the role of society

The next phase will address the implementation of these guidelines internationally. The WHO Guidelines on Transformative Medical Education are also in preparation. An exciting prospect is to make practical and institutionalize these ideas and to create global nodes of Centers of Excellence in Social Responsiveness and Accountability to guide the academic community, society, and governments.

The African Science Academy Development Initiative

As an element of civil society, science academies play a critical role in molding policies, advising the government, and "enabl[ing] citizens to better hold their democratically chosen representatives accountable by illuminating in a dispassionate fashion the science pertinent to issues of national importance."[46] How countries in the MLCs access their scientific minds both within their countries and in the diaspora is a true measure of maturity of governance and the democratic process. Several consensus studies by the various African Academies are currently underway or completed, such as studying the impact and policy formulations addressing infectious diseases such as HIV-AIDS, malaria, and tuberculosis; under-five mortality; health and nutrition; and food, water, and health security.[46]

Sub-Saharan Africa has an abundance of natural resources and scientific talent. Its economy is predicted to grow 5% to 5.5% in 2011, faster than the Organization for Economic Co-operation and Development and several other economies.[47] Recently, I had an opportunity to discuss various problems in global health and solutions from the perspective of the Africans with Gotlieb Monekosso, the father of African medical education and the emeritus director of the WHO Africa Region, while we traveled together in the last row of a bus from Mthatha to East London, South Africa. As Monekosso related, before independence, medical education in Africa was closely linked with Africa's political fortunes and misfortunes—there was no brain to drain, no research, no plans for the future. After independence, universities experienced very rapid exponential growth, with all its excitement and risks. However, universities, which Monekosso referred to as the nation's electric power generating unit, are still not used to their fullest potential. Universities are also the conscience of the nation, and paradoxically, the focal point of dissent, reaction, and sometimes conservative immobility. Because Africa is very rich in resources, it should be self-sustaining in various aspects of development.[48,49] In contrast to universities, there is a dearth of public health schools, and the Africans rightfully lament that there are "only 493 full-time faculty in public health for the entire continent...and only 42 doctoral students...the total academic public health workforce in Africa could fit into the department of epidemiology at Johns Hopkins."[50]

The 21st century can rightfully be called the century of global health, information, and knowledge because of the dramatic and complex pace and impact of globalization in several arenas. Knowledge translation is "the exchange, synthesis, and ethically sound application of knowledge—within a complex set of interactions among researchers and users—to accelerate the capture of the benefits of research...through improved health, more effective services and products, and a strengthened health care system."[51] This has become the foundation of the post-20th century society. Today it is not enough to generate knowledge; the connectivity that enables information to be widely and quickly available opens up corridors both in the real and virtual world for two-way or multiple-way sharing. Transformative education for medical, nursing, and midwifery health professionals has received increased attention a hundred years after the early reforms of the 20th century. Several recent reference groups and commissions on scaling up health education have focused on the inadequacies and imbalances of the global health workforce to meet the specific health needs of societies in both the MLCs and upper income economies.[43–45,52,53] WHO and PEPFAR are working jointly on the long-term objective of transforming the education of health professionals so that social accountability is a norm for health professional schools. The launching of the Medical Education Partnership Initiative (MEPI) (http://www.fic.nih.gov/programs/training_grants/mepi/index.htm) and Nursing/Midwifery Education Partnership Initiative (NEPI) is anchored on the development of these principles at the outset.[54] MEPI is a 5-year, $130 million commitment by the United States' government to transform African medical education and significantly increase the number of health workers in sub-Saharan Africa. The initiative is designed to support PEPFAR's goal to train and retain 140,000 new health workers and strengthen the capacity of medical education systems in Africa. MEPI has awarded grants to African institutions in 12 countries, and has 30 regional partners as well as more than 20 United States' collaborators. Two other comprehensive reports on transformation of health professional education last year, the IOM report focused on nursing education[52] and the highly influential independent Lancet Commission on the transformation of professional education to strengthen health systems in an interdependent world,[53] have added considerable weight to the urgency of transforming health professionals' education. Scaling up of general education globally should include prekindergarten, primary, and secondary schools to prepare the current and future global health workforce. The dangers of education without future prospects of employment for the graduates are being exposed during the current crises in the Middle East. This situation is not unique to that region.

GLOBAL HEALTH LAW, SOCIAL JUSTICE, AND DIPLOMACY

In the last decade, remarkable progress has been made in the fields of global health law, human rights, social justice, and diplomacy. We have previously reviewed some of these aspects under the rubric of Global Health Ethics.[7] How can rights be ingrained and made more relevant for health professional practice in global health? George and colleagues, referring to the thinking of the Indian-born Noble Laureate Amartya Sen and RC Solomon, state , "Justice is generated through a continued process of public engagement and rational analysis to incrementally improve the lives of the most vulnerable people, rather than being derived from abstract principles alone."[55–57] Furthermore George and colleagues, referring again to Sen, state, "More attention has been paid to *niti*, which denotes the development of rules and behavioral norms of justice, than to *nyaya*, the actual social 'realizations' of justice—the lives people lead, regardless of whether or not the institutional architecture and laws have been perfectly rendered."[55,56]

A recent, skillfully crafted definition, that can be called "global health law with a face," includes the goal of global health law equity and health for all as outlined by the WHO, particularly to benefit the world's poorest populations, "Global health law is a field that encompasses the legal norms, processes, and institutions needed to create the conditions for people throughout the world to attain the highest possible level of physical and mental health. The field seeks to facilitate health-promoting behavior among the key actors that significantly influence the public's health, including international organizations, governments, businesses, foundations, the media, and civil society. The mechanisms of global health law should stimulate investment in research and development, mobilize resources, set priorities, coordinate activities, monitor progress, create incentives, and enforce standards. Study and practice of the field should be guided by the overarching value of social justice, which requires equitable distribution of health services, particularly to benefit the world's poorest populations."[58]

SUMMARY

Today, the breaking down of barriers to global health development gives us an unprecedented opportunity, not only for a new intergenerational dialog, but for sustained focus and action on the evolving paradigm of global health, global health education, and emerging health-system and research agendas. The renewed focused attention and action on the Millennium Development Goals, health system strengthening, reinvention of primary care with its moral-ethical backbone and framework, action on chronic and infectious diseases, neglected tropical diseases, poverty, education, climate change, long-neglected mental health, trauma, and surgical and anesthesia needs will certainly change how we view health and education. We continue to advocate for a comprehensive definition and compass of "global health with a face" that is beyond a discipline or goal, has a moral underpinning, and is accepted worldwide. The hard lessons we have learned teach us that all of these activities in the field and vision of global health must be integrated and shared among all sectors for sustained human development and the social good of all humankind.

ACKNOWLEDGMENTS

This work was supported by funding from Kaiser Permanente, and the author wishes to thank Naomi L. Ruff, PhD, ELS, for copyediting assistance.

REFERENCES

1. Velji AM, editor. International health. Infect Dis Clin North Am 1991;5(2).
2. Velji AM, editor. International health, beyond the year 2000. Infect Dis Clin North Am 1995;9(2).
3. Velji A, editor. Global Health, global health education, and infectious disease: the new millennium, part I. Infect Dis Clin North Am 2011;25(2).
4. Velji A, editor. Global Health, global health education, and infectious disease: the new millennium, part II. Infect Dis Clin North Am 2011;25(3).
5. Grant JP. Reaching the unreached: a miracle in the making. Asia Pac J Public Health 1991;5(2):154–62.
6. Alsan MM, Westerhaus M, Herce M, et al. Poverty, global health and infectious disease. Infect Dis Clin North Am 2011;25(3), in press.
7. Velji AM, Bryant JH. Global health ethics. In: Markle W, Fisher M, Smego R, editors. Understanding global health. Columbus (OH): McGraw Hill; 2007. p. 295–317.
8. Crisp N. Global health capacity and workforce development: Turning the world upside down. Infect Dis Clin North Am 2011;25(2):359–67.
9. Frenk J, Gómez-Dantés O, Knaul FM, et al. Globalization and Infectious Diseases. Infect Dis Clin North Am 2011;25(3), in press.
10. World Health Organization. Sound choices: enhancing capacity for evidence-informed health policy. Geneva (Switzerland): World Health Organization; 2007. Available at: www.who.int/alliance-hpsr. Accessed January 2, 2011.
11. Sommer A. Global health leadership. A continuing US challenge. West J Med 1992;157(1):71–3.
12. Velji A. Eight years and counting—what can Americans do? [editorial]. West J Med 1992;157(1):84.
13. Henry J. Kaiser family foundation. The U.S. Global Health Initiative. Menlo Park (CA): Henry J. Kaiser Family Foundation; 2011. Available at: http://www.kff.org/globalhealth/8116.cfm. Accessed February 2, 2011.

14. Bliss KE. Key players in global health: how Brazil, Russia, India, China, and South Africa are influencing the game. Washington, DC: Center for Strategic and International Studies; 2010.
15. Almeida C, Campos RP, Buss P, et al. Brazil's conception of South-South "structural cooperation" in health. RECIIS 2010;4(1):55–65.
16. Buss P. 19th Global Health Education Consortium's Distinguished Service Award acceptance speech. Available at: http://globalhealth.kff.org/multimedia/2010/April/10/GHEC-Keynote.aspx. Accessed February 16, 2011.
17. Bryant JH, Velji AM. Global health and the role of universities. Infect Dis Clin North Am 2011;25(2):311–21.
18. Debas H, Coates T. The new paradigm of the 21st century: University of California and Global Health Institute. Infect Dis Clin North Am 2011;25(3), in press.
19. Cornia GA, Jolly R, Stewart F. Adjustment with a human face. Oxford University Press. Oxford (United Kingdom): Clarendon Press; 1987.
20. White KL. Healing the schism: epidemiology, medicine, and the public's health. New York: Springer-Verlag; 1991.
21. Murray CJL, Lopez AD. The global burden of disease: a comprehensive assessment of mortality and disability from diseases, injuries, and risk factors in 1990 and projected to 2020. Boston: Harvard School of Public Health; 1996.
22. World Health Organization. The world health report 2000: health systems: improving performance. Geneva (Switzerland): World Health Organization; 2000.
23. Taylor LH, Latham SM, Woolhouse ME. Risk factors for human disease emergence. Philos Trans R Soc Lond B Biol Sci 2001;356(1411):983–9.
24. Antibiotic Resistance: Promoting Critically Needed Antibiotic Research and Development and the Appropriate Use ("Stewardship") of these Precious Drugs. Testimony before the House Committee on Energy and Commerce Subcommittee on Health. Washington, DC, 2010. Available at: http://www.idsociety.org/WorkArea/linkit.aspx?LinkIdentifier=id&ItemID=16656. Accessed January 25, 2011.
25. Chavez G, Delahanty K, Cahill C, et al. Recommendations for Reducing Morbidity and Mortality Related to Healthcare-Associated Infections in California: Final Report to the California Department of Health Services 2005. Available at: http://www.cdph.ca.gov/services/boards/Documents/HAIAWGReporttoDHSFinal.pdf. Accessed January 25, 2011.
26. Allegranzi B, Nejad SB, Combescure C, et al. Burden of endemic health-care-associated infection in developing countries: systematic review and meta-analysis. Lancet 2011;377(9761):228–41.
27. Rosenthal VD. Health-care-associated infections in developing countries. Lancet 2011;377(9761):186–8.
28. Rosenthal VD, Maki DG, Jamulitrat S, et al. International Nosocomial Infection Control Consortium (INICC) report, data summary for 2003-2008, issued June 2009. Am J Infect Control 2010;38(2):95, e2–104.
29. Hotez PJ, Molyneux DH, Fenwick A, et al. Control of neglected tropical diseases. N Engl J Med 2007;357(10):1018–27.
30. Garg N. Neglected Diseases and Access to Medicines. Infect Dis Clin North Am 2011;25(3), in press.
31. Samb B, Desai N, Nishtar S, et al. Prevention and management of chronic disease: a litmus test for health-systems strengthening in low-income and middle-income countries. Lancet 2010;376(9754):1785–97.
32. Alleyne A. Global health: the Twenty-First century global health priority agenda. Infect Dis Clin North Am 2011;25(2):295–7.

33. World Health Organization. Everybody's business: strengthening health systems to improve health outcomes: WHO's framework for action. Geneva (Switzerland): World Health Organization; 2007. Available at: http://www.who.int/healthsystems/strategy/everybodys_business.pdf. Accessed January 02, 2011.
34. World Health Organization. Primary health care now more than ever: the world health report 2008. Geneva (Switzerland): WHO; 2008.
35. Luboga S, Macfarlane SB, von Schreeb J, et al. Increasing access to surgical services in sub-saharan Africa: priorities for national and international agencies recommended by the Bellagio Essential Surgery Group. PLoS Med 2009;6(12):e1000200.
36. Alleyne GA. The challenge and prize for international health organizations in the Americas. Salud Publica Mex 1997;39(5):480–5.
37. Searing L. Global health: a conversation with Susan Scrimshaw, PhD. Leadership in Public Health 2000;5(2):17.
38. Velji AM. Global Health Education Consortium (GHEC): 20 years of leadership in Global Health and Global Health Education. Infect Dis Clin North Am 2011;25(2):323–35.
39. Palsdottir B, Neusy A. Network of innovative schools. Infect Dis Clin North Am 2011;25(2):399–409.
40. Pliny the elder. Available at: http://www.quotationspage.com/quote/24429.html. Accessed December 10, 2010.
41. Farquhar C, Nathanson N. The Afya Bora Consortium: an African-US partnership to train leaders in global health. Infect Dis Clin North Am 2011;25(2):399–409.
42. Summary of Proceedings, Infectious Diseases Summit: Building Healthcare Leadership in Africa: Accordia Global Health Foundation Alliances to Fight Infectious Diseases in Africa; 2009. Available at: http://www.accordiafoundation.org/sites/www.accordiafoundation.org/files/2009%20Infectious%20Diseases%20Summit%20Proceedings.pdf. Accessed January 11, 2011.
43. Mullan F, Frehywot S, Chen C, et al. The sub-Saharan African Medical School Study: data, observation, and opportunity. Available at: http://www.samss.org/samss.upload/wysiwyg/SAMSS%20Report_FinalV2_120110b.pdf. Accessed January 11, 2011.
44. Mullan F, Frehywot S, Omaswa F, et al. Medical schools in sub-Saharan Africa. The Lancet 2010. DOI: 10.1016/S0140-6736(10)61961-7.
45. International Reference Group. Global Consensus for Social Accountability of Medical Schools, 2010. Available at: http://healthsocialaccountability.org/. Accessed January 25, 2011.
46. The African Science Academies development initiative: progress and promise: the national academies. Available at: http://www.nationalacademies.org/asadi/progressreport.pdf. Accessed December 10, 2010.
47. Okonjo-Iweala N. Promoting smart and responsible investment in Africa. Presented at 2010 China Mining Congress and Expo. 2010. Tianjin (China). Available at: http://web.worldbank.org/WBSITE/EXTERNAL/NEWS/0,contentMDK:22765931~pagePK:64257043~piPK:437376~theSitePK:4607,00.html?cid=3001_2. Accessed February 18, 2011.
48. Monekosso GL. Strategies for developing innovative programs in international medical education. A viewpoint from Africa. Acad Med 1989;64(5 Suppl):S27–31.
49. Monekosso GL. African universities as partners in community health development. J Community Health 1993;18(3):127–36.
50. Ijsselmuiden CB, Nchinda TC, Duale S, et al. Mapping Africa's advanced public health education capacity: the AfriHealth project. Bull World Health Organ 2007;85(12):914–22.

51. Canadian Institutes of Health Research. Knowledge translation strategy 2004-2009. 2008. Available at: http://www.cihr-irsc.gc.ca/e/26574.html. Accessed February 23, 2011.

52. Committee on the Robert Wood Johnson Foundation Initiative on the Future of Nursing, Institute of Medicine. The future of nursing: leading change, advancing health Washington, DC: National Academies Press; 2011. Available at: http://books.nap.edu/openbook.php?record_id=12956. Accessed January 25, 2011.

53. Frenk J, Chen L, Bhutta ZA, et al. Health professionals for a new century: transforming education to strengthen health systems in an interdependent world. Lancet 2010;376(9756):1923-58.

54. World Health Organization. Scaling up nursing and medical education: report on the WHO/PEPFAR planning meeting on scaling up nursing and medical education. Geneva, 13-14 October 2009. Geneva (Switzerland), 2009. Available at: http://www.who.int/hrh/resources/scaling-up_planning_report.pdf. Accessed January 25, 2011.

55. George A, Chopra M, Seymour D, et al. Making rights more relevant for health professionals. Lancet 2010;375(9728):1764-5.

56. Sen A. The idea of justice. New Delhi: Penguin Books; 2009. Cited by: George A, Chopra M, Seymour D, Marchi P. Making rights more relevant for health professionals. Lancet May 22 2010;375(9728):1764-5.

57. Solomon RC. A passion for justice: emotions and the origins of the social contract. Lanham (MD): Rowman & Littlefield; 1995. Cited by: George A, Chopra M, Seymour D, Marchi P. Making rights more relevant for health professionals. Lancet May 22 2010;375(9728):1764-5.

58. Gostin LO, Taylor AL. Global health law: a definition and grand challenges. Public Health Ethics 2008;1(1):53-63.

The University of California Global Health Institute Opportunities and Challenges

Haile T. Debas, MD[a],*, Thomas J. Coates, PhD[b,c]

KEYWORDS

- Global health • Interdisciplinary • Education • Research
- Governance

The mission of the University of California Global Health Institute (UCGHI) (http://www.ucghi.universityofcalifornia.edu/)[1] is as follows: "Recognizing the long-standing and emerging challenges to global health, the University of California Global Health Institute will create multi-campus, trans-disciplinary centers of expertise to address these challenges through a novel problem-based and action-oriented structure. By integrating the vast expertise of faculty on the ten campuses, this unprecedented University-wide initiative will focus on producing leaders and practitioners of global health, conducting innovative and important research, and developing international collaborations to improve the health of vulnerable people and communities in California and world-wide."

In just a few years, the University of California (UC) has taken major steps in creating a unique transdisciplinary, multicampus academic global health model in the rapidly evolving field of global health. After 3 years of planning funded by the UC Office of the President (UCOP) and the Bill and Melinda Gates Foundation, the UCGHI was launched in November 2009 and has since evolved into an alliance of resources across the 10 campuses unequalled in its breadth and depth of faculty expertise and capacity to lead the global health movement. UC's strength in a range of

This work is supported by a grant from the Bill and Melinda Gates Foundation.

The authors have no conflict of interest to disclose.

[a] University of California Global Health Institute, University of California, 3333 California Street, Suite 285, San Francisco, CA 94143-0443, USA

[b] University of California Global Health Institute, San Francisco, CA, USA

[c] UCLA David Geffen School of Medicine, 9911 West Pico Boulevard, Suite 955, Los Angeles, CA 90035, USA

* Corresponding author.

E-mail address: hdebas@globalhealth.ucsf.edu

Infect Dis Clin N Am 25 (2011) 499–509

doi:10.1016/j.idc.2011.06.001

0891-5520/11/$ – see front matter © 2011 Published by Elsevier Inc.

disciplines from agriculture and engineering to health sciences and economics gives the university a comparative advantage over the 260 US and Canadian universities that have created global health programs in the past decade. The UCGHI, linked closely with existing campus global health programs, expands the interdisciplinary reach in research, education, and service to be a catalyst to the growth of the global health discipline on all 10 campuses. It is a model emblematic of a future envisioned in the 2010 report of the UC Commission on the Future: University of California in the 21st Century (http://ucfuture.universityofcalifornia.edu/).[2]

THE PLANNING PROCESS

The idea for the UC-wide global health initiative was conceived as a result of discussions of the 2005 UC Long-Range Guidance Committee, which concluded that major universities have to have global reach if they are to be competitive in the twenty-first century. The UCOP then provided funding to begin the initial planning process. Subsequent planning was accomplished over a 3-year period, thanks to a generous planning grant from the Bill and Melinda Gates Foundation. Planning was undertaken by several committees made up of faculty, administrators, and students representing the 10 campuses of the university and with the guidance of an External Scientific Advisory Committee. The initial plan was to form a UC-wide School of Global Health, but when the California economy collapsed in 2008, the vision was scaled back to establish, instead, an institute with 3 multicampus centers of expertise (COEs). It is hoped that UCGHI will serve as the nucleus of a future UC School of Global Health.

VISION

The vision is that the institute will represent a paradigm shift from traditional academic programs. The institute is designed to be problem based and not discipline based and is an interdisciplinary and transdisciplinary program bringing together faculty and trainees not only from the health sciences disciplines but also from nonhealth sciences, such as agriculture, business, economics, engineering, law, the social and behavioral sciences, and veterinary science. The unparalleled academic resources of the UC are thus engaged to address major global health problems. The program unifies faculty and students from all 10 campuses of the university. The programs of UCGHI are action oriented and go beyond those of traditional academic programs, which focus on education, research, publication, and dissemination. In addition, UCGHI strives to implement research and policy projects on a large scale. UCGHI is designed to be value adding and will collaborate with, but not attempt to replicate, the existing schools and programs.

SIGNIFICANCE OF THE UC GLOBAL HEALTH INITIATIVE

No university is better situated than the UC to be a leader in global health. The global health sector is a significant contributor to the economy of California. A recent study conducted by the UCGHI faculty showed that the global health sector supports 350,000 high-quality jobs in California, which generates nearly $20 billion in wages and salaries in the state per annum (http://www.ucghi.universityofcalifornia.edu/planning/reports.aspx).[3] California citizens need to be prepared to participate in and expand this workforce. With California's large number of immigrants and proximity to the Mexican border and the Asia Pacific region, the health of California is increasingly intersecting with the health of the world. The growing burden of disease in lower-income countries and potential infectious disease outbreaks focus attention on how diseases can spread rapidly in an increasingly globalized world. The expertise of the UC faculty provides solutions to these critical problems.

Global health is a national priority and is high on the policy and research funding agenda of the federal and state agencies as well as private foundations (http://www.iom.edu/Reports/2008/The-US-Commitment-to-Global-Health-Recommendations-for-the-New-Administration.aspx).[4] Much of the increase in funding for global health from the United States and other agencies can be attributed to the response of donor countries and foundations to the human immunodeficiency virus (HIV)/acquired immune deficiency syndrome (AIDS) epidemic. The response has shed light on the fact that many other diseases, both infectious and chronic, contribute to substantial mortality in the developing world. Other conditions such as eye problems, mental health difficulties, food insecurity, lack of educational and economic opportunity, and lack of effective pain control contribute to lowered quality of life and reduced economic output and security. The major world problem of climate control and global warming and the many ripple effects on food and health have yet to be felt. Lack of adequate person power in the developing world only makes all the problems worse, because there are not the personnel needed not only in the health sector but also in other related sectors whose efforts affect health.

Students are demanding education and degrees in global health, as well as research and service opportunities, in increasingly large numbers. Today's students are citizens of the world in ways that never happened with prior generations. They can be in quick, rapid, and inexpensive communication with people all over the world. Less expensive travel makes it possible to see the world. Students more and more are in contact with families in their country of origin, and those relationships nourish and cherish their desire to do something about the problems they see in those countries of origin. And it is no secret that disparities have increased in the United States among immigrant populations and traditionally underserved segments of the population. Students are motivated to contribute to solutions and want to learn how that can be done.

The UCGHI is already galvanizing the expertise in global health across the UC system, with hundreds of the UC faculty currently engaged in research and educational activities through the 3 COEs. The UCGHI has the opportunity to bring more students and faculty together in multidisciplinary teams to provide transformative solutions to the greatest health challenges the world is facing today.

THE STRUCTURE AND GOVERNANCE OF THE UCGHI

The UCGHI is directed by Haile T. Debas, MD, and codirected by Thomas J. Coates, PhD.

The UCGHI consists of an administrative core, 3 COEs, an educational program, and Information, Communication, and Education Technology (ICET) (**Fig. 1**).

The administrative core, hosted at University of California, San Francisco (UCSF), handles all administrative functions, including coordinating the system-wide activities of the UCGHI. The director (Debas) is at the UCSF campus and the codirector (Coates) at UC Los Angeles. The administrative core supports the External Scientific Advisory Committee and the Leadership Committee. The administrative core handles all communications for the UCGHI (including the Web site), manages all financial administration, and raises funds on behalf of the UCGHI. It is responsible for all communications with the UCOP and for establishing and monitoring milestones and activities. The administrative core is also responsible for developing and implementing the educational programs of the UCGHI, managing system-wide global partnerships, organizing UC Global Health Day, stimulating grant submissions from the COEs, facilitating best

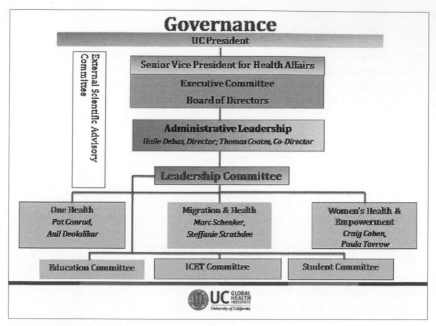

Fig. 1. Organizational chart.

practices for international research administration, and implementing the recommendations of the External Scientific Advisory Committee, the Executive Committee, and the Board of Directors.

The External Scientific Advisory Committee, chaired by Harvey Fineberg, MD (president of the Institute of Medicine), meets annually to provide strategic direction and advice and review the progress of the UCGHI and the COEs. **Box 1** presents the External Scientific Advisory Committee members.

The Executive Committee is chaired by John Stobo, MD (UCOP senior vice president for health affairs) with members including Michael Drake, MD (chancellor, UC Irvine), Stephen Shortell, PhD (dean, UC Berkeley School of Public Health), and Haile Debas, MD (director, UCGHI). The Executive Committee meets monthly and provides input into the development and operation of the UCGHI in between meetings of the Board of Directors.

The Board of Directors, chaired by John Stobo, MD, consists of the Executive Committee plus 1 member nominated by the chancellor of each campus. The Board of Directors is providing direction and input into the planning and development of the UCGHI. **Box 2** presents the members of the Board of Directors.

The Leadership Committee meets semimonthly by telephone and quarterly in person and is responsible for day-to-day operations of the UCGHI, providing leadership on research, education, and partnership development. The Leadership Committee is chaired by Haile T. Debas, MD, and cochaired by Thomas J. Coates, PhD. Membership includes the codirectors of each of the 3 COEs, the education cochairs, and the ICET cochairs (**Box 3**).

The ICET Committee is cochaired by James Kahn, MD (UCSF) and David Ernst, PhD (UCOP). The ICET Committee provides vision and leadership for planning of the UCGHI by developing a roadmap for how ICET can support and enable the UCGHI's mission and activities (**Box 4**).

Box 1
External Scientific Advisory Committee

Harvey Fineberg, MD

   President, Institute of Medicine (Chair)

Jo Ivey Boufford, MD

   President, New York Academy of Medicine

Luisa Cabal

   International Legal Program at the Center for Reproductive Rights

Wyatt Hume, DDS, PhD

   Provost, United Arab Emirates University

Jeffrey Koplan, MD, MPH

   Vice president, Global Health, Emory University

Ramanan Laxminarayan, PhD, MPH

   Center for Disease Dynamics, Economics & Policy

Onesmo K. ole-MoiYoi, MD, DSC (HC), EBS

   Chairman, Kenya Agricultural Research Institute

Jaime Sepulveda, MD, MPH, DRSC, MSC

   Senior fellow, Global Health Programs, The Bill and Melinda Gates Foundation

THE COES

Three COEs form the foundation of the UCGHI transdisciplinary education, research, and partnership programs. These 3 COEs were selected after letters of intent were requested from all 10 UC campuses. The range of proposals ranged from infectious diseases, disasters and emergencies, chronic diseases, innovative technology for pediatric global health, and others. The proposals were ranked by an external committee of national and international experts in global health, and the final selection was made by the director with the assistance of the External Scientific Advisory Committee.

The COEs currently part of the UCGHI are:

- Center of Expertise on Migration and Health (COEMH), codirected by Steffanie Strathdee, PhD (UC San Diego) and Marc Schenker, MD, MPH (UC Davis), starts with the fact that migration is a global phenomenon involving hundreds of millions of people, with major social and economic impacts on countries of origin and destination. In the United States, California is by far the most affected by the population movements. The COEMH is the first multidisciplinary, university-based program in the world devoted to systematically studying the health consequences of international population movements and developing more effective strategies to address them. Training the next generation of health care researchers and practitioners to understand and deal more effectively with California's immigrant and refugee communities is a vital necessity. The research agenda at the COEMH focuses on 4 key areas: behavioral and socioeconomic determinants of health, health outcomes in the migrants' communities of origin and destination, child health, and health care delivery and policy. Forty scholars at all 10 UC campuses serve on the center's core faculty.

Box 2
Board of Directors

The Board is led by an Executive Committee:

John D. Stobo, MD (Chair)

Senior vice president, Health Sciences & Services, UCOP

Haile T. Debas, MD

Codirector, UC Global Health Institute

Michael V. Drake, MD

Chancellor, University of California, Irvine

Stephen M. Shortell

Dean, UC Berkeley School of Public Health

With faculty representation from all 10 campuses, including:

Cherie Briggs

Ecology, Evolution & Marine Biology, University of California, Santa Barbara

Mary Croughan, PhD

Executive director, Research Grant Programs Office, UCOP

Steven C. Currall, PhD

Dean, Graduate School of Management, University of California, Davis

Sir Richard Feachem, KBE, FREng, DSc(Med), PhD

Professor of Global Health, University of California, San Francisco

Joshua Graff-Zivin, PhD

International Relations & Pacific Studies, University of California, San Diego

Sheldon Greenfield, MD

Executive director, Center for Health Policy Research, UC Irvine School of Medicine

Eva Harris, PhD

Professor of Infectious Diseases and Vaccinology, director of Center for Global Public Health, UC Berkeley School of Public Health

Patrick E. Mantey, PhD

Director, Information Technologies Institute, director, CITRIS Santa Cruz

Manuela Martins-Green, PhD

Department of Cell Biology and Neuroscience, University of California, Riverside

Claire Panosian, MD

UCLA Program in Global Health, University of California, Los Angeles

Jan Wallander, PhD

School of Social Sciences, Humanities and Arts, University of California, Merced

R. Sanders Williams, MD

President, J. David Gladstone Institutes

Box 3
Leadership Committee

Directors

    Thomas J. Coates, PhD, UC Los Angeles

    Haile Debas, MD, UC San Francisco

Centers of excellence codirectors

    One Health: Water, Animals, Food, and Society

        Patricia Conrad, DVM, PhD, UC Davis

        Anil Deolalikar, PhD, UC Riverside

    Migration and Health

        Marc Schenker, MD, MPH, UC Davis

        Steffanie Strathdee, MD, PhD, UC San Diego

    Women's Health and Empowerment

        Craig Cohen, MD, PhD, UC San Francisco

        Paula Tavrow, PhD, MSc, MALD, UC Los Angeles

ICET Committee cochairs

    David Ernst, JD, UCOP

    Jim Kahn, MD, UC San Francisco

Education Committee cochairs

    John Ziegler, MD, MSC, UC San Francisco

    Wayne Cornelius, PhD, UC San Diego

Box 4
ICET Committee

David Ernst, UCOP (cochair)

Jim Kahn, UC San Francisco (cochair)

Dipak Basu, NetHope

Opinder Bawa, UC San Francisco

Jim Davis, UC Los Angeles

Laine Farley, California Digital Library

Mara Fellouris, UC San Francisco

Mara Hancock, UC Berkeley

Mike Minear, UC Davis

Paula Murphy, UC San Francisco

Frank Rijsberman, Google Foundation

David Sessions, Walmart International

Chris Thomas, Intel

- Center of Expertise on One Health: Water, Animals, Food, and Society (COEOH), codirected by Patricia Conrad, DVM, PhD (UC Davis) and Anil Deolalikar, PhD (UC Riverside), creates linkages between human, animal, and environmental health. Forging these bonds helps to promote a global and species-spanning understanding of health and disease. The mission of the COEOH is to assess and respond to global health problems arising at the human-water-animal-food interface and to design, implement, and evaluate practical, cost-effective, and sustainable solutions that focus on the foundation of health in collaboration with local partners. Research at the COEOH focuses on reducing the rate of disease resulting from malnutrition, unsafe water, and animal-borne and vector-borne diseases, with the aim of designing, implementing, and evaluating health interventions at the national, regional, community, and household levels. Many global health problems related to One Health are relevant to California; for example, food, proximity to animals, water contamination, water scarcity, and how the combination of these factors leads to illnesses.
- Center of Expertise on Women's Health and Empowerment, codirected by Paula Tavrow, PhD (UC Los Angeles) and Craig Cohen, MD, MPH (UCSF), believes that advances in women's health globally are impeded by poverty, limited access to educational and economic opportunities, gender bias and discrimination, unjust laws, and insufficient state accountability. These forces intersect to restrict access to vital women's health services and the information that women need to improve their lives. By prioritizing women's health concerns, rights, and empowerment, this COE is uniquely poised to catalyze societal-level changes that will yield improvements in the well-being of women on a global scale.

All 3 COEs bring together experts from different disciplines, develop innovative and transformational solutions for major global health challenges, translate discoveries into large-scale action, establish partnerships, train future leaders, and build capacity in the global health workforce. Faculty from all 10 campuses are involved in the COEs' activities and research.

THE EDUCATIONAL MISSION OF THE UCGHI

The UCGHI is the first UC multicampus program that includes, in addition to research, the missions of teaching, service, and partnerships. The UCSF Global Health Sciences Program created a master's degree in global health and the first degrees were awarded in 2008 (http://globalhealthsciences.ucsf.edu/education/).[5] This 1-year master's program forms 1 anchor of the educational vision of the UCGHI.

The UCGHI has also started planning for a proposed 2-year research-oriented master's degree in global health, which will seek to prepare students for leadership roles in global health, including international health policy, health care delivery, nongovernmental organizations serving limited-resource populations in the United States and abroad, and research and development. The UCGHI Master of Science (MS) program will offer both breadth and depth and will provide broad training to satisfy core global health competencies, including quantitative and qualitative research methods, epidemiology, biostatistics, social and behavioral determinants of health, the economics of health, cost-effectiveness analysis, global health practice, policy development, and leadership. Students will also be able to pursue a substantive specialization in 1 of 3 areas: Migration and Health, One Health, and Infectious Diseases and Therapies. The opportunity to develop such a specialty portfolio will enhance students' career prospects and will be one of the program's major strengths.

Training will be broadly interdisciplinary, drawing on faculty in health sciences, environmental sciences, and social and behavioral sciences. For all students, including those not wishing to pursue a specialization track, the availability of nonhealth sciences electives (eg, in the social and behavioral sciences, ecology, engineering, and so forth) will be another attraction. As the UCGHI MS degree is intended to be a research-oriented academic degree (vs a professional degree), there will be a substantial field research requirement, with fieldwork to be done abroad or among immigrant/refugee populations and other low-resource communities in California, and a required thesis. The real-world experience gained through these field placements will be a key element of students' training.

Faculty for the program will be drawn from 3 consortium campuses and other UC campuses, whose faculty will participate through distance learning, guest lecturing, thesis mentoring, or fieldwork supervision. The goal will be to engage faculty from all 10 campuses in the training of UCGHI MS students. For example, for training in the Migration and Health track, faculty at 5 nonconsortium campuses can be invited to participate: faculty in UC Merced's PhD program in psychology (approval pending) whose work relates to the mental health of migrants; experts on the sociology of immigration, immigrant education, and immigration law at UC Berkeley, UC Irvine, and UC Los Angeles; and specialists on community organizations among California's Latino populations at UC Merced and UC Santa Cruz. For the One Health track, faculty from UC Berkeley, UC Merced, and UC Santa Cruz who focus on water issues, nutrition, and environmental health will be asked to participate. For the Infectious Diseases and Therapies track, relevant faculty at UC Berkeley, UC Irvine, UC Los Angeles, and UCSF can be tapped. In particular, UC Los Angeles and UCSF have Centers for AIDS Research with large numbers of faculty working in HIV-related research.

The 1-year master's degree option includes 30 units of coursework and a thesis. A second master's degree option is proposed to be 2 years in duration (six quarters), with flexible options to potentially shorten the time required for completion to approximately 18 months for students already enrolled in professional degree programs (eg, medicine, veterinary medicine, law, business).

The program may be completed concurrently with a PhD program in another discipline, such as anthropology, economics, environmental sciences, political science, psychology, public health, and sociology. Requirements can be designed so that concurrent PhD students could receive credit for some of the graduate courses they have already taken and thus complete the core UCGHI MS requirements in less time.

THE USE OF TECHNOLOGY IN THE UCGHI

A distributed institute requires technology to support distance collaboration and teaching. The ICET core of the UCGHI is planning and implementing such technologies to support not only collaboration within California but also collaboration with international partners. The ICET priorities are supporting distance teaching, collaborative research across UCGHI, and support for UCGHI international partnerships. The following are in the planning phase for implementation when resources become available:

1. Learning management system
2. Lecture capture
3. Videoconferencing/distance learning platforms
4. Curriculum management tools

5. Web-based cases
6. Collaboration tools
7. Course evaluation

THE UCGHI AS A MODEL FOR THE UNIVERSITY OF THE FUTURE

The next steps in the development of the UCGHI involve achieving the following 6 objectives:

1. Develop and implement a system-wide strategy to provide the organizational infrastructure for global health research, education, outreach, and fundraising at all 10 UC campuses.
2. Bring students and faculty together in multidisciplinary teams to provide transformative solutions to the greatest health challenges facing the world today.
3. Train future leaders in global health using online technology applications.
4. Develop and sustain global partnerships.
5. Develop systems to facilitate international research and training.
6. Raise funds to support the infrastructure and the research, education, and partnership needs of the UCGHI.

It is no secret that the State of California is strapped for funds, and Governor Brown's 2011 budget includes a $500 million reduction in funding for the university. In response to the impending budget cuts, University President Yudof convened the UC Commission on the Future (COTF) to determine ways of reforming the university with an eye toward maintaining quality while encouraging efficiencies to preserve precious funds. The UCGHI will implement several recommendations of the UC Commission on the Future: University of California in the 21st Century (http://ucfuture.universityofcalifornia.edu/presentations/cotf_final_report.pdf).[2] It is multi-campus, multidisciplinary, and largely virtual. The multicampus and multidisciplinary programs of the UCGHI demonstrate that "research and training will be cost effective while actually creating some academically richer opportunities for the participants." Specifically, the UCGHI addresses the following COTF recommendations:

- Continue timely exploration of fully online instruction for undergraduates, as well as for self-supporting programs and in university extension. The UCGHI is already implementing online instruction in its extension courses and makes extensive use of videoconferencing in its master's program. A 2-year multicampus master's degree and planned undergraduate programs will make even fuller use of online instruction. In the next 5 years, it is proposed to train future global health leaders using online technology and applications (objectives 3 and 5).
- Facilitate multicampus research and doctoral/postdoctoral training. The UCGHI is already facilitating multicampus research through its 3 COEs and has competed successfully for a multicampus postdoctoral training program in Women's Health and Empowerment and a research program in Migration and Health. It will continue to facilitate multicampus research and expand doctoral and postdoctoral training (objectives 3 and 5).
- Collaborate with external partners to expand sponsored internships, fellowships, and visiting faculty. The UCGHI has partners on all continents and active exchange programs with academic, governmental, and nongovernmental programs all over the world. Undergraduate and master's students participate in these relationships during field studies. During the next 5 years, global partnerships will be developed and sustained (objective 4).

- Increase graduate student enrollment to meet long-range planning goals and research mission prescribed in the master's plan. The UCGHI coordinates with the UCSF master's program and is now actively planning a 2-year research master's degree in global health. It is proposed to initiate planning for doctoral programs in global health. All these programs will be multicampus and multidisciplinary (objectives 3 and 5).
- Expedite implementation of UC's initiative on system-wide administrative reforms, with the goal of $500 million in annual savings. The UCGHI has demonstrated that a central administration can stimulate and facilitate global health research and education throughout the UC system in a highly cost-effective manner. System-wide strategies will be developed and facilitated to provide the organizational infrastructure for global health research, education, and fundraising, exploiting synergies across the UC campuses (objective 1).
- Accelerate development of self-supporting programs and increase the income derived from these programs to $250 million per year in 5 years. The UCGHI already has 30 students enrolled in a self-supporting 1-year master's program at UCSF and proposes a 2-year self-supporting multicampus research master's that will enroll at least 30 additional, and possibly significantly more, students. A doctoral program will follow (objectives 3 and 5).
- Raise UC-wide ambitions for private fundraising. The UCGHI is already actively involved in UC-wide fundraising. It is proposed to raise funds to support the infrastructure and the research, education, and partnership needs of the UCGHI (objective 6).

SUMMARY

The creation of the UCGHI represents a paradigm shift in structure and function. Its 3 COEs (Migration and Health, One Health, and Women's Health and Empowerment) not only involve all 10 of the UC campuses but also bring together a wide range of disciplines from both the health and nonhealth sciences. They have created truly interdisciplinary and transdisciplinary programs that are addressing complex global health challenges of the twenty-first century, training future global health leaders, and forging international academic partnerships. The metrics by which UCGHI will judge itself will include not only the usual metrics for academic success but, just as importantly, the actual impact its programs make on the health and welfare of poor people everywhere.

REFERENCES

1. University of California Global Health Institute Website. Available at: http://www.ucghi.universityofcalifornia.edu/. Accessed February 4, 2010.
2. University of California Website. Available at: http://ucfuture.universityofcalifornia.edu/. Accessed February 4, 2011.
3. University of California Global Health Institute Website. Available at: http://www.ucghi.universityofcalifornia.edu/planning/reports.aspx. Accessed February 4, 2011.
4. Institute of Medicine Website. Available at: http://www.iom.edu/Reports/2008/The-US-Commitment-to-Global-Health-Recommendations-for-the-New-Administration.aspx. Accessed February 4, 2011.
5. University of California, San Francisco Global Health Sciences Website. Available at: http://globalhealthsciences.ucsf.edu/education/. Accessed February 4, 2011.

Global Health: The Fogarty International Center, National Institutes of Health: Vision and Mission, Programs, and Accomplishments

Joel G. Breman, MD, DTPH[a,*], Kenneth Bridbord, MD, MPH[b],
Linda E. Kupfer, PhD[a], Roger I. Glass, MD, PhD[b]

KEYWORDS

- Fogarty International Center • NIH
- Research training in poor countries
- Infectious and noninfectious diseases training

The Fogarty International Center (FIC) is 1 of the 27 institutes and centers (ICs) of the United States National Institutes of Health (NIH), a component of the Department of Health and Human Services (DHHS). The FIC supports basic, clinical, and applied research and research training for US and foreign investigators working in low-income and middle-income countries (LMICs). Since its establishment by Congress in 1968, more than 3600 scientists globally have received long-term (≥ 6 months) research training and research awards through FIC programs, mostly scientists and public health leaders from the poorest nations; tens of thousands more have received shorter-term training.

To implement its programs, FIC partners with more than 20 ICs at NIH, numerous US Government agencies, the World Health Organization (WHO), the Bill & Melinda Gates Foundation and other foundations and, most importantly, LMICs, to develop,

The authors have nothing to disclose.

[a] Fogarty International Center, National Institutes of Health, 16 Center Drive, Bethesda, MD 20892, USA

[b] Fogarty International Center, National Institutes of Health, 31 Center Drive, Bethesda, MD 20892, USA

* Corresponding author.

E-mail address: joel.breman@nih.gov

Infect Dis Clin N Am 25 (2011) 511–536

doi:10.1016/j.idc.2011.06.003

0891-5520/11/$ – see front matter Published by Elsevier Inc.

fund, and implement programs of common interest and mutual benefit. More than 400 extramural research training and research projects involving more than 100 US universities are operating in more than 100 LMICs (**Fig. 1**). The FIC also convenes small and large conferences so that the most eminent authorities can address critical global health research problems such as polio eradication, the impact of climate on disease outbreaks, setting disease control priorities in developing countries, confronting the global epidemiologic and demographic shift, defining the research agenda for stopping the spread of *Plasmodium falciparum* resistance to artemisinin compounds, and strengthening research capacity in LMICs. In addition to extramural activities, within FIC there is a research division focusing on quantification of epidemiologic trends tied to influenza, diarrheal diseases, malaria, and other infectious diseases (IDs). Other divisions within the FIC define FIC global health research policies, strategies, and programs; track and evaluate the success of FIC trainees and activities; promote international collaborations of all NIH ICs; and, administer the global health programs.

Global health research is now one of the NIH director's priorities; this commitment has increased enthusiasm and investment in global health research across the campus. The FIC director's role as the NIH Associate Director for International Research enables Fogarty to encourage the mobilization of the NIH investment to focus strategically on priority global health issues. President Barack Obama and Secretary of State Hillary Clinton have identified global health as a top international

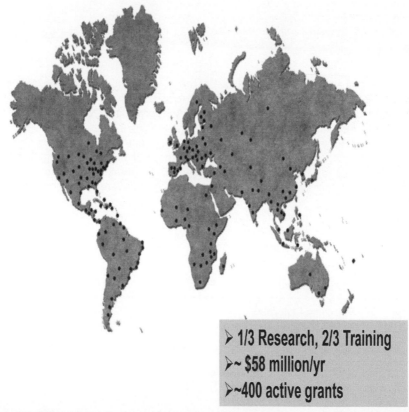

> 1/3 Research, 2/3 Training
> ~ $58 million/yr
> ~400 active grants

Fig. 1. FIC, NIH-supported major extramural training and research sites, 2010. (*From* National Institutes of Health, Bethesda, MD.)

priority within the administration's new Global Health Initiative,[1] which focuses on IDs and maternal-newborn and child health.

Why this focus on young children and mothers? A recent review of mortality of children less than 5 years old has shown that worldwide mortality in children younger than 5 years has dropped from 11.9 million deaths in 1990 to 7.7 million deaths in 2010; yet, 3.1 million (40%), 2.3 million (30%), and 2.3 million (30%) of these deaths occur in the neonatal (<1 month), postneonatal (1 month to 1 year), and 1-year to 5-year periods, respectively.[2] Many if not most of these deaths are caused by preventable infections. In addition, there are an estimated 350,000 maternal deaths yearly during pregnancy or childbirth and these deaths are also avertable.[2,3]

THE DISEASE CONTROL PRIORITIES PROJECT AND THE FIC STRATEGIC PLAN, 2008 TO 2012

A landmark set of encyclopedic studies was published in 2006 by the Disease Control Priorities Project (DCPP) addressing global health and global health research priorities and the cost-effectiveness of interventions to address common health conditions in LMICs. The DCPP was an alliance of the FIC/NIH, World Bank, WHO, Population Reference Bureau (for dissemination), and the Bill & Melinda Gates Foundation (as funder), with goals to quantify the global burden of diseases by geographic region, assess epidemiologic and demographic trends and projections, and compute the cost-effectiveness of interventions to manage, control, and prevent those diseases.[4-8] The FIC served as the Secretariat for the DCPP. The DCPP analyses showed that during the latter half of the twentieth century, life expectancy increased dramatically throughout the world to greater than 60 years in all regions, except for sub-Saharan Africa (SSA), where life expectancy at birth was 46 years in 2001 (**Fig. 2**). Chronic and noncommunicable diseases have become more prominent in all regions, including the poorest as well as the richest, where cardiovascular diseases, mental illness, and cancers are also major problems (**Table 1**).[4,5] Perinatal conditions (birth trauma, infections, respiratory distress) are among the top 5 causes of disability adjusted life years (DALYs) in all but one LMIC region (Europe and Central Asia). Even with the demographic and epidemiologic shift, IDs comprise close to 30% of the disease burden in LMICs (**Table 2**).

Although SSA countries have only 13% of the population of LMICs, they have 25% of the DALYs, and 54% of all the IDs; countries in South-East Asia (SEA) comprise 27% of the LMIC population, 29% of all DALYs, and 27% of the IDs. Within SSA and SEA regions, IDs contribute 59% and 31% of the entire disease burden, respectively (see **Table 2**).[4-9] The top 6 IDs comprise almost 25% of all DALYs in LMICs (**Table 3**); SSA has the highest human immunodeficiency virus (HIV)/AIDS, malaria, measles, and sexually transmitted disease burdens and SEA leads in respiratory infections and diarrheal diseases.[9]

A map of the world with size of the country and regions reflecting infectious and chronic disease deaths is shown in **Fig. 3** (http://www.worldmapper.org); SSA and SEA are most prominent in this projection for deaths caused by IDs. By virtue of their large populations, countries in SEA have a dual burden of disease and deaths.

Best buys in health were calculated in the DCPP by a comprehensive set of cost-effectiveness analyses addressing more than 300 conditions for which proven personal and community-based interventions are available; the best buys expressed as DALYs averted per dollar invested include both chronic and communicable diseases (**Box 1**).[7] These conditions are addressed by several of the FIC programs. Assisting LMICs in setting their own priorities based on local analytical exercises,

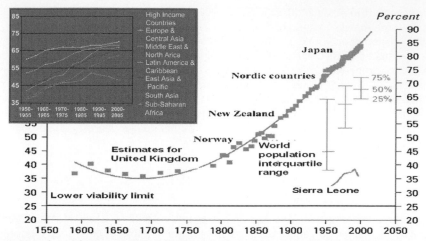

Fig. 2. Trends in life expectancy at birth: globally and by geographic (World Bank) region, 1550 to 2050. (*Courtesy of* World Bank Publications, Washington DC; with permission. Available at: http://www.dcp2.org.)

including best buys, was a major goal. Several countries are using DCPP materials and methods. India and South Africa have begun extensive national priority setting and health-sector planning exercises; these have been based on field research, health information, analysis, consensus meetings, and policy development actions, which are leading to disease reduction programs.[10,11] Both countries have a large dual burden of disease.

The goals and priorities of the FIC Strategic Plan, 2008–2012, were informed by and derive in great part from the extensive reviews and analyses in the DCPP and from US and LMIC stakeholders. As a research and training institution, the FIC vision is "a world in which the frontiers of health research extend across the globe and advances in science are implemented to reduce the burden of disease, promote health, and extend longevity for all people." The FIC achieves this vision through: facilitating and conducting global health research; building partnerships between and strengthening research institutions in the United States and abroad; and, training the next generation of scientists to understand, control, and prevent diseases, especially those in LMICs. FIC specific goals and priorities in the plan are shown in **Box 2**[12]; new goals address the shifting global burden of disease and disability and continue to address the unfinished agenda of IDs, research and research training, and implementation research to better deliver and scale up efficacious and locally feasible interventions.

FIC PROGRAMS

FIC programs address IDs, noninfectious diseases, and a variety of cross-cutting themes. The FIC extramural research training and research programs are listed in **Box 3**; the research training programs (usually D43s in NIH award classification) most often run for 5 years and are renewable through recompetitions. They have leadership development in science and public health as a primary goal. The FIC and NIH research programs (usually R01s, R03s, and 21s) do not have training as a primary goal per se but substantial numbers of LMIC scientists have emerged as leaders, benefitting directly from these collaborations. The FIC research training programs alone have trained more than 3600 scientists for periods from 6 months or longer to 4 years; 50% of the trainees have been associated with the HIV/AIDS

Table 1
Leading causes of DALYs in LMICs and high-income countries by geographic (World Bank) region, 2001

Rank	South Asia (GNI:$450) LE 63	Sub-Saharan Africa (GNI:$460) LE 46	East Asia and the Pacific (GNI:$900) LE 69	Europe and Central Asia (GNI:$1970) LE 69	Middle East and North Africa (GNI:$2200) LE 68	Latin America and the Caribbean (GNI:$3580) LE 71	High-income Countries (GNI:$26,500) LE 78
1	Perinatal conditions	HIV/AIDS	Cerebrovascular diseases	Ischemic heart disease	Ischemic heart disease	Perinatal conditions	Ischemic heart disease
2	Lower respiratory infections	Malaria	Perinatal conditions	Cerebrovascular diseases	Perinatal conditions	Unipolar depressive disorders	Cerebrovascular diseases
3	Ischemic heart disease	Lower respiratory infections	Chronic obstructive pulmonary disease	Unipolar depressive disorders	Traffic accidents	Homicide and violence	Unipolar depressive disorders
4	Diarrheal diseases	Diarrheal diseases	Ischemic heart disease	Self-inflicted injuries	Lower respiratory infections	Ischemic heart disease	Alzheimer's and other dementias
5	Unipolar depressive disorders	Perinatal conditions	Unipolar depressive disorders	Chronic obstructive pulmonary disease	Diarrheal diseases	Cerebrovascular diseases	Tracheal and lung cancer

Abbreviations: GNI, gross national income per capita (US$); LE, life expectancy at birth (average male and female, years).
Courtesy of World Bank Publications, Washington DC; with permission. Available at: http://www.dcp2.org. *Data from* Lopez AD, Mathers CD, Ezzati M, et al, editors. Global burden of disease and risk factors 2006. World Development Indicators; 2006.

Table 2
Disease burden in DALYs: LMICs by geographic (World Bank) region, 2001

Region	Population in millions (%)	For all diseases, no. in millions (%)	For infectious and parasitic diseases, no. in millions (%)	Infectious diseases burden in region,%[a]
Sub-Saharan Africa	668 (13)	345 (25)	173 (54)	59
South Asia	1,388 (27)	409 (29)	88 (27)	31
Middle East/North Africa	310 (6)	66 (5)	7 (2)	16
East Asia/Pacific	1,850 (35)	346 (25)	37 (12)	14
Latin America/Caribbean	526 (10)	104 (8)	10 (3)	13
Europe/Central Asia	477 (9)	117 (8)	5 (2)	6
Total	5,219 (100)	1,387 (100)	320 (100)	29

Columns under header: **Disability-Adjusted Life Years (DALYs)**

[a]includes respiratory infections

Mathers et al, 2006, in Lopez et al, *Global Burden of Disease and Risk Factors*

DCPP DISEASE CONTROL PRIORITIES PROJECT

Courtesy of World Bank Publications, Washington DC; with permission. Available at: http://www.dcp2.org.

programs; the Global Infectious Diseases Program, and the International Bioethics Education and Career Development Program have trained more than 400 persons each. Over 95% of reporting is complete for degree status of trainees: 46% received diplomas or certificates; 31% received master's degrees; 13% received doctorate degrees; 8% were post-doctoral students; and, 2% received bachelor's degrees. All research training programs by beginning and ending dates, number of grants given, and persons trained since the first major grant program began in 1988, including numbers of foreign and US trainees are in **Table 4**. The number of trainees by country is shown in **Table 5**. China, Brazil, South Africa, and India have had more

Table 3
Infectious burden, LMICs by geographic (World Bank) region, 2001

Disease	Disease Burden In LMICs DALYs, %	Disease burden by region, %					
		SSA	SA	ME/NA	EA/P	LA/C	E/CA
Respiratory inf.	6.3	36	40	4	14	4	3
HIV/AIDS	5.1	79	10	1	4	3	1
Diarrheal disease	4.2	37	38	4	15	4	1
Malaria	2.9	89	6	2	3	1	.1
TB	2.6	22	38	2	30	3	4
Measles	1.7	59	28	2	10	0	1
STD	0.7	40	39	4	9	5	2
	23.5						

SSA = Sub Saharan Africa; SA = South Asia; ME/NA = Middle East/North Africa; EA/P = East Asia/Pacific; LA/C = Latin America/Caribbean; E/CA = Europe/Central Asia

Mathers et al, 2006, in Lopez et al, *Global Burden of Disease and Risk Factors*

Courtesy of World Bank Publications, Washington DC; with permission. Available at: http://www.dcp2.org.

than 200 trainees each. In addition, tens of thousands of others have benefitted from shorter training experiences supported by the FIC and partners, including those tied to laboratory skills and technology transfer. Thousands more scientists and public health workers have been mentored and trained by the FIC trainees on their return home, and these in turn are training others. Thus, the FIC programs are a gift that keeps on giving.

The FIC proposed budget for fiscal year (FY) 2011 is about $73 million 0.24% of the NIH budget, of which $58 million is targeted toward the extramural research training programs. The FIC extramural budget grew substantially from 1988 to 2003 ($10 million to $50 million) but has flattened over the past 7 years; cofunding from partners

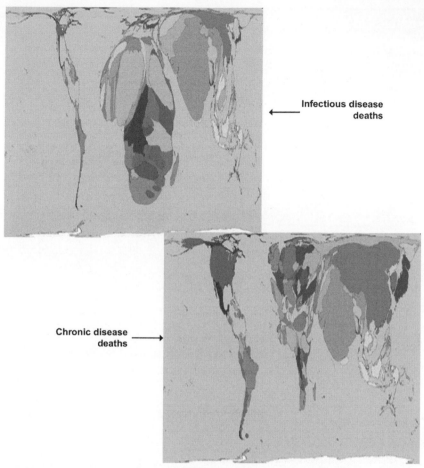

Fig. 3. Deaths caused by infectious and chronic (noninfectious) diseases by geographic region and country, 2002 to 2005. (*From* Worldmapper. © Copyright SASI Group (University of Sheffield) and Mark Newman (University of Michigan). Available at: http://www. worldmapper.org/)

has provided more than 20% of FIC support over the past decade with a notable increase in FY 2009 and FY 2010 largely because of the American Recovery and Reinvestment Act and the Medical Education Partnership Initiative (MEPI) (discussed later) (**Fig. 4**). From 1988 to 2010, FIC programs have invested more than 1 billion dollars, including cofunding, on global health research training, research, and capacity building in LMICs through partnerships with US institutions. A few examples of FIC programs follow.

IDs Programs

The AITRP, launched in 1988 in response to the HIV/AIDS epidemic, was the first FIC research training program to focus on LMICs and has remained the focus of FIC Extramural Programs; the AITRP has been the template for other Fogarty research training programs. Specific FIC programs have addressed the ecology of IDs (a research program), malaria, tuberculosis, and global IDs (non-HIV/AIDS), and biodiversity conservation/drug discovery from natural products (a research program).

Box 1
Top 10 best buys in health using disease burden and cost-effectiveness analysis

- Prevent neonatal mortality
- Ensure healthier mothers and children
- Promote good nutrition
- Reduce deaths from cardiovascular disease
- Stop the AIDS pandemic
- Stop the spread of tuberculosis
- Control malaria
- Combat tobacco use
- Reduce fatal and disabling injuries
- Ensure equal access to high-quality health care

Data from Refs.[4–6]

The AITRP

Since 1988, more than 1500 long-term trainees from more than 90 LMICs at greatest risk have benefited from more than $200 million FIC dollars invested in the AITRP; close to 90% of these trainees have returned to their home country and assumed important positions combating HIV/AIDS and related conditions (**Fig. 5**). Almost two-thirds of the trainees have been involved in PhD or postdoctoral advanced training in patient diagnosis, management, and prevention and undertaking basic virology, pathogenesis, and immunologic studies.[13–24] What follows are a few examples of research and training conducted as part of the AITRP program.

- The Botswana-Harvard AIDS Institute Partnership (BHP), established in 1996, addresses prevention of mother-child transmission, the genomic analysis of the HIV virus, vaccine development, and virus resistance and patient adherence to antiretroviral drugs; the BHP Reference Laboratory is in a training facility building in Gaborone supported by the AITRP and other donors.
- A Brazilian trainee linked to the University of California, Berkeley, AITRP has become Director of the National STI/HIV/AIDS Program and President of the National AIDS Commission.
- Decreasing HIV/AIDS transmission by circumcision of HIV-infected men was shown by FIC-supported scientists from Uganda and John Hopkins University.[22]
- The recently published and highly publicized study reporting the effectiveness of a vaginal gel in preventing HIV/AIDS transmission in South Africa was the result of several collaborations between the AITRP-supported Center for the AIDS Program of Research in South Africa, Cape Town, and Columbia University.[17,18]
- Because HIV predisposes patients to opportunistic infections, tuberculosis (and drug-resistant tuberculosis) is a closely related area of training and investigation in the AITRP and other FIC cooperative initiatives.[15,16,23]

GID

This program builds sustainable research capacity in LMICs in Asia, Africa, and Latin America that suffer from malaria and other infectious conditions, including neglected

---

Box 2
The FIC, NIH, strategic plan: goals and priorities, 2008 to 2012

- Goal I: Mobilize the scientific community to address the shifting global burden of disease and disability
  - Strategic priorities
    - Expand Fogarty's investment in noncommunicable diseases research and research training
    - Continue to invest in IDs research and research training
- Goal II: Bridge the training gap in implementation research
  - Strategic priorities
    - Support and expand the development of research training programs for implementation research
    - Support the application of implementation research to the recommendations from the DCPP
- Goal III: Develop human capital to meet global health challenges
  - Strategic priorities
    - Expand programs to provide early global health research experiences for US health science students and junior faculty
    - Sustain research training for future generations of foreign health scientists
    - Expand research support for foreign researchers to promote pathways to independence
- Goal IV: Foster a sustainable research environment in LMICs
  - Strategic priorities
    - Support the development of research hubs in LMICs
    - Bolster the development of expertise and use of information and communication technologies in support of research and research training programs
    - Sponsor the development of Fogarty alumni networks
- Goal V: Build strategic alliances and partnerships in global health research and training
  - Strategic priority
    - Forge partnerships based on mutual interest and complementary strengths

From National Institutes of Health, Bethesda, MD.

---

tropical diseases[25,26]; special focus is given to conditions that affect young children and pregnant women. As of 2004, the program had helped train more than 400 students at the undergraduate, graduate, and postdoctoral levels. Some examples of the science and training conducted under the GID program follow.

- Grantees from the University of Maryland working with colleagues in Mali and Malawi have discovered genetic markers useful for detecting resistance of *Plasmodium falciparum* to antimalarial drugs.[27]
- Scientists from the University of California, San Francisco, working with Ugandan Colleagues[28] have studied effective drug combinations, including artemisinin-based combination therapies for managing malaria.
- Principal investigators (PIs) from Cornell University and the University of California, Berkeley, have been working with PIs from the Foundation Oswaldo Cruz in

---

Box 3
FIC, NIH: Research and research training grants, 1988 to 2011

Research Training Grants

- AIDS International Training and Research Program (AITRP)
- Chronic, Non-communicable Diseases and Disorders Across the Lifespan: Fogarty International Research Training Award (NCD-LIFESPAN)
- Fogarty International Clinical Research Scholars & Fellows (FICRS-F)
- Fogarty International Collaborative Trauma and Injury Research Training Program (TRAUMA)
- Framework Programs for Global Health (FRAME)
- Global Infectious Disease Research Training Program (GID)
- Global Research Training in Population Health (POP)
- Independent Scientist in Global Health Award (ISGHA)
- Informatics Training for Global Health (ITGH)
- International Research Ethics Education and Curriculum Development Award (BIOETH)
- International Clinical, Operational, and Health Services Research and Training Award (ICOHRTA)
- International Implementation, Clinical, Operational, and Health Services Research Training Award for AIDS and Tuberculosis (IICOHRTA-AIDS/TB)
- International Collaborative Genetics Research Training Program (GENE)
- International Malaria Clinical, Operational & Health Services Research Training Programs Planning Grants (MALARIA ICOHRTA)
- International Research Scientist Development Award for US Postdoctoral Scientists (IRSDA)
- International Training and Research in Environmental and Occupational Health (ITREOH)
- Medical Education Partnership Initiative (MEPI)
- Millennium Promise Awards: Non-communicable Chronic Diseases Research Training Program (NCoD)

Research Grants

- Brain Disorders in the Developing World: Research Across the Lifespan (BRAIN)
- Dissemination and Implementation Research in Health
- Ecology of Infectious Diseases (EID)
- The Japan Society for the Promotion of Science (JSPS)
- Fogarty International Research Collaboration Award (FIRCA)
- Global Research Initiative Program for New Foreign Investigators (GRIP)
- International Cooperative Biodiversity Groups (ICBG)
- International Tobacco and Health Research and Capacity Building Program (TOBAC)
- Stigma and Global Health Research Program (STIGMA)[a]

[a] Not active in 2011.
From National Institutes of Health, Bethesda, MD.

Table 4
FIC, NIH, research training grants: number of grants and persons trained in LMICs and in the United States, 1988 to 2010

Program	Years of the Program	Year of First Training (as Reported in CareerTrac)	Number		
			Grants	Training Experiences for Long-term Foreign Trainees	Training Experiences for Long-term US Trainees
AIDS international Training and Research Program (AITRP)	1988–present	1989	29	1559	22
International Training and Research In Environmental and Occupational Health (ITREOH)	1995–present	1995	14	187	1
Global Research Training in Population Health (POP)	1995–2010	1996	12	232	0
Global Infectious Disease (GID)	1997–present	1996	41	405	1
Actions for Building Capacity (ABC)[a]	1998–2003	1997	7	48	0
Maternal & Child Health (MCH)	1999–2004	1998	10	64	0
Informatics Training Programs (International Training in Medical Informatics & Informatics Training in Global Health)[b]	1999–present	1999	11	87	0
International Malaria Research Training (MALAR)[a]	1999–2003	2000	4	15	0
International Bioethics Education and Career Development (BIOETHICS)	2000–present	2001	18	415	1

International Clinical, Operational and Health Services Research and Training Award (I CHORTA)	2001–2010	2001	15	169	1
International Implementation, Clinical, Operational, and Health Services Research Training Award for AIDS and Tuberculosis (II CHORTA-AIDS/TB)	2002–present	2002	10	174	0
International Collaborative Genetics Research Training (GENE)	2002–2009	1999	6	31	4
Scholars and Fellows Programs (Fogarty International Clinical Research Scholars Program & FIC/ELLISON Fellowships)[c]	2003–present	2004	1	215	212
Trauma and Injury Research Training Program (TRAUMA)	2004–present	2004	9	71	0
Total			187	3672	242

[a] Folded into the Global Infectious Diseases Program in 2004.
[b] Medical Informatics folded into Informatics Training for Global Health in 2003.
[c] FIC/ELLISON folded into FICRS in 2003.
From National Institutes of Health, Bethesda, MD.

Table 5
Countries and number of long-term trainees in research training programs supported by the FIC, NIH: 1988 to 2011

#	Country		#	Country		#	Country	
1	CHINA	290	28	BOTSWANA	29 ⎤	54	ETHIOPIA	8 ⎤
2	BRAZIL	273	28	TURKEY	29 ⎦	54	HUNGARY	8 ⎬
3	UNITED STATES[a]	241	30	POLAND	28	54	NICARAGUA	8 ⎦
4	SOUTH AFRICA	228	31	ROMANIA	26	57	BELARUS	7 ⎤
5	INDIA	217	32	MOZAMBIQUE	25	57	CONGO (DRC)	7
6	UGANDA	186	33	GHANA	22 ⎤	57	EL SALVADOR	7 ⎬
7	PERU	170	33	MALI	22 ⎦	57	MONGOLIA	7
8	ARGENTINA	169	35	CAMEROON	20 ⎤	57	TAIWAN	7 ⎦
9	KENYA	138	35	INDONESIA	20 ⎦	62	BOLIVIA	5 ⎤
10	HAITI	122	37	PHILIPPINES	18	62	CROATIA	5
11	ZAMBIA	108	38	UKRAINE	17	62	ESTONIA	5 ⎬
12	MEXICO	105	39	CZECH REPUBLIC	15 ⎤	62	LESOTHO	5
13	NIGERIA	100	39	HONDURAS	15 ⎬	62	NEPAL	5 ⎦
14	RUSSIA	81	39	VENEZUELA	15 ⎦	67	ECUADOR	4 ⎤
15	THAILAND	79	42	CAMBODIA	14 ⎤	67	LATVIA	4
16	TANZANIA U REP	67	42	COTE D'IVOIRE	14 ⎦	67	NAMIBIA	4
17	MALAWI	54	44	LAOS	13 ⎤	67	SUDAN	4 ⎬
18	VIETNAM	52	44	SENEGAL	13 ⎦	67	UNITED KINGDOM	4 ⎦
19	BANGLADESH	47	46	ARMENIA	12 ⎤	72	BURKINA FASO	3 ⎤
20	COLOMBIA	45 ⎤	46	ZAIRE/DROC	12 ⎬	72	GUATEMALA	3
20	ZIMBABWE	45 ⎦	46	NOT STATED[b]	12 ⎦	72	KAZAKHSTAN	3 ⎬
22	GEORGIA	44 ⎤	49	DOMINICAN REP	11	72	SRI LANKA	3 ⎦
22	PAKISTAN	44 ⎦	50	JAMAICA	10	76	BARBADOS	2 ⎤
24	URUGUAY	40	51	EGYPT	9 ⎤	76	GERMANY	2
25	COSTA RICA	34	51	LITHUANIA	9 ⎬	76	MOLDOVA	2 ⎬
26	CHILE	32 ⎤	51	SLOVAKIA	9 ⎦	76	SERBIA & MONTENEGO	2
26	RWANDA	32 ⎦				76	SIERRA LEONE	2 ⎦

[a]Reflects Clinical Scholars Program

[b]12 Trainees provided no "Country of Origin"

TOTAL 3639

From National Institutes of Health, Bethesda, MD.

Salvador and Rio de Janeiro, Brazil, studying leishmaniasis, schistosomiasis, human T-lymphotropic virus 1, meningitis, and other emerging pathogens of the urban and rural poor.[29]

EID

This research program, partnered with the National Science Foundation, funds interdisciplinary research that elucidates ecological and biologic mechanisms that govern the complex relationships tied to environmental changes and transmission dynamics of IDs. Activities focus on the development of predictive models for the emergence and spread of diseases in humans and other animals, and to create and enhance strategies to prevent or control them.

- One project focusing on a parasitic disease of coral reefs is among the first to show conclusively that climate is a driver for ID in marine ecosystems. The same project has adapted an RNA-based biosensor for field diagnosis of *Aspergillus*.

The FIC Intramural Program-International Epidemiology and Population Studies (DIEPS) focuses on the study of the determinants, spread, and burden of IDs using

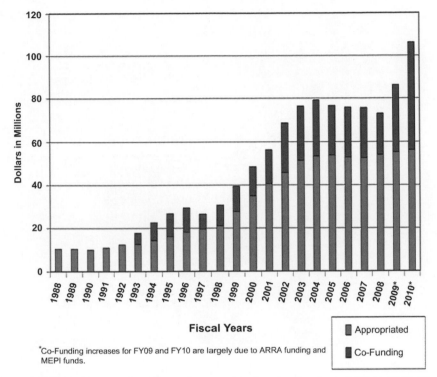

Fig. 4. FIC, NIH, extramural programs (appropriated and cofunding), 1988 to 2010. (*From* National Institutes of Health, Bethesda, MD.)

descriptive and analytical approaches, with a focus on mathematical modeling. The Multinational Influenza Seasonal Mortality Study (MISMS), Research and Policy for Infectious Disease Dynamics (RAPIDD), and Malnutrition and Enteric Diseases (Mal-ED) Network programs are collaborating globally to understand, describe, predict and prevent epidemics.

MISMS investigators analyze national and global mortality patterns associated with global influenza virus circulation using modern molecular and modeling approaches.[30–35] Collaborations have been established with more than 30 countries, many in the southern hemisphere, where influenza patterns had been described sparsely. Information is disseminated via yearly meetings, interactive workshops, and a Web site (http://www.origem.info/misms/index.php). Recent seasonal influenza trends, epidemics, and basic reproduction numbers in Brazil have been reported by MISMS investigators.[30] The MISMS network is funded in great part by the Office of Global Affairs, DHHS.

RAPIDD researchers make mathematical modeling relevant to policy makers responding to ID outbreaks through analysis and forecasting. Of particular interest are animal-human relationships manifesting in zoonoses. Selected IDs addressed include emerging infections (hantavirus, Nipah virus), monkeypox, and rotavirus.[36–40] This program is supported by the Department of Homeland Security.

The new MAL-ED Network is describing the complex interrelationships between enteric infections and malnutrition in young children in 8 LMICs in Asia, Africa,

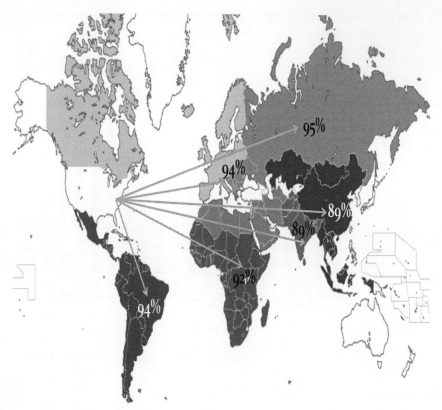

Fig. 5. Return rate of FIC, NIH, trainees, 1988 to 2010. (*From* National Institutes of Health, Bethesda, MD.)

and Latin America. Countries have initiated longitudinal cohort studies using standardized protocols to describe the global pattern of nutritional and enteric factors influencing early childhood development. This large project is comanaged by FIC and the Foundation for the NIH and is funded by the Bill & Melinda Gates Foundation.

Continuing a long history of convening authorities to discuss critical issues in public health policy, the FIC has sponsored several consensus symposia in recent years dealing with IDs.

- In 2007, a meeting titled "Polio Immunization: Moving Forward" was coorganized with the National Institute of Allergy and Infectious Diseases (NIAID). This meeting advised research on inactivated and live polio vaccines and other topics in support of the polio eradication initiative.[41]
- In 2010, in Rio de Janeiro, FIC coorganized a historic symposium "Smallpox Eradication after 30 Years: Lessons, Legacies, and Innovations" with the Sabin Vaccine Institute and the Foundation Oswaldo Cruz, Rio de Janeiro. Emphasis at the symposium was placed on the relevance of smallpox eradication for other programs.[42] A special issue of *Vaccine* will be devoted to the papers presented at this meeting, which will focus on the newer disease control and eradication programs inspired by the triumph of smallpox eradication.

- Also in 2010, the FIC and NIAID coorganized a meeting "Artemisinin Resistant Malaria: Addressing Research Challenges, Opportunities, and Public Health Challenges." The research and control agendas and types of collaborations needed to stop the spread of artemisinin resistance are being disseminated widely.

NONINFECTIOUS DISEASE AND CROSS-CUTTING PROGRAMS

Several analyses of the trends in global disease burdens have indicated that cardiovascular diseases (heart attacks, stroke, hypertension), brain disorders and mental illness (depression, schizophrenia), cancer (lung, cervical, gastrointestinal, breast), trauma/injuries (motor vehicle, war), tobacco use, and lifestyle choices (nutrition-obesity-diabetes, hypertension), and others comprise most health problems in rich and poor countries alike (see **Table 1**).[4–7,43] Acute and chronic environmental and occupational health problems are emerging as major challenges globally, especially in eastern European countries; the FIC has trained close to 200 scientists to deal with these increasing air, water, and land pollution hazards (see **Table 4**).[44] FIC has added recently several research and research training programs (see **Box 3**, **Table 4**) in response to the changes in demographics and epidemiologic burdens. FIC programs are beginning to stress dissemination and implementation research. Evaluation, social science, and management research will be emphasized.[45] The ultimate goal of implementation research is to deliver effectively and scale-up proven interventions.

NCD-LIFESPAN

This new program is training scientists in the diagnosis, management, and understanding of noninfectious, chronic diseases. Cardiovascular, nutritional, neuropsychiatric, metabolic, and tobacco-related diseases are in this category.[46–52]

TRAUMA

This program supports research training on the diagnosis, prevention, or treatment related to injury and trauma in LMICs. The importance of this new program was shown recently in Cairo, where those trained at the Ain Shams hospital in emergency care in collaboration with the University of Maryland saved lives during the recent turbulent political events in Egypt.

FRAME

The FIC has supported the burgeoning development of multidisciplinary global health coalitions and curricula at US universities. Schools of medicine, public health, nursing, veterinary medicine, and dentistry have joined with faculties of journalism, communications, law, arts, sciences, and others to respond to the growing interest of undergraduates and graduates in global health issues. Major foci of these new programs are to define global health, develop curricula, expand faculty interest and competence, and promote interdisciplinary global health research opportunities for students and faculty.

FICRS-F

This resoundingly successful cofunded program offers a 1-year, carefully mentored, clinical research training experience for doctoral students and postdoctoral candidates from the United States; the scholars (mainly medical students; residents and fellows are newly added) are paired during their training with colleagues from LMICs where they will work. The research training sites are established at NIH-funded and vetted sites in 26 LMICs in Africa, Asia, and South America. Vanderbilt University now manages this program, which has trained more than 400 young scientists (>200 from the United States and >200 from abroad) who aspire to a career in clinical research and global health (see **Tables 4** and **5**).

FICRA

The FIRCA program fosters international research partnerships between NIH-supported scientists and their collaborators in LMICs; the program benefits the research interests of both collaborators and increases and enhances research capacity at the LMIC site. Only scientists who have an eligible NIH grant may apply. Special consideration is given to proposed research that addresses significant global health problems, particularly those problems of high relevance to the foreign country or region; social and behavioral science and chronic diseases are special focus topics.

GRIP

GRIP was established by FIC in 2002 to promote productive reentry of NIH-trained foreign investigators into their home countries. The specific goal of the initiative was to provide funding opportunities on returning home for the increasing pool of foreign investigators and health professionals with state-of-the-art knowledge of research approaches to address local problems. GRIP uses the research (R01) funding mechanism. Since 2002, GRIP awards have been made to 77 investigators at 60 institutions in 22 countries.

MEPI

It is estimated that SSA has only 600,000 health care workers for a population of 682 million; relatively few of these are physicians.[53–55] The new MEPI is supporting 13 institutions in 12 SSA countries that, in partnership with the Health Resources and Services Administration, receive support from the US President's Emergency Plan for AIDS Relief (PEPFAR). The US and African academic partners will develop, expand, and enhance models of medical education focusing on front-line health care providers. These models are intended to support PEPFAR's goal of increasing the number of new health care workers by 140,000, strengthen existing medical education systems, and build clinical and research capacity in Africa as part of a retention strategy for faculty of medical schools, especially clinical professors. MEPI intends to provide up to $130 million in grants over 5 years to African institutions in a dozen countries, forming a network of about 30 regional partners, country health and education ministries, and more than 20 US collaborators.

Eleven programmatic awards, largely funded by PEPFAR, will expand and enhance HIV/AIDS medical education and research training. Eight smaller non-HIV/AIDS awards, funded by the NIH Director's Common Fund, with additional support from several NIH institutes, will encourage the development of expertise in maternal and child health, cardiovascular diseases, cancer, mental health, surgery, and emergency medicine. Over a 5-year period, MEPI intends to provide up to $10 million for each programmatic award, up to $2.5 million for each linked project, and up to $1.25 million for each pilot grant.

FOGARTY SUCCESS STORIES

In addition to successes mentioned earlier, FIC trainees have made numerous scientific advances, attained leadership positions, and received honors during and since their training. A few examples of these achievements are described briefly in **Box 4**.

SUCCESSFUL TRAINING FOR RESEARCH IN LMICS: THE FOGARTY MODEL

There is a great need to develop a larger health workforce in LMICs. Over the past 23 years the FIC has developed a successful model for training scientists and public health workers in research and leadership and their application to local problems. Close to 90% of long-term trainees have returned to their home countries and many have become national and international leaders.

Over the years, FIC has developed strategies that ensure the programs succeed in building capacity in LMICs. Experience with the development of these research training programs has led to a series of principles FIC uses to develop successful research collaboration training programs (**Box 5**). In general, Fogarty investments are long-term, made for 5 years, renewable by recompetition to 10 or more years; focus on institutional strengthening, including addressing managerial and administrative skills; require that US institutions twin with foreign research centers, emphasizing local priorities and involvement; require that the United States and other northern country grantee or the LMIC have an underlying research grant (R01 or equivalent) supported by NIH or another funder; this gives the collaboration a solid research base and intellectual and financial support from other NIH research organizations, including ICs. Further, Fogarty launched a program to expand opportunities for NIH-trained foreign scientists to obtain competitive reentry (GRIP) awards of about $50,000 per year to begin an independent research program in their home country.

Principles for encouraging LMIC scientists to return to their countries and decrease the brain drain are also addressed by the PIs during the training programs.[56] One principle is to include an agreement between the trainees, their institutions, and the co-PI, in the United States and home country, for the trainee to return to the home country. Mentors often secure positions for successful trainees when they return, increasing their likelihood of success.

Whereas institutions have rich research environments, networks, and cachet, highly motivated individuals create ideas, inventions, and innovations that advance science and public health. We have developed a 12-step program to develop leaders in science (**Fig. 6**). In distinction from richer countries, many scientists from LMICs frequently have the opportunity to present their analyses and views to decision makers, are actively involved in developing disease management and prevention guidelines, and have a strong influence on priority setting, decision making and allotment of funds for research, and public health and development programs. It is not uncommon for an FIC-trained leader to lead a national control or elimination program. Leaders in science and public health from rich and poor countries are increasingly faced with ethical issues tied to their research and its application. The FIC ethics research program is addressing this cross-cutting area.[57]

The importance of good mentoring in FIC programs must be stressed. Good mentoring is a long-term relationship between trainees and senior investigators, between trainees and persons with special experience and skills, and between trainees themselves. As research institutions in LMICs have become stronger in staff and other resources, collaborations between LMICs have blossomed; many trainees from northern, rich countries are now being mentored by scientist grantees

Box 4
Selected Fogarty success stories

- Fogarty grantee Dr Walter Curioso from the University of Washington and Peru's Cayetano Heredia University found cell phones to be highly useful in research targeting Peru's sex workers. Health workers must be able to communicate with the patients regarding side effects and complications of medications. Traditionally, a paper-based system was used, but Dr Curioso tapped into Peru's extensive mobile phone network and generated an 80% reporting success rate.

- Fogarty-funded tobacco research provided information critical to the recently implemented law in Syria banning public smoking. According to grantee Dr Wasim Maziak, founder of the Syrian Center for Tobacco Studies, who is based at the University of Memphis, Tennessee, "The inclusion of water pipe smoking restrictions in the ban is clear evidence of our direct involvement in public policy."

- Former Fogarty trainee at Yale University, Dr Johnson Ouma, studied tsetse fly genetics in Kenya. Dr Ouma's research investigated the movement and control of tsetse population, and his findings were recently published in *PLoS Neglected Tropical Diseases.*

- Dr Irmansyah was recently appointed as Indonesia's Director of Mental Health after completing a year-long Fogarty-funded fellowship at Harvard University, where he received training in genetics research.

- Dr Agnes Moses is a graduate of AITRP at the University of Witwatersrand in South Africa. Dr Moses helped to make tremendous strides in HIV/AIDS disease management. She organized a program aimed at reducing mother-to-child disease transmission in Malawi. She also published articles in the journal *AIDS* about her work treating pregnant HIV-positive women and was honored by the Elizabeth Glaser Pediatric AIDS Foundation.

- Dr Veronica Rajal, a clean-water scientist and Professor at the National University of Argentina at Salta, was trained at University of California at Davis. Her work on a complex water filtration technique combining polymerase chain reaction and hollow fiber ultrafiltration was published in *Water Research.* Dr Rajal, in addition to her work in clean water and sanitation, is also working on capacity building; she is developing a master's program in environmental engineering.

- A team of researchers funded by AITRP and led by Dr Quarraisha Abdul Karim from South Africa and Columbia University found microbicide gel, when used regularly by women, reduced the risk of HIV transmission by up to 54% in South Africa.

- Dr Ronald Gray, a Fogarty grantee working at Johns Hopkins University, found that male circumcision can reduce the risk of male HIV infection by approximately 60%. The 2-year study, which looked at more than 5,000 men in rural Uganda, is poised to be at the forefront of a new era for HIV prevention.

- Dr Kawengo Agot, a former AITRP trainee at the University of Washington and GRIP awardee from Kenya, became the PI on an $11 million cooperative agreement with the National Center for HIV, Viral Hepatitis, STDs and Tuberculosis Prevention at the Centers for Disease Control and Prevention entitled "HIV Prevention and Care Services for Young People in Kenya."

- Thanyawee Puthanakit, a 2002 graduate of the Johns Hopkins' AITRP, served as a scientific board member of the HIV/AIDS Treatment Program for the Thailand Ministry of Public Health and the WHO.

- Saul Johnson, an AITRP trainee from South Africa who completed his MS from Columbia University, participated in numerous important monitoring and evaluation studies in the Southern African region. He was an advisor and research manager for the consortium that managed the Khomanani Campaign, the South African Government's mass media campaign directed to HIV/AIDS between 2001 and 2006. He also assisted the Global Fund to monitor HIV programs in Namibia, Swaziland, Angola, Malawi and Zimbabwe, among others.

- Carlos Diaz Granados was a former AITRP trainee at Emory University in Atlanta, Georgia. On his return to Colombia, he led the development for the first evidence-based guidelines for the management of HIV infection in Colombia. These guidelines were endorsed by the Colombian Ministry of Social Protection (Health) and the Colombian Association of Infectious Diseases.

- Lilian Ferrer is a former AITRP trainee at University of Illinois who is now in charge of the Office of International Affairs at Pontificia Universidad Católica de Chile. Other duties include having served on the review panel for grant applications for the Chilean Ministry of Health and as a member of the scientific committee for the first Chilean Congress in Public Health.

- Dr Maria Amelia Veras of Brazil received an AITRP Fogarty scholarship to attend the University of California Berkeley School of Public Health from 1999 to 2001. She is a member of the Epidemiology Advisory Board of the National STI/AIDS Program and works as a consultant for the Brazil Ministry of Health and to the Angolan National AIDS Program.

- Dr Chuan Shi joined the ICOHRTA Fogarty training program in 2009 at Harvard University. With the knowledge and skill acquired from the training, he finished a functioning assessment instrument for schizophrenia in China and tested its reliability and validity in 2010.

- Dr Jean "Bill" Pape is the founding director of Groupe Haïtien d'Étude du Sarcome de Kaposi et des Infectieuses Opportunistes (GHESKIO), the world's first HIV/AIDS clinic; Dr Pape is a longtime NIH grantee in Haiti. GHESKIO was named the recipient of the 2010 Gates Award for Global Health. The organization has provided continuous medical care in Haiti since 1982, never once shutting its doors or charging fees. A Haitian physician, Dr Pape graduated from Weill Cornell Medical College in 1975 and returned to Haiti in 1979. He is an international leader in the fight against AIDS and the provision of health care for the resource-poor. In recognition of his achievements, he has received the Legion d'Honneur from the French government and the Carlos Slim 2010 Global Health Award and has been elected a member of the US Institute of Medicine.

From NIH; with permission.

---

from and in LMICs. Most encouraging is that many young scientists trained by the FIC programs have gone on to publish in internationally renowned journals, win research awards (including R01s), and establish their own independent laboratories, where they can mentor the next generation of research scientists in their own and other countries.

Box 5
Principles of successful FIC research and research training programs

- Respond to national and global priorities
- Collaborating institutions develop twinning partnerships
- Mutually beneficial to collaborators
- Long-term commitment (>5 years) by FIC
- Durable national commitment
- Training linked directly to innovative research
- Selection of trainees and research projects by collaborating LMIC institutions
- Flexibility in types of training and research and management mechanisms
- Over time center of gravity shifts to the lower-income countries
- Research capacity strengthening tied to public health
- Program outcomes: scientific and public health leaders
- Long-term and multigenerational institutional and individual partnerships

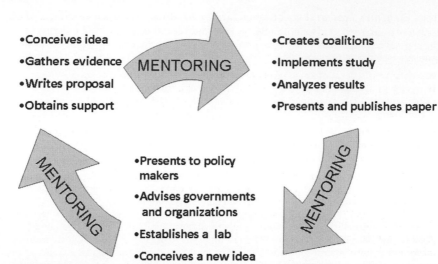

Fig. 6. What a superior trainee scientist must do: the 12-step program for developing successful trainees. (*Courtesy of* World Bank Publications, Washington DC; with permission. Available at: http://www.dcp2.org.)

SUMMARY

Since 1988, more than 1 billion dollars have been invested, including cofunding, on global health research training, research, and capacity building in FIC programs targeting LMICs through partnerships with US institutions. Through these efforts, FIC has supported a large cadre of scientists in becoming global health leaders. We have defined several characteristics of successful capacity-building initiatives, including institutional strengthening, twinning of research centers, focus on local problems, active mentorship, mutual benefit to all partners, and, innovation in research. FIC's ID programs, such as AITRP, GID, and EID, have made breakthroughs in drug development and testing, genetic marker research, and understanding and managing patients with neglected tropical diseases. Intramural epidemiology and population studies programs have made important contributions by defining global mortality patterns associated with influenza, and investigating animal-human relationships manifesting in zoonoses and the complex relationships between enteric infections and malnutrition in children. FIC-funded noninfectious disease programs have expanded global health teaching and training in the United States. Several new programs, such as TRAUMA and NCD-LIFESPAN, promote research on the heavy toll caused by noncommunicable diseases and injuries. FIRCA, GRIP, and MEPI foster capacity building and institutional strengthening in LMICs. The wide variety of programs, projects, and initiatives supported by FIC reflect FIC's goals of providing comprehensive training and tools to investigators to ultimately, and sustainably, build capacity in global health research and lesson the burden of disease worldwide.

ACKNOWLEDGMENTS

We thank FIC scientist-program managers and support staff for their capable stewardship of the research training and research programs: these are Josh Rosenthal, Flora Katz, Xingzhu Liu, Jeanne McDermott, Kathleen Michels, Myat Htoo Razak,

Barbara Sina, and Yvonne Njage; Mark Miller, Ellis McKenzie, Cecile Viboud, and Sta-cey Knobler for research and leadership contributions in infectious diseases; and James Herrington, Karen Hofman, Letitia Robinson, Nalini Anand, and Rachel Sturke for coordinating global science strategy, policy, and planning at NIH; we are grateful for assistance in preparation of the manuscript from Mantra Singh, Celia Wolfman, Erica Schonman, Natalie Engmann, Danielle Bielenstein, Ann Puderbaugh, Farah Bader, and Vikash Parekh. Our special gratitude goes to the many FIC PIs in the United States and abroad and their trainees who are responsible for the achievements result-ing from FIC support, and for training the next generation of leaders in science and public health. We thank Gerald Keusch, former Director of the FIC, who had an impor-tant role in the development of many initiatives mentioned in this article.

REFERENCES

1. Secretary of State Hillary Rodham Clinton. The global health initiative: the next phase of American partnership in health. Speech. Available at: http://www.state.gov/secretary/rm/2010/08/146002.htm. Accessed August 16, 2010.
2. Rajaratnam JK, Marcus JR, Flaxman AD, et al. Neonatal, postneonatal, childhood, and under-5 mortality for 187 countries, 1970–2010: a systematic analysis of prog-ress towards Millennium Development Goal 4. Lancet 2010;375(9730):1988–2008.
3. Paxton A, Wardlaw T. Are we making progress in maternal mortality. N Engl J Med 2011;364:1990–3.
4. Jamison DT, Breman JG, Measham G, et al, editors. Disease control priorities in developing countries. 2nd edition. New York: Oxford University Press; 2006.
5. Lopez AD, Ezzati M, Mathers CD, et al, editors. Global burden of disease and risk factors. New York: Oxford University Press; 2006.
6. Jamison DT, Breman JG, Measham AR, et al, editors. Priorities in health. New York: Oxford University Press; 2006.
7. Laxminarayan R, Mills AJ, Breman JG, et al. Advancement of global health: key messages from the Disease Control Priorities Project. Lancet 2006;367:1193–208.
8. Hotez PJ, Remme JH, Buss P, et al. Combating tropical infectious diseases: report of the Disease Control Priorities Project in Developing Countries. Clin Infect Dis 2004;38:871–8.
9. Breman JG, Jamison D, Alleyne G, et al. Infectious diseases and the disease control project. In: Serageldin I, Masood E, El-Faham M, editors. Changing lives, biovision, Alexandria 2006. Alexandria (Egypt): Biblioteca Alexandrina; 2007. p. 81–94.
10. Jha P, Laxminarayan R. Choosing health: an entitlement for all Indians. Toronto: Center for Global Health Research, University of Toronto; 2009.
11. Hofman K, Tollman SM. Health policies and practice: setting priorities for health in 21st century South Africa. S Afr Med J 2010;100(12):798–800.
12. FIC strategic plan reflects the collective wisdom of the Fogarty staff, the Fogarty Advisory Board, and the hundreds of stakeholders who provided advice and comments at national and international meetings or through the Fogarty Web site. A full copy of the strategic plan is available at: http://www.fic.nih.gov/About/Documents/stratplan_fullversion.pdf. Accessed July 11, 2011.
13. Atashili J, Kalilani L, Seksaria V, et al. Potential impact of infant feeding recom-mendations on mortality and HIV-infection in children born to HIV-infected mothers in Africa: a simulation. BMC Infect Dis 2008;8:66.
14. Dunkle KL, Stephenson R, Karita E, et al. New heterosexually transmitted HIV infections in married or cohabiting couples in urban Zambia and Rwanda: an analysis of survey and clinical data. Lancet 2008;371(9631):2183–91.

15. Gupta A, Nayak U, Ram M, et al. Postpartum tuberculosis incidence and mortality among HIV-infected women and their infants in Pune, India, 2002–2005. Clin Infect Dis 2007;45(2):241–9.

16. Harris JB, Hatwiinda SM, Randels KM, et al. Early lessons from the integration of tuberculosis and HIV services in primary care centers in Lusaka, Zambia. Int J Tuberc Lung Dis 2008;12(7):773–9.

17. Karim QA, Kharsamy AB, Naidoo K, et al. Co-enrollment in multiple HIV prevention trials–experiences from the CAPRISA 004 Tenofavir gel trial. Contemp Clin Trials 2011;32(3):333–8.

18. Karim QA, Karim SS, Frohlich JA, et al, on behalf of the CAPRISA 004 Trial Group. Effectiveness and safety of tenofovir gel, an antiretroviral microbicide, for the prevention of HIV infection in women. Science 2010;329(5996):1168–74.

19. Morris MB, Chapula BT, Chi BH, et al. Use of task-shifting to rapidly scale-up HIV treatment services: experiences from Lusaka, Zambia. BMC Health Serv Res 2009;9:5.

20. Potter D, Goldenberg RL, Chao A, et al. Do targeted HIV programs improve overall care for pregnant women? Antenatal syphilis management in Zambia before and after implementation of prevention of mother-to-child HIV transmission programs. J Acquir Immune Defic Syndr 2008;47(1):79–85.

21. Turan JM, Miller S, Bukusi EA, et al. HIV/AIDS and maternity care in Kenya: how fears of stigma and discrimination affect uptake and provision of labor and delivery services. AIDS Care 2008;20(8):938–45.

22. Wawer MJ, Makumbi F, Kigozi G, et al. Circumcision in HIV-infected men and its effect on HIV transmission to female partners in Rakai, Uganda: a randomized controlled trial. Lancet 2009;374(9685):229–37.

23. Zhao M, Li X. Transmission of MDR and XDR tuberculosis in Shanghai, China. PLoS One 2009;4(2):e4370.

24. Mpontshane N, Van den Broeck J, Chhagan M, et al. HIV infection is associated with decreased dietary diversity in South African children. J Nutr 2008;138(9):1705–11.

25. Jones KE, Levy NG, Storeygard A, et al. Global trends in emerging infectious diseases. Nature 2008;451:990–3.

26. Berriman M, Haas BJ, LoVerde PT, et al. The genome of the blood fluke *Schistosoma mansoni*. Nature 2009;460(7253):352–8.

27. Laufer MK, Takala-Harrison S, Dzinjalamala FK, et al. Return of chloroquine-susceptible falciparum malaria in Malawi was a re-expansion of diverse susceptible parasites. J Infect Dis 2010;202(5):801–8.

28. Nankabirwa J, Cundill B, Clarke S, et al. Efficacy, safety, and tolerability of three regimens for prevention of malaria: a randomized, placebo-controlled trial in Ugandan schoolchildren. PLoS One 2010;5(10):e13438.

29. Riley LW, Ko AI, Unger A, et al. Slum health: diseases of neglected populations. BMC Int Health Hum Rights 2007;7:2e.

30. Alonso WJ, Viboud C, Simonsen L, et al. Seasonality of influenza in Brazil: a traveling wave from the Amazon to the subtropics. Am J Epidemiol 2007;165:1434–42.

31. Chowell G, Bertozzi SM, Colchero MA, et al. Severe respiratory disease concurrent with the circulation of H1N1 influenza. N Engl J Med 2009;361(7):674–9.

32. Chowell G, Viboud C, Simonsen L, et al. The reproduction number of seasonal influenza epidemics in Brazil, 1996–2006. Proc Biol Sci 2010;277(1689):1857–69.

33. Ghedin E, Laplante J, DePasse J, et al. Deep sequencing reveals mixed infection with pandemic influenza A (H1N1) virus strains and the emergence of oseltamivir resistance. J Infect Dis 2011;203(2):168–74.
34. Gordon A, Saborío S, Videa E, et al. Clinical attack rate and presentation of pandemic H1N1 influenza A and B in a pediatric cohort in Nicaragua. Clin Infect Dis 2010;50(11):1462–7.
35. Viboud C, Miller M, Olson D, et al. Preliminary estimates of mortality and years of life lost associated with the 2009 A/H1N1 pandemic in the US and comparison with past influenza seasons. PLoS Curr 2010;RRN1153.
36. Lloyd-Smith JO, George D, Pepin KM, et al. Epidemic dynamics at the human-animal interface. Science 2009;326(5958):1362–7.
37. Pepin KM, Lass S, Pulliam JR, et al. Identifying genetic markers of adaptation for surveillance of viral host jumps. Nat Rev Microbiol 2010;8(11):802–13.
38. Pitzer VE, Viboud C, Simonsen L, et al. Demographic variability, vaccination, and the spatiotemporal dynamics of rotavirus epidemics. Science 2009;325(5938): 290–4.
39. Pulliam JR, Dushoff J. Ability to replicate in the cytoplasm predicts zoonotic transmission of livestock viruses. J Infect Dis 2009;199(4):565–8.
40. Rimoin AW, Mulembakani PM, Johnston SC, et al. Major increase in human monkeypox incidence 30 years after smallpox vaccination campaigns cease in the Democratic Republic of Congo. Proc Natl Acad Sci U S A 2010;107(37): 16262–7.
41. Ehrenfeld E, Glass RI, Agol VI, et al. Immunisation against poliomyelitis: moving forward. Lancet 2008;371:1385–7.
42. Breman JG, De Quadros C, Dowdle WR, et al. The role of research in viral disease eradication and elimination: lessons for malaria eradication. PLoS Med 2011;8(1):e1000405.
43. Daar AS, Singer PA, Persad DL, et al. Grand challenges in chronic non-communicable diseases. Nature 2007;450(22):494–6.
44. Bridbord K, Breman JG, Primack K, et al. Building global environmental health capacity through international scientific cooperation and partnerships. Int J Occup Environ Health 2006;12:295–9.
45. Madon T, Hofman KJ, Kupfer L, et al. Implementation science. Science 2007;318: 1728–9.
46. Gaziano TA, Young CR, Fitzmaurice G, et al. Laboratory-based versus non-laboratory- based method for assessment of cardiovascular disease risk: the NHANES I Follow-up Study cohort. Lancet 2008;371(9616):923–31.
47. Boivin MJ, Bangirana P, Byarugaba J, et al. Cognitive impairment after cerebral malaria in children: a prospective study. Pediatrics 2007;19(2):E360–6.
48. Fernald LC, Gertler PJ, Hou X. Cash component of conditional cash transfer is associated with higher body mass index and blood pressure in adults. J Nutr 2008;138(11):2250–7.
49. Anjana RM, Lakshminarayanan S. Parental history of type 2 diabetes mellitus, metabolic syndrome, and cardiometabolic risk factors in Asian Indian adolescents. Metabolism 2009;58(3):344–50.
50. Hoddinott J, Maluccio JA, Behrman JA, et al. Effect of a nutrition intervention during early childhood on economic productivity in Guatemalan adults. Lancet 2008;371(9610):411–6.
51. Jha P, Jacob B, Gajalakshmi V, et al. A nationally representative case-control study of smoking and death in India. N Engl J Med 2008;358(11):1137–47.

52. Pradeepa R, Anitha B, Mohan V, et al. Risk factors for diabetic retinopathy in a South Indian Type 2 diabetic population–the Chennai Urban Rural Epidemiology Study (CURES) Eye Study 4. Diabet Med 2008;25(5):536–42.
53. Collins FS, Glass RI, Whitescarver J, et al. Developing health workforce capacity in Africa. Science 2010;330(6009):1324–5.
54. Mullan F, Frehywot S, Omaswa F, et al. Medical schools in sub-Saharan Africa. Lancet 2010;377(9771):1113–21.
55. Mullan F, Frehywot S. Non-physician clinicians in 47 sub-Saharan African countries. Lancet 2007;370(9605):2158–63.
56. Kupfer L, Hofman K, Jarawan R, et al. Strategies to discourage brain drain. Bull World Health Organ 2004;82(8):616–23.
57. Ajuwon AJ, Kass N. Outcome of a research ethics training workshop among clinicians and scientists in a Nigerian university. BMC Med Ethics 2008;9:1.

The Asia Pacific Academic Consortium for Global Public Health and Medicine: Stabilizing South-South Academic Collaboration

Walter K. Patrick, MD, MPH, PhD[a,b,]*

KEYWORDS

- South-South • Academic collaboration
- Development assistance for health
- Asia Pacific Academic Consortium for Public Health
- Developmental strategies

The north-south distinction refers to the socioeconomic division that exists between the economically developed, industrialized countries, collectively known as the north, and the low-income and middle-income countries, the south. Although north-south exchange or cooperation programs are common, the dynamics of north-south linkage have been traditionally described as unidirectional dependence, with growth in the south being determined primarily by developments in and priorities of the north. On the contrary, south-south cooperation refers to cooperative activities between newly industrialized southern countries and others in the south to find solutions to common development challenges including those related to health and health care.[1] For instance, health technology transfer has some unique characteristics, including discontinuous changes and multiplier effects, in that relatively low-tech or mid-level interventions such as immunization and drug treatment of selective conditions can have dramatic results in improvement of life expectancies initially.[2] Then a plateau

[a] Global Health and Medicine, John A. Burns School of Medicine, University of Hawaii, Honolulu, HI, USA
[b] Asia Pacific Academic Consortium for Public Health (APACPH), Department of Public Health Science, John A. Burns School of Medicine, University of Hawaii at Manoa, 1960 East West Road, Honolulu, HI 96822, USA
* Dean's Suite, Room 224D, John A. Burns School of Medicine, University of Hawaii, 651 Ilalo Street, Honolulu, HI 96813.
E-mail address: walterp@hawaii.edu

Infect Dis Clin N Am 25 (2011) 537–554
doi:10.1016/j.idc.2011.05.005
0891-5520/11/$ – see front matter © 2011 Elsevier Inc. All rights reserved.

is reached when increasing risks of technology (eg, drug resistance, cost, and inadequate care) increase disease burdens and have a negative effect unless overall improvement in basic needs and infrastructure is ensured. High-end technology transfer without development in health infrastructures and basic social needs can be counterproductive without equity and distributional aspects of health policy.[3]

In 1978, the Third World Non-Aligned Group of nearly 120 nations urged the United Nations (UN) to establish a Special Unit for South-South Cooperation (SSC) within the UN Development Program. Despite uneven progress, 3 decades later, the organization reviewed experiences, trends, and achievements at the SSC Developmental Expo.[4] Several commentaries emphasized the slow progress on issues of social justice and poverty reduction but identified some dramatic achievements related to some of the millennium development goals (MDGs) (ie, health improvement through overall development and provision of primary care services). Emerging south-south collaborations and the expanding role of countries like Brazil, South Africa, India, Malaysia, Korea, and China were highlighted. These emerging donor countries are also in transition following the pattern of Japan, which was both donor and recipient of aid in the 1960s,[5] and later became a major aid provider, a trend shown among Asia Pacific Academic Consortium for Public Health (APACPH) members from East and South Asia. The African-South American (ASA) collaboration had grown to 62 countries and, although primarily focusing on energy and trade, has begun to focus on issues of peace, security, and health needs such as in human immunodeficiency virus (HIV)/AIDS relief and poverty reduction. The level of assistance from emerging donors like China, India, Brazil, and others has grown to nearly 10% of overall development assistance.[6] The nonaligned summit observed that SSC has been relatively successful in reducing south dependence and in creating a shift in the international balance of power.[7] Brazil's form of south-south development aid, which is less conditional and more acceptable, has been called a "global model in waiting."[8]

The emerging south in Asia shows 2 levels in transition: the East Asian Tigers (S1 countries) and the Southeast Asian countries (S2 countries) like Malaysia and Thailand, which have grown economically and moved up in overall human development indices.[9] The distinctions and locations of the geographic south, therefore, are now less categorical and definitions are more blurred. International technological dualism (unequal developments in the area of science and technology between rich and poor countries postulated in the 1970s[10]) has also been challenged with the growing technological achievements and scientific publications in south countries like India, China, and Malaysia. Similarly, the digital divide, referring to the major gap in information and communication technology development,[11] does not seem to hold true in the emerging south, such as Korea, Malaysia, Hong Kong, Thailand, and Taiwan. Furthermore, the use of advanced medical technologies in these countries is as high or in some cases even higher and more cost-effective than in the north.[12] Despite this paradox, it was estimated that 88% of all Internet users are from industrialized countries that comprise only 15% of the world's population.[11,13]

In that sense, the Internet, hailed as a "great equalizer,"[14] a revolutionary technological tool to transfer information on a global scale, has not served the poorer countries and has effectively protected the richer nations in pandemics like severe acute respiratory syndrome (SARS) and H1N1.[15] The dream "for poorer villages and isolated communities to have a well-placed computer to serve like a communal well providing essential information about epidemics and medical services for villagers"[16] is still a far cry for the poorer south. The transference of health technology in specific disease entities through vaccines and drugs (the medicalization model of health assistance) has been remarkably successful. On the other hand, the limited research resources for health problems in the south with emphasis on research interests of the north adds a barrier to enhancement of south-south academic partnerships and maintains the north-south gradient of expertise and dependence.[17] However, research of complex conditions such as HIV/AIDS, malaria, diabetes, heart disease, and cancers, which are deeply rooted in poverty, environment, lifestyles, and occupation require long-term commitment and a research strategy that promotes south universities' competency and leadership in examining conditions and contexts beyond medical constructs and solutions. The emerging interest in social determinants of health and noncommunicable diseases (NCDs) has the potential to promote south-south partnerships relevant to local conditions and needs. In addition, south-south collaboration between higher-education institutions often has more shared interest in research priority, capacity building, and problem-based research training. Under conditions requiring social participation and reform, south involvement and leadership in human resource development is essential. However well meaning and altruistic it may be, the steep north-south gradient in the medicalization model needs to be flattened in partnerships with leading universities in the south. This initiative of using the expertise of lead universities in the south to support more regional and national networks and private partners within countries is a strategic lesson that APACPH learnt in its early years. Similar to land grant universities in the United States and universities in Canada and South America, south universities have a strong orientation for service and a common bond of social responsibility. That tradition has a sound basis in creating a global nexus to promote south-south partnerships. Future educational reforms advocated for health professionals[18] and problem-solving research recommended in global health practice[19] have the potential to increase relevance and support for a multiple-level societal and policy involvement for health. In such endeavors north consortia support to south-south partnerships would be valuable.

HEALTH AS A HUMAN RIGHT: THE SOCIAL RESPONSIBILITY OF UNIVERSITIES

Health as a human right and primary health care as a means of promoting health for all globally[20] are underlying values of APACPH. Most universities and agencies with well-established global health track records essentially contribute to the World Health Organization (WHO) ideal, but each institution interprets according to its own priorities, assets, and expertise, largely enhanced through consortia arrangements.[21] In the late 1970s, postcolonial national movements and underlying cultural values in voluntarism for health improvement such as the Sarvodaya Shramadana movement[22] served as a rallying point for university collaboration in Asia. The Cold War era that made health assistance a key strategy to influence foreign nations also attracted US universities to participate largely in family planning and maternal and child health (MCH) programs abroad. These trends in social responsibility, voluntarism, and health assistance to promote equity provided the context and climate for the founding of APACPH. The synergy and support of international organizations such as WHO, the United Nations Children's Fund (UNICEF), and the World Bank, and financial support of the US Agency for International Development, shaped the early directions of APACPH. The peace dividends for health in the post–Cold-War period of the 1990s provided additional stimulus in child survival programs, including control of diarrheal disease and upper respiratory infection.[23,24] Often priorities and issues that APACPH selected were those advocated by member institutions in the south. For example, activities and policy changes to improve the neglected female child although challenging were initiated by the Institute of Medicine of Nepal.[25,26] Similarly, priority for the health of indigenous people was also strongly advocated by member institutions such as

Curtin University, Australia, Kalinga Institute of Industrial Technology (KIIT), India, and the University of Hawaii, all of which have a long-standing tradition in working with indigenous populations.[27] It was the inherent commitment and experience of members on issues of common concern that brought them together rather than the opportunity to access donor resources. Using seed grants these small groups have generated external resources and support from their own institutions to further common goals. The south member, KIIT, the largest educational complex globally for indigenous people, is planning in partnership with a select group of north and south members in APACPH to develop a unique training-oriented, service-oriented, and research-oriented global health graduate program for indigenous people. Successes in common but challenging problems such as these have brought cohesion and convergence among APACPH members. It has ensured expertise through joint efforts. The negative effects of such a model are many: waning motivation, delays in start-up, and breakdown in supplies and services as resources are diminished. Sub-regional networks of 3–5 members addressing common problems are adjusting to these challenges by: tapping partner resources for projects in advance, pacing implementation of projects, supporting local initiatives and providing reinforcement through other related activities (eg, agriculture, nutrition, family planning, urban and indigenous people's development). These sub-regional clusters through such mechanisms have been successful in seeking additional resources from national and global agencies.

CHALLENGE IN GLOBAL HEALTH: ALTRUISM AND EQUITY

Conflicts between intrinsic values and operational challenges often lead to compromises in global health practice. Health as integral to human development has been universally recognized from ancient times in the Asia Pacific region, as noted in the Asoka Edicts (269–231 BC), reflecting the notion of a benevolent monarch safeguarding health of the people. This personal individualistic approach has expanded across Asian societies largely through communal perspectives, religious concepts, and charitable practices of dhana (Hinduism-Buddhism), zakat (Islam), and tithe in Christianity. The establishment of hospitals and clinics, such as the world's oldest hospital in Mihintale, Sri Lanka,[28] evolved out of that perspective: the highest value in that culture is the physician-king, embodying the state's responsibility for health and well-being of people. During the colonial era, missionaries expanded the caring traditions beyond national borders, taking care of the sick and those stigmatized by diseases such as leprosy (Hansen disease). Remnants of leprosy hospitals and settlements can be seen dotted across the coastline of Asia, including the one established by Father Damien in Kalaupapa, Hawaii.[29] The work of Mother Teresa and her order in India and more than 120 other countries is a striking reminder of the evolution of missionary health care in Asia.[30] Missionary zeal and altruism remain underlying values among global health practitioners, carrying that imprimatur of charity without the overt intent to proselytize. In the poorer countries adequate care is the luxury afforded to the upper strata of society. This observation is also true to a certain extent even in affluent countries such as the United States, where there are nearly 45 million uninsured people.[31] The dilemma of balancing human rights and cost of care polarizes politics, making health care reform a constant challenge.[31] Hence, health as a universal human right, although acknowledged in the constitution of WHO (1946) and in numerous international treaties, has been mostly symbolic for the needy urban and rural populations. Ideologies, values, practices, and prejudices, not merely the lack of resources, still maintain the disparities in health for significant segments of the global population.[32] In this dilemma one realizes that health equity is the central challenge for universities in global health.

GLOBAL HEALTH AND UNIVERSITY CONSORTIA

Medical voluntarism is prevalent in the United States and is often linked to religious organizations and universities with a long-standing tradition of providing development assistance for health (DAH).[33] The emergence of university consortia as a composite that is greater in the sum of its expertise and resources than individual members is a more recent phenomenon. It is estimated that less than 100 consortia are in the United States, of which about 20% to 30% are involved in global health. Several of them are well established and linked to prestigious universities with 5 to 10 institutional members. APACPH and the Global Health Education Consortium (GHEC) are the more established consortia, which have been functioning for nearly 25 and 20 years, respectively. Consortia are dynamic, even unstable at stages in their development, and are constantly challenged for resources. Leadership issues are not uncommon and are more linked to resources than policy, country, or affiliations. Economics of scale and complementarities of skills in organizations tend to form partnerships or mergers, providing resources and stability. The recently founded Consortium of Universities for Global Health (CUGH, 2008) is one of the larger university alliances in the United States. Besides the traditional fields of medicine, nursing, and public health, CUGH has the potential of accelerating advocacy for global health and involving several other disciplines such as engineering, law, agriculture, veterinary medicine, and social sciences. Responding to the increase in DAH funding in the United States, there has been a striking increase in the overall number of universities and their top leadership promoting university-wide involvement in global health (CUGH, 2009).[34] Global health training in universities across the United States has accelerated, and this trend is a giant step in bringing contentious professions to serve synergistically together in DAH. Some of these developments may be cosmetic and opportunistic but nevertheless they have provided stimulus and momentum to a field that was overwhelmed by global crises, burnout, and a growing paralysis because of lack of resources.

DAH

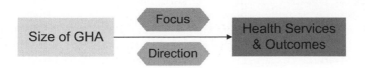

The size of DAH can support or overwhelm recipient countries and control the focus and direction of their health programs. Many south countries in Asia depended on DAH for basic health services.[35] The size of DAH for particular diseases can also distort the pattern of health development in terms of overall health needs and maintenance of health services.[36] Historical evidence of the failure of vertical eradication programs is easily forgotten with the growing potential and efficacy of vaccine-related prevention and mass drug treatment models. Under such circumstances, collaborating south universities become compliant to north interests in the focus of research and selective short-term benefits. Long-term sustainable outcomes requiring investment in infrastructures are often sacrificed.[37]

There are several ethical and strategic concerns that DAH needs to address. One obvious concern is that with the massive DAH, there is a likely convergence of donor interests and a concurrent trend of north university leadership to spearhead that effort.

This situation has been common in the past, with focus on a few selected diseases and selective approaches. The theoretical justifications, although valid in restricted contexts, have been found wanting in a broader social and health context or in long-term outcomes. South voices can be silenced to compliance and disadvantage. Many global health practitioners and scientists have questioned in hindsight the usefulness and limitations of selective programs. In a recent commentary both ethical and strategic concerns on DAH were addressed.[38] Therefore it is critical that south coalitions are supported to realistically address underlying problems (the social and economic constructs in health) rather than the short-term measures that a developed country can successfully implement based on supporting systems and levels of development in sanitation, child care, and nutrition. That has been the perennial challenge not only in global health in poor countries but in the health improvement of the disadvantaged communities in affluent countries. The continuum in DAH from altruism through enlightened self-interest to soft medical diplomacy or hard mercenary or military opportunism is full of ethical dimensions in which the recipients of aid can be manipulated to become passive, coerced, or corrupted, often having little to say. The value of north consortia is their transparency and capacity to support and empower collegial south universities to address problems realistically and help them serve as ombudsmen for health and build south-south consortia that will help not only to solve emergencies but also to build processes to maintain and sustain health improvement.

Historically, colonization of the south had a predominantly military and mercenary perspective in providing health care. Even although such an overt polarization is not visibly articulated, bilateral aid arrangements still follow that model, with variations and compromises tempered with the missionary medicine approach. University consortia have overcome such tendencies and constantly show humanitarian aspects in their global health contributions, supporting the proposed notion of enlightened self-interest for global health involvement (**Fig. 1**).[39] Detractors, critics, and reasonable purists will continue to have reservations, realizing the conditions of need and the size of DAH. The need for repackaging, refinement, and justification for DAH is a continuously challenging process both nationally and internationally. Major epidemics like smallpox and the recent SARS and swine flu push the panic button to invest in protecting others outside our borders to protect us. Then one realizes that all of us are intimately connected in issues of health through germs, food, water, and air. Yet the realization that global health is linked to violence, war, disasters, and economic poverty is not easy, unless touched by killer tornadoes (United States, 2011) or the Asian tsunami (2004), which drowned a village thousands of miles away, or a nuclear disaster (Japan, 2011), which caused thousands to be evacuated. The application of benefit-accrued models such as in the eradication of smallpox is valid. To promote their acceptance in the context of NCDs has been challenging certainly in the United States, especially in the poorer communities, where structural changes as well as behavioral and medical interventions are needed. The challenges will be similar, or even greater, in developing countries. Successes in reducing NCD burden in developing countries with poor living conditions may not be so prominent as those for emerging infectious diseases. However, initiatives such as tobacco control (China) and oral cancer prevention (India, Sri Lanka, Taiwan) offer leverage to initiate and

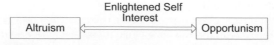

Fig. 1. The DAH model.

expand to comprehensive strategies through south-south partnerships. University consortia have shown effectiveness in meeting local health needs through research, training, and service networks. The shift of balance from the visibility of pandemics and disasters to the major burden of NCD and its multidimensional nature is a major conceptual shift from treatment to prevention and socioeconomic changes. That paradigm shift will require a collective educational response of universities both in the south and in the north to acknowledge and address monster problems that are buried in the iceberg of NCDs, where the diseases are manifestation of multiple conditions that are significantly rooted in the context of where and how people live. The models of comprehensive preventive health in the prominent NCDs such as cancers, obesity, diabetes, cardiovascular diseases, and mental health are rudimentary in contrast to the ballooning needs in the south. China illustrates the tragic impact of the ballooning effect of smoking and tobacco use, diminishing its major health and economic gains.

Other forms of justification for DAH are the potential to serve in medical diplomacy that has been increasingly used in disaster relief.[40] Unlike the military, most universities are ill equipped as first responders in the global disaster arena. They are more efficient in providing disaster preparedness training and facilitating postdisaster long-term rehabilitation and reconstruction. However, disaster assistance with high visibility on the global stage is a temptation for universities and consortia to show their commitment at high cost and low effectiveness. Yet universities that have a primary mission to global humanitarian service as a long-standing tradition and expertise can be successful. For example Tzu Chi University, an APACPH member, is well prepared for disaster relief through its foundation as well as its global networks and partners. Such networks, often religious, tend to overcome access barriers such as political barriers that were evident during the Nargis cyclone, which killed more than 138,000 and displaced more than 2 million people in Myanmar. One of the unspoken realities in DAH is the politics in aid with bilateral agreements that dominate, and military and trade priorities that predominate. Even thoughtful aid administrators have little flexibility in overriding their governmental earmarks. Visibility in aid and more visibility in DAH have become an inevitable phenomenon, if not the key component in DAH, because it provides leverage to raise funds but also places pressure on showing immediate success. In the process there is systemic distortion (ie, all inputs go into 1 health problem: a clearly definable disease and its elimination; a distortion of overall reality). For example, the eradication of malaria was not possible by use of pesticide or mass drug administration alone without significant improvements in environment and human habitation. There are few places where there is total drug resistance and pesticide resistance. The need for balanced comprehensive approaches seems logical but of course more expensive and not so immediate. That is the paradox and motivating energy in DAH. Various scientific models justify the validity of the approaches advocated, not adequately recognizing external environments and other problems not of their immediate concern. Yet lessons in failure because of tunnel vision are not easily seen much less learnt in DAH as competing interests, technology, and visibility for success take priority.

In this aid environment, DAH has built high-tech hospitals to placate leaders of aid receipt. However, these high-profile institutions drain the services of doctors and nurses from much-needed urban and rural areas. This pharaoh effect of visible aid that does more for the donor than for recipients is seen in deteriorating hospitals in the Pacific islands, lacking maintenance or staffing.[41] As recipient countries and donors become more realistic, there is better rationalization and use of DAH such as in overall health improvement, addressing highly visible problems using low-cost interventions. Review of major aid agencies of DAH programs show that, although they have a distinct focus in their health assistance programs, more often they are competitive and duplicative rather than complementary. Although reinforcement is a useful paradigm in sustaining health improvement, one of the serious problems seen during the family planning era of the 1970s to 1980s in Asia was that the villages were flooded with paid community volunteers creating competing systems staffed with poorly paid government workers, a phenomenon that is repeating itself in parts of Africa. The driving force for instant success and visibility by donors in poor countries is a tragedy that is often repeated; raising expectations without the commitment or resources to sustain efforts through improved local systems. Political agendas predominate in DAH. However, as countries providing assistance gain experience and recipient countries gain skills in negotiation, DAH packages with greater flexibility and relevance emerge from building hospitals to supporting infrastructures, outreach, transport, disease prevention, and health education, as is increasingly seen in the aid provided by Japan and other emerging donor countries. University consortia, especially south-south consortia, can provide leadership to such policy determinations in infrastructure building and outreach. The University of Sabah Medical School, in partnership with APACPH member universities that were involved in rural/island health, established a Center of Excellence in Rural Health in 2008 to provide visibility and credibility on rural health research and training.

Direct emergency assistance through the military is common, especially for health, and is an immediate response in most countries but is often delayed in the United States. However, military assistance seems more prompt and more acceptable internationally during major disasters such as the Indian Ocean tsunami, when US Navy Hospital Ship *Mercy* significantly contributed to posttsunami relief in Asia.[42] Whatever the range of often overlapping motivations is, the resurgence of interest in global health has led to a dramatic increase in course offerings, joint projects, and programs across medical, public health, and nursing schools. There is a vision for health professionals to have a global perspective in caring-curing skills to serve in global settings. US universities, especially as consortia, not only have the potential, but the collective experience to make that expectation a reality. Expansion of global health training into a formal federally funded global health corps has been suggested.[43] Medical residency programs, including pediatrics, geriatrics, disaster management, and emergency medicine, are providing greater emphasis on global health training and overseas placements.[44,45] Consortia such as GHEC have provided long-standing leadership in education and promoting interinstitutional partnerships with south consortia. Interuniversity collaborations at national and regional levels continue to further evolve in North America, Latin America-Caribbean nations, and recently in Europe. The influx of DAH funds from government and foundation sources seems to be a key catalyst.[46] What is exciting about the expansion in government and philanthropic engagement in global health is that several models to support south-south partnerships are likely to evolve as the emerging south countries take leadership to access more effectively global health resources. In the development of APACPH sustained support for national and regional networks was found to be a key step in capacity building (see **Fig. 1**).

There is much that DAH and university participation can reaffirm, whether in the north or south, especially through consortia. Raising common concerns to the common problems among vulnerable populations levels the playing fields for all. In that process, a fundamental lesson that APACPH learnt was that university consortia need to continue to bridge north-south boundaries and bring relevance to the passion to serve. This essence of global health, the sense of a common humanity, the drive that keeps a doctor, a nurse, or a health worker struggling to keep a child alive, to help a mother with a safe delivery, to prevent a cancer death (whether rich or poor, whether in hospital or a village clinic, or a home) is the same motivation that bridges the gaps between altruism and opportunism in global health.

GLOBALIZATION: ERA OF DISASTERS AND PANDEMICS: THE CNN EFFECT

The World Wide Web and the instant sharing of tragedies, disasters, and pandemics alike on a global scale through television images and multimedia have brought a high degree of awareness of the widely prevalent pathetic human conditions both in the upper-income, middle-income, and low-income countries. Along with popular concerns during catastrophes, the increased participation of celebrities, major philanthropists, and government has created an unprecedented climate for global contributions to specific health causes such as HIV/AIDS, tuberculosis, and malaria.[46] The global media lens has shown that disasters often define and expose vulnerabilities of health systems for elderly people (Katrina, 2005; Japan, 2011) and the chronicity of neglect in sanitation (postearthquake disaster and cholera outbreak in Haiti). The stark differences and inequalities in health have become globally apparent through television lenses. In this complex developmental melee, universities serve as conduits for knowledge, technical expertise, and resources. They have made major contributions in selectively directing the improvements for global health. Instant communication and the dramatic increase in disaster reporting have accelerated the focus on health. On the negative side are tendencies for trivializing tragedy and demanding unrealistic results. The last decade has seen a significant increase in disasters. There were 385 disasters between 2000 and 2009, an increase of 233% from 1980 to 1989 and of 67% from 1990 to 1999.[39] Hurricane Katrina (2005) and a string of megadisasters and pandemics in the Asia Pacific region have filled media screens and brought home instantly how globally connected we are. In this era of disasters and pandemics, the south universities and research centers have been in the spotlight, either blamed or recognized. During that time, north-south collaboration has enhanced the credibility and expertise of institutions in the south in outbreak surveillance, infection control, and disaster management. Disasters and pandemics in the last decade have also created a stimulus for networking among APACPH members. The first APACPH Collaborating Center of Excellence for Injury Prevention and Disaster Management was established in 2005 in the Taipei Medical University, with links to the National Emergency Medical Center and the emergency medicine departments at 3 university hospitals and the School of Public Health. In addition, 3 other member universities, 2 from the south and 1 from the north, served as additional partners in training, research, and emergency relief. The Collaborating Center has provided training for educators and experts from the south in fields including disaster management in pandemics (SARS) and humanitarian relief in various contexts (Asian tsunami, earthquakes, and typhoons in Taiwan, Indonesia, China, and the Philippines). Taiwan, as the typhoon corridor in the North Pacific, being regularly exposed to earthquakes, monsoonal floods, and the largest number of typhoons every year, is geographically well located for the study of natural disasters.[47] The Center of Excellence also serves as a research center where Masters and doctoral students, health professionals, and health and hospital administrators have been trained. Research has identified several recurring problems: loss of communication and data early in disasters, leading to the impression of the loss of truth as the first symptom in any disaster; surveillance; crisis communication; and crisis management. The Collaborating Center of Excellence model developed by APACPH serves further to promote south-south exchanges and build credibility and expertise through such networks. The model has been expanded to address other needs in the Asia Pacific region such as the epidemic of oral cancer associated with betel nut and tobacco chewing, and rural/island health. The Center for Peace and Health devoted to reduction of conflicts and violence through health initiatives has also been established.

As the focus in health generally shifts to emergencies in the global arena (epidemics and disasters), the less visible problem of NCDs has been neglected. The growing burden of NCDs in the south has since been recognized by APACPH. University presidents and senior academic leadership have become actively involved in highlighting the problem of NCD. There is growing recognition that education for health needs to begin at the core undergraduate level for personal behavioral issues (drugs, smoking diet, and violence) as well as to gain skills in cultural competencies and understanding of community structures and policies. Therefore university-wide educational reform for global health at undergraduate level with a focus on interdisciplinary partnership at the graduate level is being planned. The key and integrating strategy is to focus on community-level applied problem-solving research. These directions are based on university president consultative meetings with senior faculty and administrators during 2008 to 2011. Presidents and Global Health Conference declarations have documented support for these and follow-up actions.[48,49]

CASE STUDY OF APACPH IN N-S PARTNERSHIPS

APACPH was founded in Kauai in 1984 with 5 university members represented by deans of medical and schools of public health. As a buildup to the formation of the consortium, many University presidents, and ministers of health and law from founding member countries attended the signing ceremony. National and international nongovernmental organizations (NGOs) including the US Centers for Disease Control, WHO, UNICEF, and the World Bank were represented. The founding mission and values were to emphasize health as human right and primary health care as a priority in the achievement of health equity.[50,51] The founding Dean from the School of Public Health in the University of Hawaii was Dr Jerrold Michael. The organization has grown slowly and deliberately to 67 members in 21 countries in 25 years. East to West it now spans from the University of Kazakhstan in Alma Ata (now Almaty), to George Washington University in the United States; north to south it extends from Tokyo University Medical School to Auckland University School of Public Health.[52] Six stages in the development of APACPH have been identified (**Fig. 2**).

In the formative first decade, the newly established organization focused on vision and mission (stage 1); development of leadership through the WHO Collaborating Center for Leadership (stage 2); and small-scale research, service, and intervention projects for vulnerable populations (stage 3), which enhanced the social responsibility of south universities as well as faculty and student participation from the north. In this decade, resources mainly came from the north.

The growth and development in the second decade show the growing leadership influence from the emerging south: East Asia and Southeast Asia, the economically advanced group of countries where largely self-supporting regional offices and networks were established (stage 4). The setup of regional office enables selected countries in the region to initiate national network building (eg, Thailand, China, and Indonesia).

During the maturation and stabilization of the third decade, Centers of Excellence were established, using a senior partnership of the south with selective expertise and some limited resources coming from the north (stage 5). The establishment of a Web-based International Cyber University for Health (ICUH), and enhanced university leadership (presidents) have created a synergy for global health in partnership with

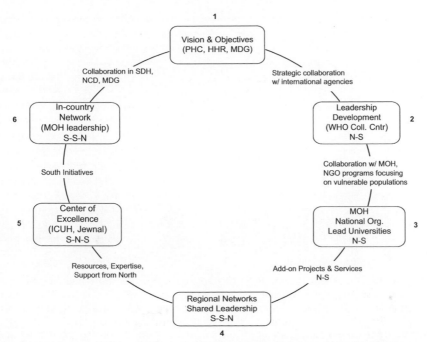

Fig. 2. Six stages in the establishment of south-north collaboration within APACPH.

the ministries of health and global health agencies. Such partnerships have initiated university-wide educational reforms for global health (President's Declaration on Global Health, Taiwan, 2009; President's Declaration on Non-Communicable Diseases, Bali, 2010). The development and strengthening of national networks of south-south universities with a collective focus on local problems is the priority at this stage of development in APACPH.

The predominance of the emerging south within the S-N-S organization is as follows. To date 23.5% of APACPH membership is represented by north universities, and 76.5% is made up of universities from 3 groups of south countries: S1 (12.5%), S2 (22%), and S3 (42%) using the country classification created by the World Bank **(Fig. 3)**.[53]

KEY CATALYSTS IN THE DEVELOPMENT OF THE SOUTH-SOUTH-NORTH COLLABORATIVE MODEL

Four key catalysts in the development of the south-south-north collaborative model were identified.

1. Leadership that began as a genuinely shared north-south leadership, not merely tokenism, developed into a cohort of senior and sustained leadership of the south with a consultative expert role for the north. The leadership development model strongly endorsed in the early stages had its problems. The quick turnover of academic leadership such as deans and presidents in Asia, sometimes every 2 years in some countries, made it necessary to build a tier of support. The stature of the early leadership cohort and the support of global leaders of WHO and

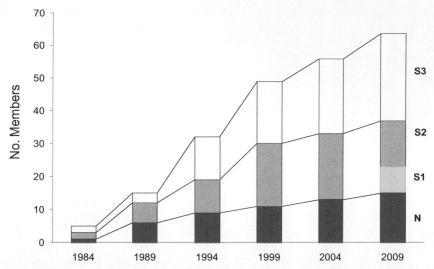

Fig. 3. APACPH membership growth in its first 25 years. Note. S1: south membership from countries in East Asia; S2: south membership from economically advanced countries in Southeast Asia; S3: south membership from economically slower developing countries in the south. Initially there was rapid growth of northern members, providing resources initially from the United States and later from Japan and Australia during the first decade; The growth of the south membership from East Asia (S1) and Southeast Asia (S2) enhanced resource support in the second decade. More active recruitment of low-income countries (S3) through regional networks is seen in the later phases, with in-kind matching contribution from them in the third decade.

UNICEF, as well as regional and national leaders, maintained the momentum in the first decade.

2. Resources were primarily from 1 source in the north (United States) in the initial stages. Subsequently, multiple funding sources were developed from other north members including Japan and Australia. In the later stages, the emerging south countries in East Asia (S1) and Southeast Asia (S2) assumed the major responsibility for funding through the Regional Center and Centers of Excellence.

3. The era of disasters and pandemics provided rapid exposure to the expertise and creativity of faculty and professionals and capacity of institutions in Asia to respond to these challenges. The ability to respond promptly to local conditions also gave leverage to south partners. The high-tech with high-touch cultural competencies in times of need with humanitarian response served to build credibility and trust, even under politically sensitive conditions among members. The APACPH Collaborating Centers in Injury Prevention and Disaster Management, Oral Cancer Prevention, Rural and Island Health, and Peace and Health brought together the expertise and commitment to address issues of common concern with resources largely coming from the lead university in the south and collaborating partners and donors from the north.

4. APACPH is a small organization but its visibility and impact have been enhanced by several factors as follows.

   a. The *Asia Pacific Journal of Public Health*, the first English journal in public health in Asia (1986). The journal offices are in the University of Malaya, which provides editorial support for an international team of editors. Besides providing global visibility the journal from its inception served to encourage excellence and focus on promising researchers from the south. The editorial team in partnership with major publishing houses has conducted workshops on research and publishing for junior faculty and students.

b. ICUH was founded in 2003 in collaboration with Yonsei University and was established to use the World Wide Web to advance public health and medical training for students and health professionals from countries with limited resources and access to undergraduate and graduate courses such as Mongolia and Vietnam. ICUH offers a focused course in 3 areas: disaster management in response to natural disasters and pandemics; public health certificate courses; and Masters of Public Health courses. Additional efforts were made to provide the courses in the region's native language.

c. The recent 42nd APACPH Global Health Conference held in Bali focused on NCDs. NCDs have become the major public health priority in APACPH with a focus on research, service, and partnership with national and global health agencies and ministries of health. The Global Health Conference also serves as an Asia Pacific forum for health policy issues and recognition of leadership largely from the south. Regional conferences and national activities continue to maintain the momentum and strengthen the network at the national level.

d. The Early Career Network (ECN) was established in 2006 after the Asian tsunami and has evolved to a small but dynamic network that serves as support groups to relief operations. They have now begun to work closely with the Collaborating Centers and in the conduct of international meetings and photography exhibitions. An important function served by ECN is to bridge the gap between university education and professional practice and maintain commitment to global health issues.

With a flat, shared leadership organizational structure and limited resources of the south-north-south model, several strategies have evolved to maintain the stability of the organization. A central rotating secretariat usually managed by a north university with significant decentralization of operations to officers and regional offices has been progressively developed. The decentralization process was initiated to enhance participation of the south as well as to restrict bureaucratic overgrowth. Consequently the responsibility to provide service and to raise funds was assumed by key institutions in the south. The Centers of Excellence, ICUH, and the journal office are largely self-supporting, maintained by respective south universities, providing an expanded resource pool for the organization. The ECN of young professionals is also south driven. Besides these organizational strategies, resource contribution shifted from the north to the emerging south in the latter part of the first decade, with a growing responsibility of the south members in the second decade to contribute significantly in kind and in local expenses including the funding and management of major conferences (see **Fig. 2**). The partnership with local and global NGOs and ministries of health provided the third stabilizer. The fourth component in this stabilization process is the ongoing development of the south national network of members and NGOs, and the access to resources.

PRIORITY FOR VULNERABLE POPULATIONS

The classic model for health assistance has been an N-S conduit, the prevalence of which has produced dependence, control, exploitation, and reciprocal corruption of the donor and recipient systems. The early efforts of the consortium was to disperse a large number of small grants on operational research and problem-solving capacities related to infectious disease control, MCH, and family planning. The emphasis was to use simple techniques and culturally appropriate strategies to ensure sustainability. These practices also leveled the academic exchanges between the north and south. During the epidemics and pandemics of SARS, avian flu, Nipah virus, swine flu, and H1N1, APACPH members provided leadership in research training and services, showing south competency. The north members supplemented the efforts through technical support and other resources. The south leadership was critical in promoting health equity and addressing sensitive issues such as neglect of female children, abuse of elderly people, and stigmatized health conditions such as HIV/AIDS. In poor countries, efforts to control or eradicate major infectious diseases by medication alone without addressing underlying social conditions and investing on infrastructure have limited success. Success requires a comprehensive primary health care approach, with involvement of key ministries besides health. In this challenge, APACPH has supported lead institutions and national and regional networks to network with NGOs to achieve common goals. For instance, the Collaborating Centers of Excellence for Oral Cancer Prevention in Asia Pacific emerged as a response to the fast-growing problem of oral cancer (in epidemic proportions in some countries) related to betel nut chewing in Asia.[54] The center is linked to cancer prevention and humanitarian organizations that rehabilitate individuals with major disfigurements and stigma. These challenges have also helped revitalize the organization's own values and commitment to redefine collectively what is unacceptable for health in the south societies as well as what is feasible with limited resources. In the context of oral cancer, the reduction of betel nut chewing is our top priority. Similarly, networks based on problem-solving efforts such as in injury prevention, indigenous health, and peace through health initiatives are being promoted. The model of health as a bridge to peace is being expanded in curricula, conferences, and publications.[55,56]

SUMMARY

Twenty-five years is a benchmark for any organization, more so in fragile international partnerships. Limited resources, rapid turnover in leadership in south universities, growing disinterest in north universities as control and power shifts to the south, slow membership growth and uneven resource support, which is largely voluntary, and organizational changes have all had a negative effect to various degrees. Despite those limitations, there is an overall sense of achievement particularly in the ability of the south's capacity to take over and manage APACPH successfully and contribute through the collective partnership. The boundaries of north and south have really almost completely blurred. From small beginnings, the annual conferences have grown to become a major global health event attracting university presidents, ministers, global health organizations, and local communities together in reinforcing policy initiatives and improving efficacy. The development of Collaborating Center and ICUH has created small but vibrant networks. In-country networks and south-south partnerships have stabilized as membership levels reached a healthy functional level of 3 to 5 in-country members. An ongoing strategy to revitalize in-country and regional networks is built in through national and regional conferences and partnership in national public health and medical organizations. Member university presidents have also begun to use APACPH networks and the Global Health Conferences to foster the social responsibility of universities whether in indigenous health, urbanization, or MDG-related goals. There have been sustained efforts to recognize and retain south leadership. Over the past 25 years, a total of 65 APACPH awards for excellence in leadership, research, teaching, and services have been given to leaders from the south. A Global Health Ambassadors program to retain the influence of leadership has been instituted. Capacity building has been slow but sustained, and has become south driven. Nearly 100 faculty and students received scholarships for their Masters and doctoral studies in the first 10 years through the WHO Collaborating Center at APACPH member universities, mostly in the north. It is estimated that more than 1000 faculty and students have been supported in short-term programs at member universities in the last 20 years. More than 60% of that support came from south universities, including the 4 APACPH Collaborating Centers. Each year, 10 to 15 APACPH travel grants are awarded to students and junior faculty to attend annual and regional conferences. APACPH members provide additional matching awards. The APACPH Global Health Conferences have therefore become a real opportunity for learning and exchange. Global health leaders and university presidents from many countries add their perspectives on global health equity across nations, the founding values of APACPH, reenergizing the commitment to primary health care and the MDGs. These acts of rededication of the social responsibility of universities to local and global communities touch the cornerstone of the social and environmental constructs in health. The beliefs and actions that emerge are value laden. In imperfect organizations like a university consortium there have been significant compromises and accommodation both by the north and the south. Yet the common goals and core activities have been revitalized by the members, especially the leadership of young global health professionals, whose dedication in serving the populations in need will sustain the collaboration.

REFERENCES

1. Tejasvi A. South-south capacity development: the way to grow? SSRN eLibrary; 2010. Available at: Social Science Research Network (SSRN). Accessed March 03, 2011.
2. United Nations Development Programme. Human Development Report. New York, 2009.
3. Gwatkin DR. Health inequalities and the health of the poor: what do we know? What can we do? Bull World Health Organ 2000;78:3–18.
4. United Nations Development Programme. Global south-south development expo 2010 executive summary. Geneva (Switzerland): United Nations; 2010.
5. Furuoka F, Oishi M. From aid recipient to aid donor: tracing the historical transformation of Japan's foreign aid policy. Electron J Contemp Jpn Stud; July 12, 2010.
6. United Nations Economic and Social Council. Trends in South-South triangular development cooperation: background study for the Development Cooperation Forum. New York, NY: April 2008.
7. Asher J, Daponte B. A hypothetical cohort model of human development. Human development research paper, vol. 40. New York: United Nations Development Programme; 2010.
8. Brazil's foreign-aid programme: speak softly and carry a blank cheque: in search of soft power, Brazil is turning itself into one of the world's biggest aid donors. But is it going too far, too fast? The Economist. Magazine Article: World Politics; 2010.
9. United Nations Development Programme. Human Development Report. New York, 2010.

10. James J. Bridging the global digital divide. Northampton (MA): Edward Elgar Publishing; 2003.
11. Pick JB, Azari R. Global digital divide: influence of socioeconomic, governmental, and accessibility factors on information technology. Inform Tech Dev 2008;14:91–115.
12. Hutubessy RC, Hanvoravongchai P, Edejer TT. Diffusion and utilization of magnetic resonance imaging in Asia. Int J Technol Assess Health Care 2002; 18:690–704.
13. World Summit on the Information Society. Bull Am Soc Inform Sci Tech 2004;30: 26–9.
14. Webster C. The World Wide Web–the great equalizer of the internet; 1995. Available at: http://pcinews.com/business/pci/hp/columns/equalizer.html. Accessed March 03, 2011.
15. Morse SS. Global infectious disease surveillance and health intelligence. Health Aff (Millwood) 2007;26:1069–77.
16. Norris P. Digital divide: civic engagement, information poverty, and the Internet worldwide. Cambridge (MA): Cambridge University Press; 2001.
17. Edejer TT. North-South research partnerships: the ethics of carrying out research in developing countries. BMJ 1999;319:438–41.
18. Frenk J, Chen L, Bhutta ZA, et al. Health professionals for a new century: transforming education to strengthen health systems in an interdependent world. Lancet 2010;376:1923–58.
19. IOM. The US Commitment to Global Health: Recommendations for the Public and Private Sectors. Washington (DC): Committee on the US Commitment to Global Health, Institute of Medicine; 2009.
20. Declaration of Alma-Ata. International Conference on Primary Health Care. Alma-Ata (Kazakhstan): World Health Organization; 1978.
21. Barringer BR, Harrison JS. Walking a tightrope: creating value through interorganizational relationships. J Manag 2000;26:367.
22. Colletta N, Ewing R Jr, Todd T. Cultural revitalization, participatory nonformal education, and village development in Sri Lanka: the Sarvodaya Shramadana Movement. Comp Educ Rev 1982;26:271–85.
23. Gupta S, Clements B, Bhattacharyaand R, et al. The elusive peace dividend. Finance Dev 2002;39:49–51.
24. UNICEF. Plan of action for implementing the world declaration on the survival, protection and development of children in the 1990s. World Summit for Children 1990. New York: UNICEF; 1990.
25. APACPH. Declaration Katmandu on neglected female children. In: The Annual Conference of Asia Pacific Academic Consortium for Public Health. Katmandu (Nepal): APACPH; 1988.
26. Patrick WK. Evening the score: the neglected girl child of Asia. Asia Pac J Public Health 1990;4:93–7.
27. APACPH. APACPH priority for health of indigenous populations. Executive board meeting of Asia Pacific Academic Consortium for Public Health. Colombo (Sri Lanka): APACPH; 2010.
28. Muller-Dietz HE [Not Available]. Hist Hosp 1975;10:65–71 [in German].
29. Daws G. Holy man: Father Damien of Molokai Honolulu. Honolulu (HI): University of Hawaii Press; 1984.
30. Kolodiejchuk B. Mother Teresa: come be my light: the private writings of the "Saint of Calcutta". New York: Doubleday Broadway Publishing Group; 2007.
31. IOM. America's uninsured crisis: consequences for health and health care. Washington, DC: Institute of Medicine Board on Health Care Services; 2009. p. 215.

32. Marmot M. Closing the gap in a generation: health equity through action on the social determinants of health. Report of the WHO Commission on Social Determinants of Health. Geneva (Switzerland): World Health Organization; 2008.

33. Kerry VB, Auld S, Farmer P. An international service corps for health–an unconventional prescription for diplomacy. N Engl J Med 2010;363:1199–201.

34. Crane J. Scrambling for Africa? Universities and global health. Lancet 2011;377: 1388–90.

35. World Health Organization. World health statistics 2009. Geneva (Switzerland): World Health Organization; 2009.

36. MacKellar L. Priorities in global assistance for health, AIDS, and population. Popul Dev Rev 2005;31:293–312.

37. Magnussen L, Ehiri J, Jolly P. Comprehensive versus selective primary health care: lessons for global health policy. Health Aff (Millwood) 2004;23:167–76.

38. Esser DE. More money, less cure: why global health assistance needs restructuring. Ethics Int Aff 2009;23:225–34.

39. Howson CP, Fineberg HV, Bloom BR. The pursuit of global health: the relevance of engagement for developed countries. Lancet 1998;351:586–90.

40. IOM. America's vital interest in global health. Washington, DC: Board on International Health; 1997.

41. Patrick WK. The dynamics of international health assistance in emerging new donor countries: lessons to be unlearned in health economics and development: working together for change. In: The 7th International Congress World Federation of Public Health. Bali (Indonesia), 1989.

42. Tarantino D. Asian tsunami relief: Department of Defense public health response: policy and strategic coordination considerations. Mil Med 2006;171:15–8.

43. Mullan F, Panosian C, Cuff PA. Healers abroad: Americans responding to the human resource crisis in HIV/AIDS. Atlanta (GA): The National Academies Press; 2005.

44. Suchocki A, Lorntz B, Sarfaty S. The Trans-university Alliance of Institutes Networking for Global Health (TRAIN for GH) report: A Survey of US Med Schools Participation in International Health Activities: Global Health Education Council. Charlottesville (VA): The Center for Global Health at the University of Virginia; 2008.

45. Panosian C, Coates TJ. The new medical "missionaries"–grooming the next generation of global health workers. N Engl J Med 2006;354:1771–3.

46. Ravishankar N, Gubbins P, Cooley RJ, et al. Financing of global health: tracking development assistance for health from 1990 to 2007. Lancet 2009;373:2113–24.

47. Extreme events and disasters are the biggest threat to Taiwan. Government Report. Taiwan Environmental Protection Administration, 2009.

48. APACPH. APACPH University Presidents' Declaration. Paper Presented at: The 42nd Conference of Asia Pacific Academic Consortium for Public Health. Bai, Indonesia. November 24–27, 2010.

49. APACPH. APACPH University Presidents' Declaration. Paper Presented at: The 41st Conference of Asia Pacific Academic Consortium for Public Health. Taipei, Taiwan. December 3–6, 2009.

50. Arnold CW. The University of Hawaii, a School of Public Health retrospective. Asia Pac J Public Health 1989;3:86–91.

51. Michael JM. The Asia-Pacific Academic Consortium for Public Health and leadership development. Asia Pac J Public Health 1987;1:6–8.

52. APACPH. The Secretary General's report. The 25th Annual Conference of Asia Pacific Academic Consortium for Public Health. Taipei (Taiwan): APACPH; 2009.

53. Carruthers R, Bajpai J, Hummels D. Trade and logistics: an East Asian perspective. In: East Asia integrates: a trade policy agenda for shared growth. Washington, DC: The World Bank, Oxford University Press; 2004. p. 77–94. [Chapter: 5].

54. Betel-quid and Areca-nut Chewing and Some Areca-nut-derived Nitrosamines. IARC monographs on the evaluation of carcinogenic risks to humans, vol. 85. Lyon (France): World Health Organization, International Agency for Research on Cancer; 2004.

55. Patrick WK. War as a Disease: Conceptual Dimensions of Warricide. In: "Health As a Bridge to Peace". Paper Presented at: The 39th Conference of Asia Pacific Academic Consortium for Public Health Pre-Conference Workshop. Saitama, Japan, 2007.

56. Patrick WK. Globalization of Violence Peace & Health: Implications for the Healing Professions in Violence Prevention. In: "Peace and Health". Paper Presented at: The 40th Conference of Asia Pacific Academic Consortium for Public Health Pre-Conference Workshop. Kuala Lumpur, Malaysia, 2008.

Global Health in the UK Government and University Sector

Cordelia E.M. Coltart, MPH, MRCP, DTM&H,
Mary E. Black, MPH, FRCP, DTM&H,
Philippa J. Easterbrook, MPH, FRCP, DTM&H*

KEYWORDS

- Global health • United Kingdom
- Development aid • Training opportunities

The United Kingdom has had a long and rich history of engagement with global health issues, and this is reflected in its academic and international development assistance structures dating back to the British colonial era. Tropical medicine, as a discipline, arose following the scientific advances of the late nineteenth century, along with the growing need for doctors to be trained to treat tropical diseases in the colonial workforce across the British empire.[1(p1)] Founded in 1898, the Liverpool School of Tropical Medicine (LSTM) was the first institution in the world dedicated to tropical diseases. The institution's inaugural lecturer was Sir Ronald Ross (1857–1932), who went onto win a Nobel Prize in 1902 for his work on identifying the *Anopheles* mosquito as the vector for malaria transmission.[2] Six months later in 1899, the London School of Hygiene and Tropical Medicine (LSHTM) was established by the Scottish physician Sir Patrick Manson (1844–1922).[1] Both schools have evolved considerably over the years from their original focus on tropical communicable diseases and sanitation to a broader interdisciplinary approach to global health. Over the last three decades, there has also been a proliferation of UK academic and other institutions engaged in international work, in addition to contributions from multiple government agencies, non governmental organizations (NGOs), and research funding bodies.

In this article, the authors review recent global health activities in the United Kingdom in several defined areas: UK government and international aid; role of UK academic and other institutions in international partnerships; and undergraduate, postgraduate and international medical graduate training opportunities.

International Office, Royal College of Physicians, 8 Street Andrews Place, Regents Park, London NW1 4LE, UK
* Corresponding author.
E-mail address: Philippa.easterbrook@hotmail.com

Infect Dis Clin N Am 25 (2011) 555–574
doi:10.1016/j.idc.2011.08.001
0891-5520/11/$ – see front matter © 2011 Elsevier Inc. All rights reserved.

id.theclinics.com

UK GOVERNMENT SECTOR AND STRATEGY IN GLOBAL HEALTH

The establishment of the UK Department for International Development (DFID) in 1997, headed by a government minister, marked a turning point in UK's aid program. Before this, the program was managed by the Overseas Development Administration, a branch of the Foreign and Commonwealth Office, which mainly focused on economic development.[3] An initial strategic white paper was published by DFID in autumn 1997, and three others have subsequently been produced (2000, 2006, and 2009), all with similar key goals regarding the elimination of poverty, delivery of clean water, sanitation, provision of basic health care and education to the world's poorest people.

In 2009, the UK's Gross Public Expenditure on Overseas Development Assistance (ODA) totalled US $11.5 million,[4] making it the fourth largest Organisation for Economic Co-operation and Development donor. Based on preliminary data from 2010, this has increased to $13.7 million dollars,[4] and the UK ranking to second. DFID contributes the majority of UK ODA, at 86% in 2009. About 60% of the UK's ODA contribution is in the form of bilateral assistance, 36% as multilateral assistance, and 4% in administration costs. **Fig. 1** presents the UK's net ODA as a percentage of Gross National Income (GNI), in comparison with 22 other OECD countries (ranked 9) and in relation to the United Nations (UN) benchmark target obligation of 0.7%, which the UK committed to meet by 2013.

In October 2010, at a time of major economic recession and substantial cuts in the UK public sector, DFID was the only government department that had its budget increased in the UK government Comprehensive Spending Review. The UK has committed to meet the UN's target for contribution towards foreign aid by 2013 at 0.7% of GNI.[5] The UK is currently well placed to meet this target and join a small number of other successful countries. The aid budget will be prioritised towards states affected by or emerging from conflict (budget increase from 22–30% (approximately US $5.5 billion)[6] with a 40% increase for Afghanistan between 2011 and 2013),[7]

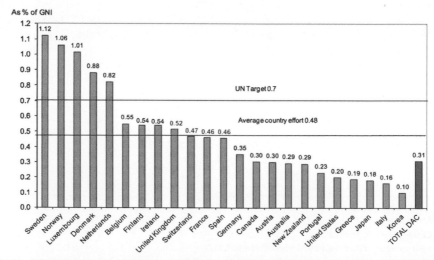

Fig. 1. Net Overseas Development Assistance (ODA) in 2009 as a percentage of the Gross National Income. (*Data from* Organisation for Economic Co-operation and Development (OECD). Preliminary data for 2009. Available at: http://www.oecd.org. Accessed March 7 2011.)

livelihood and wealth creating, and a specific health focus on malaria and maternal and child health. Fifty percent of the direct support to countries will go toward improving health, education, water, sanitation, and social protection services. In addition, DFID will spend £9.7 billion on improving health systems and services up to 2015; donate £1.6 billion towards the Global Fund to Fight AIDS, tuberculosis, and malaria; and invest approximately £400 million on global health research over five years.[8] Although the sustained budgetary commitment is to be applauded, UK and international NGOs have expressed concern about the negative consequences of what is perceived as an increasingly militarized aid strategy that aims for short-term "fixes," notably in Afghanistan.[9]

Contribution of Research Funding Agencies and NGOs

The UK contributes to the global health agenda via numerous other research and funding agencies and nongovernmental bodies.

Medical Research Council

The publicly funded Medical Research Council (MRC) established in 1913 has supported health research in developing countries for more than 80 years, with a changing focus from nutrition to infections research. 'Going global' is one of the four strategies within the 2009–2014 MRC strategic plan, with the specific objective to undertake "global health research that addresses the inequalities in health which arise particularly in developing countries."[10] In addition to funding global health through cyclical calls for grant applications, MRC is participating, together with UK DFID and the Wellcome Trust, in a joint global health trials scheme to fund late-phase trials of health interventions in low-income settings. Commitments of up to £12 million per year for the next three years have been made.

The MRC supports two major overseas units: MRC Uganda based in Entebbe and MRC Gambia. In Entebbe, the MRC/Uganda Virus Research Institute's (UVRI) Uganda Research Unit on AIDS is an internationally recognized center of excellence for research in human immunodeficiency virus (HIV) infection and related diseases. The unit was established in 1989 after a request from the Uganda government to the UK government to contribute to the understanding and control of the HIV epidemic in Uganda. An initial bilateral agreement signed between the two governments has been renewed every five years and, in 2009, was renewed up to 2019. In 2005, the MRC program was upgraded to a research unit, and it currently receives approximately £7 million of support annually, half of this as core funding from the MRC and the other half from external funders (eg, DFID). The key missions of this unit are to: (1) to conduct research to improve the control of the HIV epidemic through prevention and care both in Uganda and elsewhere in Africa, (2) to contribute to the translation of research findings into policy and practice, both locally and internationally, and (3) to support capacity building for research in Africa.

The research portfolio of MRC Gambia spans basic scientific research, clinical studies, large epidemiologic studies, and intervention trials across five main domains (bacterial diseases, genetics, malaria, nutrition, and viral diseases). There are field sites up country: Basse, Keneba, and Walikunda (in The Gambia) and Caio (in Guinea Bissau), each in a different ecological setting, providing varied research opportunities. There are approximately 200 scientists, clinicians, and senior administrative staff from many parts of the world, as well as hosting many visiting researchers, and more than 500 support staff.

The Wellcome Trust

The Wellcome Trust is a large UK-based charitable foundation that supports biomedical research and medical humanities. It devotes a significant proportion of funds to health-related research conducted outside the UK through its international funding schemes, its network of overseas programs in (Kenya, Malawi, South Africa, Thailand, and Vietnam (**Box 1**)); and four Wellcome Trust Centres for Research in Clinical Tropical Medicine (Bloomsbury [University College and LSHTM], Imperial College, LSTM, and Oxford University).[11] In 1995, an additional scheme was established to focus support for the trust's Public Health and Tropical Medicine fellowship schemes, which facilitates the recruitment and training of outstanding clinicians, to maintain the UK's strength in clinical tropical medicine and provide a UK base to support researchers engaged in projects outside the UK.

Contribution from NGOs

Other influential bodies include the Overseas Development Institute (the UK's leading independent think tank on international development and humanitarian issues)[12] and Bond (the UK membership body for NGOs working in international development with 370 members ranging from large bodies with a worldwide presence to smaller specialist organizations working in certain regions or with specific groups of people).[13] Prominent members include Action Aid,[14] the British Red Cross,[15] CARE,[16] Christian Aid,[17] Oxfam,[18] Merlin,[19] Plan UK,[20] Save the Children,[21] and Sightsavers,[22] as well as thousands of smaller voluntary organizations eg, Hearing conservation council.[23]

Health is Global: A UK Government Strategy 2008–2013

Based on the premise that global health enables the harmonization of international and domestic health concerns and the adoption of a more global outlook than that afforded by a development or foreign assistance perspective alone,[24] the UK Department of Health identified five key reasons for the promotion of global health and the development of a UK global health strategy (GHS): (1) improve global security and health protection, (2) enhance sustainable development, (3) improve trade by promoting health as a commodity, (4) maximize global public good, and (5) encourage a human rights approach to health.[25] In 2008, a government-wide GHS, "Health is Global: a UK Government Strategy 2008–2013", was launched. The strategy was based on five key areas for action (**Fig. 2**), with 10 key underlying principles (**Fig. 3**).[25]

An independent review in 2010 of the impact of this GHS in the BRICS countries (Brazil, Russia, India, China and South Africa) noted some "good examples of coherence in UK government working on the GHS in the BRICS countries, which is impressive given the short time frame." However, "the spirit of the GHS (as articulated in the GHS principles) remains poorly embedded in the main government departments that have the highest level of funding and responsibility for working overseas (DFID and Foreign and Commonwealth Office)." Three years on, it remains unclear how well the aims and targets have been achieved and implemented.[26]

The 2007 Crisp Report—Global Health Partnerships: The UK Contribution to Health in Developing Countries

In 2006, the then Prime Minister, Tony Blair, tasked Sir Nigel Crisp[27] (former chief executive of the National Health Service [NHS] and permanent secretary at the Department of Health) to carry out a review on how to optimize UK experience and expertise to improve health in developing countries. The resulting 2007 report "Global Health Partnerships: the UK Contribution to Health in Developing Countries," identified the

---

Box 1
The UK Wellcome Trust supported major overseas programs

The research programs have the following key aims:

- To conduct medical research of relevance to the country and region

- To provide opportunities for clinical and science graduates locally and abroad to gain additional experience of research by collaborating in or conducting projects

- To assist in the establishment of a vigorous local research capacity with a strong local base and international collaborative links

o The Kenya Medical Research Institute (KEMRI)–Wellcome Trust Research Programme is well known internationally for its work tackling malaria and other infectious diseases, particularly bacterial and viral childhood infections. With links to the trust since the 1940s, the program was formally established in 1989 in partnership with the KEMRI. The program conducts basic and clinical research in parallel, with results feeding directly into local and international health policy. It aims to expand the country's capacity to conduct multidisciplinary research that is strong, sustainable, and internationally competitive. The program employs more than 600 people, 95% of whom are Kenyans. Of the 100 scientists in the program, 75 are East Africans. A £9 million strategic award from the Wellcome Trust is helping to train local researchers in areas such as translational research, social science, and clinical trials. The program also has increasing links with researchers and institutions around the region, with research projects based in neighboring countries such as Somalia and Uganda.

o The Malawi-Liverpool Wellcome Trust Clinical Research Programme is based at the College of Medicine in the University of Malawi in Blantyre. It performs health research and trains clinical and laboratory scientists from Malawi and abroad. Officially established in 1995, it employs more than 200 people, including around 35 scientists, of whom the majority are Malawians. The program has strong links with the University of Liverpool, the LSTM and works closely with the Malawian Ministry of Health on Malawi's malaria, HIV, and tuberculosis control programs. The program has helped to advance malaria treatment and monitoring, notably through the development of the Blantyre Coma Score, conducted multiple trials of antimalarial therapies at different sites across the country, and described the detailed pathogenesis of cerebral malaria using a unique collection of postmortem brain material.

o The Africa Centre for Health and Population Studies, South Africa, at the University of KwaZulu-Natal performs research on population and health issues affecting a rural population with one of the highest burdens of HIV in the world. The center was established by the Wellcome Trust in partnership with the South African Medical Research Council in 1998 and employs more than 500 people, including around 25 scientists. The cornerstone of their research program is a biannual household demographic survey that since 2000 has collected data on births, deaths, marriage and migration events, as well as household economics. The survey covers a population of around 90,000 in 11,000 households. An additional annual HIV surveillance study, established in 2003, covers individuals aged 15 years and over, collecting data on HIV status, sexual behavior and relationships, and other health issues. The center also has a virology laboratory at the Medical School in Durban, with research relating to the dynamics of HIV in breast milk and population viral phylogenetics. The center works with the local department of health to run one of the region's largest rural primary-care-level antiretroviral therapy programs.

o The Mahidol-Oxford Tropical Medicine Research Unit in Thailand was established in 1979 by scientists from Mahidol University in Bangkok, Thailand, and the University of Oxford. It is part of the Wellcome Trust's Southeast Asia Major Overseas Programme Network, with the other major part of the program being based in Vietnam (Ho Chi Minh City). Field research extends across Thailand and includes the Shoklo Malaria Research Unit in Mae Sot, providing essential health care to refugee and displaced communities along the Thai-Myanmar border. Other sites are based at Ubon Ratchathani and Udon Thani in Thailand's northeast and rural north regions. The program also includes the Wellcome Trust–Mahosot Hospital–Oxford Tropical Medicine Research Collaboration, based in Laos, run in collaboration with the

Mahosot Hospital in Vientiane. The program employs around 370 people, more than 90% of whom are local staff. The program supports an internationally competitive training and career development track, from master of science to postdoctoral training, to develop research leaders both locally and internationally. The trust has provided £21.6 million of funding to the program since 2005, including around £3 million of core funding each year.

o The Vietnam Research Programme was established in 1991 in Ho Chi Minh City (hosted by the Hospital for Tropical Diseases a branch of the Oxford University Clinical Research Unit) and in 2006 in Hanoi (hosted by the National Institute of Infectious and Tropical Diseases, with close links with National Institute of Hygiene and Epidemiology and National Hospital for Paediatrics). Its research program focuses on improving the prevention, diagnosis, and treatment of infectious and noninfectious diseases. The program collaborates widely across Vietnam and with research groups in Cambodia, China, Indonesia, Malaysia, the Philippines, Nepal, Singapore, and Latin America. The Oxford University Clinical Research Unit also coordinates with the Southeast Asia Infectious Disease Clinical Research Network, a multinational group that strives to advance scientific knowledge and clinical management of infectious disease through integrated collaborative clinical research. The program has a formal training program, with 40 Vietnamese doctor of philosophy students and more than 20 masters students currently registered for degrees at Vietnamese or international universities.

Data from Wellcome Trust. Available at: http://www.wellcome.ac.uk/. Accessed February 28, 2011.

need for better coordination and more strategic international partnerships as one important strategy. In relation to medical training, the Crisp report noted that "an NHS framework for international development should explicitly recognise the value of overseas experience and training for UK health workers and encourage educators, employers and regulators to make it easier to gain further experience and training." It further recommended that "the General Medical Council (GMC) should work with the Department of Health, Royal Colleges, medical schools and others to facilitate overseas training and work experience."

In 2008, the Department of Health issued a formal response to the Crisp report and some further recommendations for implementation.[28] There was some concern expressed that although global health partnerships "were promoted to better focus health aid, their overlapping and unclear mandates in addition to a tendency to be highly issue-specific in their activities, might complicate the task of leading donors to recipient countries and managing foreign assistance for maximum impact."[29] Other recommendations regarding implementation were that better organization of health exchanges/partnerships would promote a more professional and equitable approach to the selection and induction of staff, in addition to placing global health and inequalities in the conscience of UK institutions (Wright, 2005).[30] It was further recommended that, in order to maximize and realize the full impact of these opportunities, the health links should be long term and aim to provide sustainable capacity for the developing country. With respect to placement of UK staff, it was recognized that the UK partners needed to ensure that international training or work experience fit in with the developing country's own agenda, plans, and needs and did not impose an additional burden.

There have been several outcomes to the Crisp report. First, as result of the Department of Health recommendations, the report has led to the establishment of the UK International Health Funding Links scheme, a three year program funded by DFID and managed jointly by the British Council and the Tropical Health Education Trust

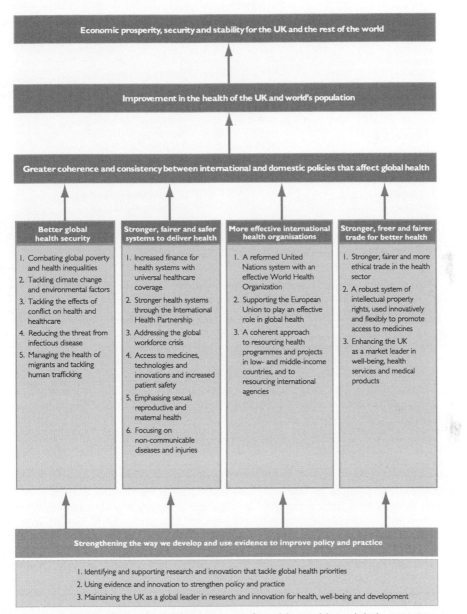

Economic prosperity, security and stability for the UK and the rest of the world

Improvement in the health of the UK and world's population

Greater coherence and consistency between international and domestic policies that affect global health

Better global health security	Stronger, fairer and safer systems to deliver health	More effective international health organisations	Stronger, freer and fairer trade for better health
1. Combating global poverty and health inequalities 2. Tackling climate change and environmental factors 3. Tackling the effects of conflict on health and healthcare 4. Reducing the threat from infectious disease 5. Managing the health of migrants and tackling human trafficking	1. Increased finance for health systems with universal healthcare coverage 2. Stronger health systems through the International Health Partnership 3. Addressing the global workforce crisis 4. Access to medicines, technologies and innovations and increased patient safety 5. Emphasising sexual, reproductive and maternal health 6. Focusing on non-communicable diseases and injuries	1. A reformed United Nations system with an effective World Health Organization 2. Supporting the European Union to play an effective role in global health 3. A coherent approach to resourcing health programmes and projects in low- and middle-income countries, and to resourcing international agencies	1. Stronger, fairer and more ethical trade in the health sector 2. A robust system of intellectual property rights, used innovatively and flexibly to promote access to medicines 3. Enhancing the UK as a market leader in well-being, health services and medical products

Strengthening the way we develop and use evidence to improve policy and practice

1. Identifying and supporting research and innovation that tackle global health priorities
2. Using evidence and innovation to strengthen policy and practice
3. Maintaining the UK as a global leader in research and innovation for health, well-being and development

Fig. 2. *From* HM Government, UK Department of Health. Health is global: a UK Government strategy 2008–13. http://www.dh.gov.uk/en/Publicationsandstatistics/Publications/PublicationsPolicyAndGuidance/DH_088702. Accessed March 7, 2011.

(THET).[31] There are now more than 100 links between UK NHS hospitals, together with their associated academic partners and organizations in developing countries. A further DFID funded initiative is the International Health Links Centre, under the auspices of the LSTM, to enhance access to health care in the developing world by

1 set out to do no harm and, as far as feasible, evaluate the impact of our domestic and foreign policies on global health to ensure that our intention is fulfilled;	**6** ensure that the effects of foreign and domestic policies on global health are much more explicit and that we are transparent about where the objectives of different policies may conflict;
2 base our global health policies and practice on sound evidence, especially public health evidence, and work with others to develop evidence where it does not exist;	**7** work for strong and effective leadership on global health through strengthened and reformed international institutions;
3 use health as an agent for good in foreign policy, recognising that improving the health of the world's population can make a strong contribution towards promoting a low-carbon, high-growth global economy;[14]	**8** learn from other countries' policies and experience in order to improve the health and well-being of the UK population and the way we deliver healthcare;
4 promote outcomes on global health that support the achievement of the MDGs[15] and the MDG Call to Action;[16]	**9** protect the health of the UK proactively, by tackling health challenges that begin outside our borders; and
5 promote health equity within and between countries through our foreign and domestic policies;	**10** work in partnership with other governments, multilateral agencies, civil society and business in pursuit of our objectives.

Fig. 3. Key principles, UK GHS 2008 to 2013. (*From* HM Government, UK Department of Health. Health is global: a UK Government strategy 2008–13. http://www.dh.gov.uk/en/ Publicationsandstatistics/Publications/PublicationsPolicyAndGuidance/DH_088702. Accessed March 7, 2011.)

promoting international partnerships that will increase the number and skills of the health workforce.[32] Both initiatives have gone some way toward creating a more coherent and systematic approach to international exchanges for NHS staff. In addition, the UK government has tripled its budget to support and expand links between NHS organizations and the developing world, with up to £5 million available from April 2011. A new health partnership scheme will fund payment of pensions and other NHS staff costs, as well as introduce a brokerage service to help match supply and demand.[33]

However, there remain significant challenges. Although the Crisp report encouraged junior doctors to gain experience abroad, the new less-flexible UK system of specialist medical training introduces barriers to prevent this happening.[34] A 2007 report entitled "*Improving health for the world's poor: what can health professionals do?*" from the international department of the British Medical in collaboration with DFID, highlights recommendations on what the BMA, other health organisations and individual health workers can do to advocate and lobby to improve global health. However, realistic practical guidance for health professionals wishing to work in developing countries remains limited.[34] As of 2011, there has been no clear response or policy following the various calls for action on how best to integrate overseas activities into UK postgraduate training programs.

UK INSTITUTIONS AND GLOBAL HEALTH PARTNERSHIPS

The proliferation of international institutional partnerships in North American and European universities has made them an important feature in the global health architecture. A similar pattern is emerging in the UK, but, to date, there has been limited discussion or debate as to the optimal role of UK universities in global health and the type of institutional partnerships with southern institutions that will meet their needs and priorities, as well as building and sustaining capacity for the future. A DFID-sponsored report in 2004 noted that global health partnerships (GHPs) are "a moving target in a changing environment" and the evaluation of their effectiveness and impact remained limited.[35] Four main categories of GHPS were identified: research and development GHPs (eg, new drug development), technical assistance or service support GHPs (providing drugs, technical assistance and support to increase access to services), advocacy GHPs (raising the profile of a particular disease or issue), and financing GHPs (providing funds for specific disease programs).[36] The authors discuss a selection of UK international institutional academic and clinical partnership projects and their activities.

Academic Partnerships

The largest number and longest established academic international partnership programs are with the London and Liverpool Schools of Tropical Medicine (LSHTM and LSTM). LSHTM is the largest institution of its kind in Europe with a mission "to contribute to the improvement of health worldwide through the pursuit of excellence in research, postgraduate teaching and advanced training in national and international public health and tropical medicine, and through informing policy and practice in these areas." In 2010, LSHTM had an operating budget of just over £100 million, research collaborations in more than 100 countries, and around 4000 students.[37,38] The LSTM is currently present in more than 60 countries worldwide, with a mission of "improving the health of the world's poorest people, helping to bring research innovation and scientific breakthroughs from the lab to those most in need."[2] An example of a recently established partnership involving both institutions, as part of a larger consortium of UK universities, is the Public Health Foundation of India.[39] This program aims to train multidisciplinary researchers who will populate the Indian Institutes of Public Health and strengthen the national public health workforce. The first cohort of students has begun training in the United Kingdom.[40] In 2010, Universities UK, the major representative body and membership organization in the United Kingdom for higher education, conducted a survey of international partnerships across its 133-member universities and colleges of higher education (Jagusiewicz E, Universities, UK, personal communication).[41] Information was sought on the largest 5 international collaborations per institution involving at least 5 members of staff and running for a minimum of 5 years to support research, training, and other capacity-building exercises internationally. A total of 44 institutions responded to the survey, reporting on 82 global health projects that met the eligibility criteria, based on 52 low- to middle-income countries. The main focus of the collaborations were research (67%), capacity building (60%), staff exchanges (46%), and students exchanges (27%). At least two-thirds of the projects were focused on small partnerships involving less that 10 people from the United Kingdom and less than 50 people from the partner institution. Funding sources of the partnerships were public (54%) or charitable (46%), whereas the private sector contributed 22% and NGOs 15%. It is recognized that this represents only a small proportion of all UK institutional international links, but information on such partnerships are not systematically documented across or within institutions.

Clinical Partnerships

The THET, a UK-based international development organization, was established in 1988 to harness the skills and expertise of UK health professionals and so help build long-term capacity of health workers in developing countries and improve the quality of services, facilities, and resources (**Box 2**).[42]

THET has successfully developed long-term partnerships between eight African countries and more than 18 UK hospitals to provide training for frontline health workers in the poorest settings and develop the institutional capacity of local health institutions. Current projects focus on Ethiopia, Somaliland, and Zambia (**Boxes 3 and 4**), but THET also has an increasing presence in Asia.

There are also many long-standing partnerships between individual hospitals and health centers in the UK and sister institutions in developing countries. A further example of a successful long-standing 20-year partnership is the staff exchange link between Hereford Hospital and Muheza in Tanzania. Each year Hereford Hospital responds to requests from Muheza and sends staff for a period of time. Over the years, these have included laboratory staff, a plumber, information technology staff, and a finance officers, as well as nurses, health visitors, radiographers, physiotherapists, and doctors. The hospital also collects and dispatches a container load of requested donated equipment. More recently, a retired physician from the Hereford hospital has worked as the medical director at Muheza. All this activity is supported by the hospital staff who give their time voluntarily and through fund raising.[27(p89)]

THET, together with the British Council, jointly manage the UK International scheme, as outlined above.

Professional Societies

Most Royal Colleges (Royal College of Physicians [RCP], Royal College of Surgeons, Royal College of Paediatrics, Royal College of General Practitioners, Royal College of Anaesthetists, Royal College of Obstetrics and Gynecology, and Faculty of Public Health) as well as various specialty societies have established active international programs and collaborations. The RCP activities in global health include both advocacy and the implementation of practical projects that focus on strengthening health systems through educational and training programs.[45] An excellent example is the ongoing collaborative initiative with the West African College of Physicians (WACP) (**Box 5**).

Box 2
THET's themes for international partnerships[42]

1. To empower frontline health workers: partners benefit from opportunities to enrich their professional and personal development, sharpen skills, learn new techniques, and broaden experiences, by harnessing the expertise and experience of UK health professionals.

2. To increase long-term sustainability: the approach creates relationships of mutual trust, respect, and solidarity. Programs build on existing systems and work in line with strategic health plans rather than creating parallel services. This work focuses on building long-term skills and capacity of health workers.

3. To develop mutually beneficial relationships: UK participants enhance skills and knowledge, deliver training and mentoring, develop problem-solving skills and the ability to think creatively. These participants improve awareness and understanding of developing health systems. Link institutions also experience an increase in staff moral.

Box 3
THET in Somaliland[43]

THET began working in Somaliland in 2000, and the link has focused on training staff to improve standards of care and providing academic support to the medical school curriculum. Work soon expanded to include health institutions, professional associations, regional health authorities, and the Ministry of Health and Labour. Achievements have included

- The Revolving Drug Fund (a source of good-quality medication available 24 hours of the day either at affordable prices or provided free to those who cannot afford to pay), the first of its kind in Somaliland.

- Setting up a blood bank and improving laboratory and pathology skills

- Supplying the first ambulance at Hargeisa Group Hospital, the main public hospital in the capital city. This vehicle played a crucial role in transporting patients during the 2007 cholera epidemic.

- Training members of the Regional Health Board to improve standard of public health facility management.

- Incorporating mental health into the training of a wide variety of health practitioners.

- Supporting the establishment of the Health Professionals Council in the development of frameworks for systems of accreditation and providing the foundation for regulation in the health sector.

The Royal College of Obstetricians and Gynecologists established a five year collaboration (2009–2014) with the LSTM and selected national governments to address the high death rate associated with pregnancy and childbirth. This includes development of an essential obstetric care and newborn care course, a diploma in reproductive care in developing countries.[47] The Royal College of Paediatrics and Child Health are collaborating with Voluntary Service Overseas (VSO) to establish several approved overseas training placements for pediatric trainees.

There is also a strong interest in global health among the new generation of junior doctors, medical students, and allied health professionals in the UK with the supported by two key organizations: Medsin and Alma Mata. Medsin is an independent student-led charity with 32 branches across universities in the UK that raises awareness of and takes action on humanitarian issues and health inequalities in the local and global communities. Formed in 1997, it comprises a network of motivated students,

---

Box 4
THET in Ethiopia[44]

THET has worked in Ethiopia for 20 years, supporting skills development of frontline health workers, such as nurses, midwives, and health officers. Programs include care of chronic disease in the community and support to health facilities in areas such as laboratory services, management, and record keeping. THET collaborates with the Ethiopian Ministry of Health and regional administrations to ensure that the work supports national health priorities and the development of health systems in the country. Major achievements include

- Training of health officers, nurses, and midwives across four regions of Ethiopia trained in clinical skills to help improve patient care

- Training of the first five surgeons to graduate outside Addis Ababa, with all five still working in the public system

- Donation of motorbike ambulances.

> **Box 5**
> **RCP London and WACP: supporting medical practice and educational opportunities in West Africa[46]**
>
> The partnership focuses on strengthening the capacity of the WACP to train future physicians in two main areas: medical education and clinical subspecialty training. The two colleges signed a formal agreement in 2008, and the WACP/RCP collaboration program for educational capacity building was launched in 2009, a three year project working alongside countries within the WACP membership, such as Nigeria, Ghana, The Gambia, Sierra Leone, Liberia, Cote d'Ivoire, and Senegal. Activities include:
>
> • Faculty development: Using the RCP expertise in training physicians as educators, WACP fellows (with teaching responsibilities) and other faculty are being trained to further develop their teaching skills, deliver educational workshops for doctors and other health care professionals, and establish a new education faculty within their college.
>
> • Clinical training: Several doctors are being trained in subspecialty areas identified as urgent priorities by the WACP. These doctors, in the formative years of their careers, receive focused subspecialty training in the UK for a three month period. Two-week teaching visits are made by leading clinicians from the UK to West African centers to demonstrate advances in their areas, appropriate for adoption in West Africa.
>
> • Learning resources: The project is reinforcing the available resources for trainees in academic centers in the region and providing the WACP accredited teaching institutions with Medical Masterclass Institutional Premier packages, the main RCP's distance-learning resource.
>
> • Joint scientific meeting: A joint conference is planned to bring the officers and staff of the colleges together, along with fellows and members, to share knowledge and expertise, celebrate success, and plan future collaboration. The conference will take place in The Gambia in November 2011.

active in curriculum issues, community projects, international exchanges, campaigns, and conferences.[48] Alma Mata, founded in 2005, is a global health network of over 1000 postgraduate medical professionals who are interested in global health issues. This organization aims to facilitate the development of clearer pathways for postgraduate education and careers in global health and provides online updates on news, events, education, lectures conferences, and careers information.[49]

EDUCATION AND TRAINING
Undergraduate Opportunities

There are currently 32 medical schools in the United Kingdom, with approximately 6300 doctors graduating each year. Since the 1970s, there has been a long-standing tradition in UK medical schools to incorporate a 6- to 8-week elective period into the curriculum during the final two years. This elective is usually spent overseas. The most comprehensive survey of medical electives in UK medical schools was undertaken in 2002; 23 (61%) of the medical schools responded, based on 2985 final year students who undertook an elective period. Most electives lasted for 6 to 8 weeks (but could be combined with scheduled medical school holidays to extend the length), and 71% took place in the final year. Overall, approximately 10% of students remained within the UK for the elective (range 3%–23%), 50% went to industrialized countries (range 44%–62%), and 40% went to developing countries (range 29%–53%). Seven medical schools provided elective destinations for students. All institutions except one offered defined aims for the elective period, including practice in a different clinical setting, gaining cultural awareness, personal and professional development, broadening horizons, and developing written and presentation skills. To complete the elective module, students were required to submit a report in 93% of the schools, fill in an assessment form in 43%, and produce a formal project report in 29%.[50]

The overseas elective is the "highlight of medical school" for many[51] and can lead to great personal and professional development. However, it is the least well researched aspect of medical school, indeed it often lacks any rigorous analysis of learning processes and expected outcomes.[50,52] This lack of analysis is mainly because it is arranged exclusively by the student, takes place outside the control and oversight of the medical school faculty, and there is usually no formal assessment associated with the placement.[52] This is in contrast to the US system where elective placements, although a more recent initiative, tend to be highly structured and well supervised. In a survey of medical students from north America, four main benefits of overseas placements were identified: improved diagnostic skills, positive attitudinal changes, increased knowledge of tropical diseases, and aiding long-term career choice.[53] In a further study conducted at the end of an international health fellowship program organized by the university of Wisconsin, participants reported additional positive benefits such as changed world views; increased cultural sensitivity; enhanced community, social, and public health awareness; enhanced clinical and communication skills; more appropriate resource use; changes in career plans; and a greater understanding of the challenges of working in areas with scarce resources.[54]

There has been no formal evaluation of the elective period across UK medical schools, but some institutions are beginning to act on this discrepancy with US-based electives. The number of structured medical elective placements are increasing, for example, the program developed and implemented by the University College London, under the auspices of the International Centre for Health and Development.[55] A few booklets exist listing various elective options, but these rapidly become out of date. Medsin plans to produce, promote, and publish on their Web site a list of effective elective periods and projects overseas in due course.[48]

Degree and Short Courses in Global/International Health

The UK offers a wide range of taught courses in various aspects of international health, as summarized in **Table 1**.

Postgraduate Training and Overseas Training Opportunities for UK Medical Graduates

In 2007, postgraduate general and specialty medical training in the UK underwent a major restructuring under a scheme called Modernising Medical Careers (MMC).[56] The current structure is that, after graduation, all medical students enter a two year foundation training scheme (foundation year 1 and foundation year 2), which aims to form a bridge between medical school and specialty/general practice training. Junior doctors then progress into specialty training schools, for example, medicine, surgery, obstetrics and gynecology, anesthetics, pediatrics, and public health as, specialty trainees (ST1–ST8) for periods ranging from five years for general practice to 10 years for some medical and surgical specialties. All conclude with acquisition of a certificate of completion of training (CCT).

Overseas placements are currently not part of structured postgraduate training but are left to individuals to arrange and obtain approval from the relevant UK training authorities. Previously, it was relatively straightforward for UK medical graduates once they had obtained full GMC registration (one year after graduation) to obtain time out of UK-based training to work abroad termed out-of-program (OOP). However, with the new MMC training structure, there are increasing restrictions, and obtaining approval to gain experience outside of the training scheme is now more difficult and may be protracted. The placement needs to be prospectively

Table 1
Selected examples of UK degree courses in Global/International Health

University	Degree	Topic
LSHTM	MSc	Biology and control of disease vectors
		Control of infectious diseases
		Demography & health
		Epidemiology
		Health policy, planning, & financing
		Immunology of infectious diseases
		Medical parasitology
		Molecular biology of infectious diseases
		Public health
		Health economics stream
		Health promotion stream
		Health services management stream
		Health services research stream
		Public health stream
		Public health in developing countries
		Tropical medicine & international health
	MSc or PGC (distance learning)	Clinical trials
		Epidemiology
		Global health policy
		Infectious diseases
		Public health
	DrPH, MPhil, or PhD	Faculty of epidemiology and population health
		Department of population studies
		Department of infectious disease epidemiology
		Department of non-communicable disease epidemiology
		Department of nutrition and public health intervention research
		Faculty of infectious & tropical diseases
		Department of disease control
		Department of clinical research
		Department of immunology and infection
		Department of pathogen molecular biology
		Faculty of public health & policy research training opportunities
		Department of global health and development
		Department of health services research and policy
		Department of social and environmental health research
	Short courses	Numerous short courses and diplomas
		Diploma in tropical medicine & hygiene
		Infectious diseases in humanitarian emergencies
		http://www.lshtm.ac.uk/prospectus/short

(continued on next page)

University	Degree	Topic
Table 1 *(continued)*		
University College London	BSc	International health
	MSc	International child health
		Global governance and ethics
		Global health and development
		Global migration
		Globalization
		International health
		International public policy
Oxford University	MSc	Global health science
Liverpool University	Master	Geographies of globalization and development
		Lifecourse, population, and mobility
		Population studies
		Research methodology in geographies of globalization and development
		Research methodology in lifecourse, population, and mobility
		Research methodology in population studies
		Tropical Medicine:
		Tropical and Infectious Disease
		Tropical Paediatrics
	Masters/Diploma/ or Cert	International Public Health
		Biology and Control of Parasites and Disease Vectors
		Humanitarian Programme Management
		Humanitarian Studies
		International Sexual and Reproductive Health
		Molecular Biology of Parasites and Disease Vectors
	Diploma	Diploma in Tropical Medicine and Hygiene
Edinburgh University	MSc	Global health academy launched in 2009
		Global health and public policy
		Health systems and public policy
		Health inequalities and public policy
		Global health and anthropology
	PhD	International public health policy
	MSC/ Diploma/ or Cert	Global health and Infectious Diseases (online)
		Global health and Non communicable diseases (online)
Leeds University	BA	International development (combined with multiple languages)
	MA	Global development
		Global development and Africa
		Global development and education
		Global development and gender
		Global development and international political economy
		Global development and political economy of international resources

(continued on next page)

Table 1 (continued)		
University	Degree	Topic
Brighton University	MA	International health promotion
	BA/MA	Globalization: history, politics, culture
Sussex University	BA	Anthropology and international development
		Economics and international development
		Geography and international development
		International development (dual accreditation with French or Spanish)
		International relations and development
		Sociology and international development
	MA	Development studies
		Gender and development
		Globalization and development
		Governance and development
		Participation, power, and social change
		Poverty and development
		Global health
		Globalization, ethnicity, and culture
		Migration studies
Glamorgan	MSc	Disaster relief health care (distance learning)
Other	—	• Expedition Medicine Courses: Approved for accreditation by the wilderness medical Society for the fellowship of the academy of wilderness medicine
		• Diploma in medical care of catastrophes: Royal society of apothecaries

Abbreviations: BA, bachelor of arts; BSc, bachelor of science; Cert, certificate; DrPH, doctor of public health; MA, master of arts; MPhil, master of philosophy; MSc, master of science; PGC, postgraduate certificate; PhD, doctor of philosophy.

recognized and approved by UK training authorities, for example, medical schools and Postgraduate Medical Education and Training Board, and deemed to be of educational value, whereby they will obtain some of the core competencies required for the designated CCT.

These increasing barriers to obtaining international experience during postgraduate medical training in the UK is in stark contrast to the US training programs, in which many of the larger institutions now embed international health into the curriculum and training structure for various residency and fellowship programs. One example of such a program is the International Emergency Medicine Fellowship program at the Beth Israel Medical Deaconess Center, where the two year rotation has multiple opportunities to obtain structured and supervised international experience and is combined with a one year master's degree in public health at Harvard.[57] A selection of training materials and curricula for these programs are available through the Global Health Education Consortium of US health care educators dedicated to global health education in health professions, schools, and residency programs.[58]

Despite the barriers, there are some recent initiatives that may facilitate the process for obtaining OOP approval for overseas activities. These include a proposal to incorporate the option for anesthetic trainees to take an OOPE between years four and five of their training program; a collaboration between the Royal College of Paediatrics and

Child Health and the VSO for a series of approved overseas placements plans for the GMC to establish a list of approved training programs and, most promising, an initiative by the Conference of Postgraduate Medical Deans (a forum for postgraduate deans to meet and discuss current issues, share best practice, and agree on a consistent and equitable approach to medical training in all deaneries across the UK) to establish a lead dean for overseas activities.

Opportunities for International Medical Graduates

With the advent of MMC, the regulations surrounding international doctors working in the UK have been tightened considerably. Eligibility criteria now preclude non–European Union doctors from applying for training posts, where previously the UK had heavily relied on these doctors, mainly from developing countries, to fill empty posts. In 2009, the UK Department of Health launched a medical training initiative (MTI), designed to allow a small numbers of international medical graduates (IMGs) to come to the UK to benefit from training and development in NHS services before returning to their home countries. In addition, several other schemes exist to support IMGs to obtain GMC registration, appropriate work visas (Tier 5) and finding posts in which to train. One such scheme is the MTI scheme run by the RCP London.[59] Representatives of the RCP London now visit selected countries (recently Sudan, Pakistan, and Sri Lanka) to interview candidates and to ensure that there is an appropriate and robust selection process. In addition, induction for IMGs into working within the UK NHS is considered vital, and there are plans to incorporate this as an assessed supernumerary component of the MTI programme.

REFERENCES

1. Cook GC. History of tropical medicine and medicine in the tropics. In: Cook GC, Zumla A, editors. Manson's tropical diseases. 22nd edition. London: W B Saunders; 2008.
2. Liverpool School of Tropical Medicine website. Available at: http://www.lstmliverpool.ac.uk/about-lstm/history-of-lstm/. Accessed February 24, 2011.
3. Department for International Development (DFID): history. Available at: http://www.dfid.gov.uk/About-DFID/History1/. Accessed February 24, 2011.
4. DFID Statistics on International Development. Available at: http://www.dfid.gov.uk/About-DFID/Finance-and-performance/Aid-Statistics/Statistic-on-International-Development-2010/SID-2010-Key-statistics/. Accessed March 7, 2011.
5. Townsend I. The UK & the 0.7% aid target, and the Draft International Development (ODA Target) Bill. House of Commons Library. Available at: http://www.parliament.uk/documents/commons/lib/research/briefings/snep-03714.pdf. Accessed August 8, 2011.
6. DFID spending review. Available at: http://www.dfid.gov.uk/Media-Room/Press-releases/2010/Spending-Review-2010/.
7. DFID. Available at: http://www.dfid.gov.uk/Media-Room/News-Stories/2010/UKs-Afghan-aid-effort-set-to-increase-by-40-Andrew-Mitchell/.
8. DFID Business plan 2010. Available at: http://www.dfid.gov.uk/Documents/DFID-business-plan.pdf. Accessed March 7, 2011.
9. Jackson A. Quick impact, quick collapse: the danger of militarised aid in Afghanistan. London: Action Aid, Afghanaid, CARE, Christian Aid, Concern Worldwide, Norwegian Refugee Council, Oxfam, Trocaire; 2010. p. 1–6.
10. Medical Research Council: global health. Available at: http://www.mrc.ac.uk/About/Strategy/StrategicPlan2009-2014/index.htm. Accessed March 1, 2011.

11. Wellcome Trust. Available at: http://www.wellcome.ac.uk/. Accessed February 28, 2011.
12. Overseas Development Institute (ODI). Available at: http://www.odi.org.uk/about/. Accessed February 28, 2011.
13. Bond: about us. Available at: http://www.bond.org.uk/pages/about-us.html. Accessed February 24, 2011.
14. Action Aid International. Available at: http://www.actionaid.org/index.aspx. Accessed February 28, 2011.
15. British Red Cross. Available at: http://www.redcross.org.uk/. Accessed February 28, 2011.
16. CARE International UK. Available at: http://www.careinternational.org.uk/. Accessed February 28, 2011.
17. Christian aid. Available at: http://www.christianaid.org.uk/. Accessed February 28, 2011.
18. Oxfam International. Available at: http://www.oxfam.org/. Accessed March 1, 2011.
19. Merlin. Available at: http://www.merlin.org.uk/. Accessed February 28, 2011.
20. Plan UK. Available at: http://www.plan-uk.org/. Accessed March 1, 2011.
21. Save the children. Available at: http://www.savethechildren.org/site/c.8rKLIXMGIpI4E/b.6115947/k.8D6E/Official_Site.htm. Accessed March 1, 2011.
22. Sightsavers. Available at: http://www.sightsavers.org/. Accessed March 1, 2011.
23. Hearing Conservation Council. Available at: http://www.hearinguk.org/. Accessed March 1, 2011.
24. Donaldson L, Banatvala N. Health is global: proposals for a UK government-wide strategy. Lancet 2007;369(9564):857–61. Available at: http://www.ncbi.nlm.nih.gov/pubmed/17350456. Accessed February 24, 2011.
25. Health is Global: a UK Government Strategy 2008–2013. Department of Health. Available at: http://www.dh.gov.uk/prod_consum_dh/groups/dh_digitalassets/@dh/@en/documents/digitalasset/dh_088753.pdf. Accessed August 7, 2011.
26. McDonald M. Annual independent review of the UK Government's global health strategy: working with Brazil, Russia, India, China and South Africa. London: Department of Health Publications; 2010. p. 1–48. Available at: http://www.dh.gov.uk/en/Publicationsandstatistics/Publications/PublicationsPolicyAndGuidance/DH_118807. Accessed February 24, 2011.
27. Crisp N. Global health partnerships: the UK contribution to health in developing countries. London: Department of Health Publications; 2007. p. 180. Available at: http://www.dh.gov.uk/en/Publicationsandstatistics/Publications/PublicationsPolicyAndGuidance/DH_065374. Accessed February 24, 2011.
28. Department of Health publications. Global health partnerships: the UK contribution to health in developing countries—the Government response. London: Department of Health; 2008. p. 72. Available at: http://www.dh.gov.uk/en/Publicationsandstatistics/Publications/PublicationsPolicyAndGuidance/DH_083509. Accessed February 24, 2011.
29. Elmendorf E. Global health: then and now. (Achieving Global Health). Available at: http://www.un.org/wcm/content/site/chronicle/cache/bypass/home/archive/issues2010/achieving_global_health/globalhealth_thenandnow?ctnscroll_articleContainerList=1_0&ctnlistpagination_articleContainerList=true. UN Chronicle; 2010. Accessed February 24, 2010.
30. Sloan J. NHS Links: a new approach to international health links. BMJ Careers 2005. Available at: http://careers.bmj.com/careers/advice/view-article.html?id=680. Accessed August 7, 2011.

31. International Health Links funding scheme. Available at: http://www.britishcouncil. org/learning-healthlinks.htm. Accessed February 24, 2011.
32. IHLC: International Health Links Centre. Available at: http://www.ihlc.org.uk/ index.htm. Accessed February 24, 2011.
33. Torjesen I. UK triples budget for building health links between NHS and developing world. BMJ 2010;341(2):c6345. Available at: http://www.bmj.com/content/ 341/bmj.c6345.full?sid=059268b8-fbf3-4fdf-907f-aab9f1e790b7. Accessed February 24, 2011.
34. Mabey D. Improving health for the world's poor. BMJ 2007;334(7604):1126. Available at: http://www.bmj.com/content/334/7604/1126.short. Accessed February 24, 2011.
35. Caines K, Buse K, Carlson C, et al. Global health partnerships: assessing the impact. London: DFID Health Resource Centre; 2004. p. 1–52.
36. Wells H. Aid instruments and the very poor: the case of global health partnerships. London: DFID Health Systems Resource Centre; 2005.
37. London School of Hygiene & Tropical Medicine (LSHTM) Global Health. Available at: http://www.lshtm.ac.uk/aboutus/director. Accessed February 24, 2011.
38. Research Assessment Exercise UK 2008. Available at: http://www.lshtm.ac.uk/ aboutus/annualreport/annual_report_2009_10.pdf. Accessed February 24, 2011.
39. Public Health Foundation of India. Available at: http://www.phfi.org/. Accessed March 6, 2011.
40. Funding highlights: Wellcome Trust. Available at: http://www.wellcome.ac.uk/ Funding/Strategic-awards/Highlights/index.htm. Accessed March 6, 2011.
41. Universities UK. Universities UK website. 2011. Available at: http://www. universitiesuk.ac.uk/Pages/Default.aspx. Accessed February 24, 2011.
42. THET: Tropical Health and Education Trust. Available at: http://www.thet.org/. Accessed February 24, 2011.
43. THET: Somaliland. Available at: http://www.thet.org/about-thet/our-programmes/ somaliland/. Accessed March 6, 2011.
44. THET: Ethiopia. Available at: http://www.thet.org/about-thet/our-programmes/ ethiopia/. Accessed March 6, 2011.
45. Global health: Royal College of Physicians UK. Available at: http://www. rcplondon.ac.uk/policy/reducing-health-harms/global-health. Accessed March 6, 2011.
46. The Royal College of Physicians (RCP) and West African College of Physicians (WACP) Partnership. Available at: http://www.rcplondon.ac.uk/international/ africa/rcp-and-wacp. Accessed August 8, 2011.
47. LSTM/RCOG International Partnership: Royal College of Obstetricians and Gynaecologists. Available at: http://www.rcog.org.uk/what-we-do/international/ partnerships/lstm/rcog-international-partnership. Accessed March 6, 2011.
48. Medsin. Available at: http://www.medsin.org/. Accessed February 24, 2011.
49. Alma Mata: Global Health Network. Available at: http://www.almamata.net/news/ content/alma-mata-global-health-network. Accessed February 25, 2011.
50. Miranda JJ, Yudkin JS, Willott C. International health electives: four years of experience. Travel Med Infect Dis 2005;3(3):133–41. Available at: http://www.ncbi.nlm. nih.gov/pubmed/17292031. Accessed February 25, 2011.
51. Dowell J, Merrylees N. Electives: isn't it time for a change? Med Educ 2009;43(2): 121–6. Available at: http://www.ncbi.nlm.nih.gov/pubmed/19161481. Accessed February 24, 2011.
52. Jolly B. A missed opportunity. Med Educ 2009;43(2):104–5. Available at: http:// www.ncbi.nlm.nih.gov/pubmed/19161477. Accessed February 24, 2011.

53. Thompson M, Huntington M, Mark K, et al. Educational effects of international health electives on U.S. and Canadian medical students and residents: a literature review. Acad Med 2003;78(3):342–7.
54. Haq C, Rothenberg D, Gjerde C, et al. New world views: preparing physicians in training for global health work. Fam Med 2000;32(8):566–72.
55. University College London Centre for International Health and Development. Available at: http://www.ucl.ac.uk/cihd/undergraduate. Accessed February 24, 2011.
56. Medical Specialty training (England). Available at: http://www.mmc.nhs.uk/. Accessed February 24, 2011.
57. International Emergency Medicine Fellowship Program, Beth Israel Deaconess Medical Center. Available at: http://www.bidmc.org/MedicalEducation/Departments/EmergencyMedicine/FellowshipPrograms/InternationalEmergencyMedicineFellowshipProgram.aspx. Accessed February 24, 2011.
58. Global Health Education Consortium. Available at: http://globalhealtheducation.org/aboutus/SitePages/Home.aspx. Accessed February 25, 2011.
59. RCP International Sponsorship Scheme, Royal College of Physicians, London. Available at: http://old.rcplondon.ac.uk/RCP-International/ISS/Pages/International-Sponsorship-Scheme.aspx. Accessed February 24, 2011.

Competencies for Global Heath Graduate Education

Judith G. Calhoun, PhD, MBA[a],*,
Harrison C. Spencer, MD, MPH, DTMH, CPH[b], Pierre Buekens, MD, PhD[c]

KEYWORDS

- Global health • Competencies • Public health
- Graduate education

Health is a necessary prerequisite for a harmonious, productive, prosperous, and peaceful world. It is indeed central to the aspiration of the world's people and of their governments and as such health is a global priority.
—T. Shilton, 2009[1]

INTRODUCTION

The multitude of social, political, technological, and economic forces currently fueling globalization (**Box 1**) are also driving the current unprecedented interest and growth in world health, health education and promotion, and global workforce development (**Box 2**).[2–4] These inflection points have drawn attention to the many imperatives and priorities for the expansion of workforce development and capacity-building, both within and across nations. Long-standing professional and geographic differences in education and training programs, licensure/certification standards, and roles and specialization requirements, however, have compromised national and international health education agenda setting. Equally impacted has been consensus building regarding the development of educational standards across the professions. Despite the repeated calls for collaboration and interprofessional education, little progress has been achieved to date in relation to these goals even within regions and individual countries. In the United States specifically, the silo-based and variable educational approaches across the health professions at large and the related

[a] Medical School, University of Michigan, 300 Huntington Drive, Suite 5100, Ann Arbor, MI 48104-1820, USA
[b] Association of Schools of Public Health, 1900 M Street NW, Suite 710, Washington, DC 20036, USA
[c] School of Public Health and Tropical Medicine, Tulane University, 1440 Canal Street, Suite 2430 New Orleans, LA 70112, USA
* Corresponding author.
E-mail address: jgcal@umich.edu

Infect Dis Clin N Am 25 (2011) 575–592
doi:10.1016/j.idc.2011.02.015
0891-5520/11/$ – see front matter © 2011 Published by Elsevier Inc.

id.theclinics.com

Box 1
Forces of globalization

- Greater international connectedness and interdependence
- Intensification of a competitive global marketplace
- Expansion of flows across countries (resources, people, goods, information, innovations)
- Escalation of dependency on intellectual capital and innovation for productivity and growth
- Greater focus on the role of prevention in health
- Increased threats of infectious disease outbreaks, natural disasters, unintentional man-made disasters, and biological and terrorist attacks
- Heightened public visibility of a global health agenda
- Societal demand and movements for greater global equity
- Incremental potential for global conflict and loss of security

---

specializations have been highlighted in all 3 of the Institute of Medicine committee reports addressing the quality chasm related to health care.[5–7]

The call for educational transformation across health professions in the United States has been uniform and resounding by leaders and researchers in educational and workforce development, foundations, health professions commissions, and professional organizations.[8–13] In addition, several international conferences and forums have promoted widespread engagement, ownership, and collaboration in

---

Box 2
Drivers of interest and growth in global health

- Increased opportunities for traveling, living, studying, and working around the world
- Innovations in information technology and communication
- Ease of communication and travel
- Emphasis on internationalization facilitated by global media
- Heightened public awareness as a matter of US foreign policy
- Greater student interest around the world regarding issues affecting health, health care, and health services
- Growing belief that health is a basic human right and a moral imperative
- New demand among undergraduates, graduate, and professional students for education and training experiences aligned with marketplace factors
- Proliferation of schools of public health across the globe, including increased global health degree-granting and certification programs
- Internationalization of health and education, expansion of free-standing institutes and centers focusing on global health and the promotion of health
- Enlightened self-interest and global health investment by the American public
- New donors with unprecedented levels of funding for global health and related areas of workforce development, research, and discovery
- Social justice movements on campuses: increased student compassion and activism fueled by world conflicts and health challenges
- Expansion of global health disciplinary frameworks beyond the health professions

global health, including the World Health Organization and the United Nations.[3] The 2009 Galway Consensus Conference, stressed greater international collaboration in the development of global health workforce capacity and competencies.[14] In early 2010, a subset of the Association of Schools of Public Health (ASPH) Global Health Committee sought to dissolve the dichotomies drawn by prior groups among global health, international health, and public health by publishing a statement asserting that "global health and public health are indistinguishable."[15] Later in 2010, a global commission of professional and academic leaders called for major reform in the training of doctors and other health care professionals to equip them for the 21st century. The commission's report, titled Health Professionals for a New Century: Transforming Education for Health Systems in an Interdependent World, was published in The Lancet, enabling it to reach a wide, global audience.[16] Related outcomes and calls from these meetings included (1) the building of shared visions; (2) catalyzing change leaders; (3) launching advocacy and dissemination action plans regarding global health education; and (4) gaining consensus on future collaborative strategies and actions for ensuring quality in education, training, and practice. Global competencies are clearly viewed as essential for global realization of these goals and global health success overall. However, existing variabilities in the development of competencies and related educational initiatives within countries and regions have been further impacted by the current economic landscape. Therefore, it is unlikely that these ambitions for educational and workforce transformation will be realized in time to influence the United Nations' 2015 Millennium Development Goals.[17]

To date there is a modicum of information regarding the development of competency models, standards setting, and specific deployments of competency-based educational program development in the health professions, both regionally and internationally. As depicted by the S curve for the adoption and use of educational transformation adapted from Rogers' framework for the diffusion of innovations, many of the educators and trainers across the entire spectrum of the global health workforce are just starting the introductory stage (phase I) of the competency journey (**Fig. 1**).[18] In contrast, newer early adopters in some professions,[19–24] oversight organizations,[19] and countries[25–28] have moved beyond debating the well-established theoretical underpinnings and merits of this evolving educational movement. These innovators are progressing in the development of competency models that serve as the basis for elevating workforce development across all levels, including university and college-based students. Sponsors of the competency movement clearly view it as an essential educational transformation for ensuring the skills and readiness of current trainees and students in world-health settings. However, other than the Centers for Disease Control and Prevention Global Health Core Competencies[29] and the University of Washington School of Public Health's competency listing for their master of public health (MPH) scholars,[2] no other models could be found in the literature specifically addressing the development of a competency model as a driver for leading international or global health education initiatives.

This article provides a brief overview of the competency-based education (CBE) movement and its impact on graduate health professions education in the United States to date. In addition, a description is provided of the current Association of Schools of Public Health (ASPH) initiatives focused on CBE and the development of a standardized global health competency model targeted at master-level students majoring in global health. These endeavors and evolving lessons serve as the basis for subsequent review and discussion regarding the evolving inflection points influencing health professions education. In addition, recommendations addressing the potential future directions in graduate health professions education are provided. Collective understanding of

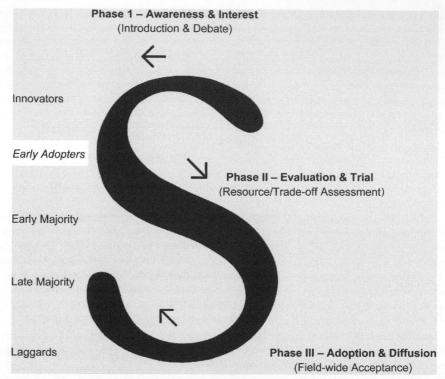

Fig. 1. S-curve framework: adoption and dissemination of educational innovations. (*Data from* E. Roger (1962, 1983)—Diffusion of innovations. 3rd Edition. New York: Free Press; 1983.)

both current macro-environmental and micro-environmental forces and future trends is essential for developing broader and more inclusive visions for a better future and the critical strategies and actions for the realization of global health.

CURRENT STATUS OF THE US COMPETENCY MOVEMENT IN GRADUATE LEVEL HEALTH PROFESSIONS EDUCATION

During the past decade, several competency models have been developed to guide health professions education and training across the wide array of professional roles, generalist and specialty positions, and postsecondary education programs both nationally and internationally.[25–28] **Table 1** provides a listing of exemplar graduate education competency modeling efforts in the United States to date that have been documented in the published literature. Other initiatives have been developed or are in current development in relation to national health and security agendas, specialty education and training programs, and individual graduate programs at various universities and colleges. However, at this writing, the specific status, potential linkages to global health, and level of education targeted for these efforts are not currently available via public search modalities. Many of these efforts to date are known to exist but have not been shared in the formally published literature.

The majority of the models listed in **Table 1** were initiated and supported by their professional associations or accrediting organizations wishing to identify the core capabilities that practitioners entering the global health workforce would need for effective practice in the decade ahead. The US Department of Education's outcomes-based educational initiatives (specifically those related to higher education and professional credentialing) have also influenced the movement at the graduate school level.[30–34] As a result, many of the accrediting and certification bodies overseeing standards for health professions educational practices and policies have required, or will soon be requiring, the identification of a specific evidenced-based competency model for guiding future program development.[35–37] Competency models are increasingly being viewed as an essential prerequisite for aligning educational program missions and vision with the types and skills of students entering their programs and the marketplaces where their students will be placed upon graduation. In addition, in line with evolving adult- and lifelong-learning principles and educational best practices, scientifically-developed and validated competency models will become the norm for directing future pedagogy, including the development and deployment of learning and assessment methods across graduate programs (**Fig. 2**).

As noted earlier, CBE deployment remains in the earliest phase for diffusion, with many barriers to its universal acceptance and widespread use. The majority of the barriers are those associated with faculty trial and evaluation, which occurs during the second phase of diffusion. Most faculties today received their graduate education during the golden decades of passive student learning, within the context of a faculty-centric paradigm. As a result, many faculty teach by transferring knowledge, predominately through lecturing and discussion methods, versus contemporary action-based learning methods. They received their teaching positions based on their specialized knowledge base and research acumen, with little or no grounding in pedagogical principles. In addition, given the reward system in higher education today with a primary emphasis on research productivity, there are few incentives for investing in teaching enhancement, nor is there interest in seeking out assistance from educational specialists or campus centers on excellence in teaching. Hence, many faculty remain more comfortable with lecturing modalities given the associated efficiencies for effort expended after initial course development.

Today's students, in contrast, are far more predisposed to the specificity and transparency afforded them in CBE. Given the economic challenges of the past decade, there is significant ambiguity regarding future employment options for the current generation of graduate students. Today's graduates are focused on their future and optimizing their potential differentiation for the work marketplaces they will be entering. They are demanding greater returns on investments than students in prior generations. In addition, they want to know how their capabilities will be enhanced through all of their learning experiences. The more relevant and similar students' educational experiences are to their future work roles, the greater their perceived preparation and readiness upon graduation. They want to be fully informed regarding what they are going to learn and achieve, the methods for such, the timeframe, and the match among the performance expectations, the learning methods, and the evaluation processes used.[38,39]

Without professional organizations, accrediting bodies, and school-wide leadership and championing of CBE, preliminary research findings indicate that most faculty would not be predisposed to adopting the associated methodologies, thereby remaining at phase I, or early entry into phase II, of the S curve of the diffusion process for this movement.[5,9]

Current Association of Schools of Public Health Competency Initiatives

Survey of competency-based education practices

In 2009, the ASPH Education Committee sponsored a faculty-student survey of the state of competency-based educational practices and challenges across US schools

Table 1
Published graduate-level health professions competency models in medicine, nursing, pharmacy, public health, and interprofessional education

Model (Sponsor)	Year	Domains/Other	Number Competencies	Number Subcompetencies	Audience
Medicine					
Accreditation Council for Graduate Medical Education Competencies (ACGME)	2002	6	24	—	Graduate medical education programs
Nursing					
Expected Outcomes and Curricular Elements of PhD Programs in Nursing (American Association of Critical Care Nurses Task Force on Research-Focused Doctorate in Nursing)	2010	3	17	—	PhD nursing graduates
Pharmacy					
Professional Pharmacists Competencies (Accreditation Council for Pharmacy Education)	2007	3 professional competencies	10	2	Graduate of pharmacy degree programs
Clinical Pharmacists Competencies (American College of Clinical Pharmacy)	2008	5	18	65	Clinical pharmacists
Public Health					
Doctor of Public Health Core Competency Model (Association of Schools of Public Health)	2007–2009	7	54	—	DrPH graduates
Master of Public Health Core Competency Model (Association of Schools of Public Health)	2004–2006	5 discipline-specific 7 cross-cutting	119	—	MPH program faculty and MPH graduates

	Year				Target audience
Public Health Preparedness & Response Core Competency Model (*Association of Schools of Public Health*)	2010	4	18	—	Mid-level public health workers (including MPH equivalent or higher degree, plus 5 years in the workforce)
Cultural Competence Education for Students in Medicine and PH (*Association of American Medical Colleges/Association of Schools of Public Health*)	2010 draft	3	35	—	Medical and PH students
Global Health Competencies (*Centers for Disease Control and Prevention*)	2008–2009	—	9	56	Global health workforce at all levels
Core Competencies for Public Health Professionals/ (*Council on Linkages*)	2009–2010	3 tiers	8	238	Entry level professional, managers, supervisors, senior managers/leaders
Competencies of Health Educators (*National Commission for Health Education Credentialing*)	2010	7 areas of responsibility	35	82	Health education specialists
Bioterrorism and Preparedness (*Columbia University*)	2002	3	9	75	PH workers targeted for bioterrorism and emergency-readiness training
Interdisciplinary Interprofessional Education Competencies (*Interprofessional Education Collaborative*)	2011	4	38	—	Allopathic medicine, dental, nursing, osteopathic medicine, pharmacy, and public health students pre-licensure/pre-certification

Abbreviations: AACN, American Association of Critical Care Nurses; DrPH, Doctor of Public Health; PH, public health.
  http://www.acgme.org/outcome/comp/GeneralCompetenciesStandards21307.pdf. Accessed July 20, 2010; http://www.aacn.nche.edu/education/pdf/PhDTask
  Force.pdf. Accessed September 6, 2010; http://www.acpe-accredit.org/pdf/ACPE_Revised_PharmD_Standards_Adopted_Jan152006.pdf. Accessed July 20, 2010;
  http://www.accp.com/docs/positions/whitePapers/CliniPharmCompTFfinalDraft.pdf. Accessed July 20, 2010; http://www.asph.org/publication/DrPH_Core_Competency_
  Model/index.html. Accessed June 17, 2010; http://www.asph.org/publication/MPH_Core_Competency_Model/index.html. Accessed July 20, 2010; http://www.asph.
  org/userfiles/PreparednessCompetencyModel-Version1.0.pdf. Accessed July 20, 2010; http://www.asph.org/document.cfm?page=836. Accessed September 6,
  2010; J. Hiland. Global Health Competencies. Centers for Disease Control and Prevention. Unpublished presentation. January, 2009; http://www.phf.org/link/
  CCs-example-free-ADOPTED.pdf. Accessed February 20, 2009; http://www.nchec.org/credentialing/responsibilities/nursing.columbia.edu/chp/pdfArchive/
  EmerPrepTrgCompetency.doc. Accessed May 6, 2008; https://www.aamc.org/download/186750/data/core_competencies.pdf. Accessed June 1, 2011.

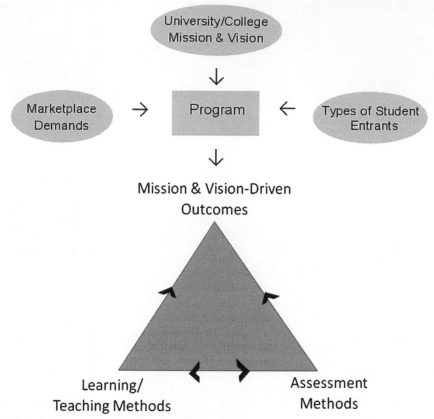

Fig. 2. Graduate education program level adoption forces and pedagogical alignments. *Data from* M. Decker—Futurecourse 2009.

of public health. A 30-item survey was sent to dean-appointed informants at all 2009 accredited US schools of public health (N = 40). The survey addressed 5 key areas: (1) faculty and student reactions to CBE in general and the MPH competency model specifically; (2) the school's approaches to dissemination, championship, and resourcing of the model; (3) strategies for promoting and increasing the awareness of the model; (4) implementation of the model in the curriculum, including the perceived adequacy of the core competencies for MPH graduates, the extent of faculty development for teaching the competencies, the degree to which course teaching and evaluation methods align with the competencies, and barriers to implementation; and (5) the state of current curricular innovation by the schools. Details regarding the findings from the study were presented at the fall 2009 annual meeting of ASPH.[40] Ninety-three percent of the accredited schools (N = 37) responded to the survey. In general, key findings included:

High levels of faculty familiarity with the model $\bar{x}$ = 3.7 on a 4 point Likert scale, with less familiarity among the students ($\bar{x}$ = 2.6)

Equal moderate levels of support across faculty and students regarding ($\bar{x}$ = 2.8 and $\bar{x}$ = 3.1 respectively): the value of CBE principles by faculty and students, and model coverage of key skills

Dean's offices and curriculum committees serving as the primary champions for competency-based educational changes

Satisfaction with the resources provided for integration of the model

Deployment of a variety of implementation strategies, including mapping of competencies to specific program curricula and alignment of teaching and evaluation methods with the competencies

Greater perceived adequacy and implementation of the discipline-specific competencies than the cross-cutting competencies

Faculty predispositions, including lack of faculty interest in, awareness of, and time for CBE principles/methods, as key barriers to implementation.

Respondents also uniformly cautioned that not enough time had elapsed for full deployment of the model and associated CBE initiatives. Findings from this survey parallel many of those found in relation to the only known multi-school analysis of graduate health professions competency-based curriculum development and integration initiatives.[9] The findings provide additional information regarding (1) the level of faculty engagement in CBE and resistance to change and (2) evidence of the types and levels of assistance required for adequate implementation–if the benefits of CBE are to be fully realized.

ASPH Global Health Competencies Model Development Project and Related Research

Advance survey

At the fall 2008 ASPH annual conference, members of the Global Health Committee discussed the increasing interest in and development of both international and global health degree and certificate programs in the United States. In February, 2009, the ASPH Global Health Committee continued these discussions, stimulated by the rapidly changing global health landscape and threats, as well as global health-related infrastructure changes underway at many leading universities. Committee members generally agreed on the increasing recognition of public health as the heart of global health. Barriers to the promotion of this perspective, however, included: (1) a lack of consensus on core global health competencies expected of master-level students, and (2) varying levels of global health instruction and practicums for students across the universities and programs providing international and global health educational experiences.[41]

Based on the February Global Health Committee retreat discussions, members decided to develop a set of core competencies for students specializing in global health at the graduate level across US programs. In preparation for the launch of model development, ASPH initiatied a survey in the summer of 2009 to determine the extent to which international and global health programs and competencies were established across 40 US schools of public health.[42] Twenty-five (63%) of the schools responded that they did have competency sets or models guiding internal or global health program planning and conduct. Of these responding schools, 20 (80%) provided copies of their specified global health program competencies. An analysis of these competencies revealed the findings outlined in **Table 2**. One school (#13) was eliminated from the final analysis as their submission addressed goals of the program, rather than actual behaviorally-stated expectations for specific student learning outcomes—competencies.

As noted in **Table 2**, there is great variability across the 20 schools that submitted a listing of their competencies. In some cases, the statements regarding their perceived competencies were more similar to instructional learning objectives versus

Table 2
Status of competency models adoption across accredited schools of public health

A School #	B Type of Program		C # Domains/Other Categories	D # Competencies/ Other Categories	E Taxonomic Domain & Level			F Selection/Development Process
	Master	Doctoral			Cognitive		Affective	
					High	Low		
1	✓	–	10	85	75	5	4	In development
2	✓	–	4 tracks of study	6	6	–	–	In development
3	✓	✓	7 tracks	62	62	–	–	Unknown
4	✓	✓	–	6	6	–	–	Unknown
5	✓	✓	6 tracks	42	39	3	–	Unknown
6	✓	–	–	6	6	–	–	Unknown
7	✓	–	–	13	10	3	–	Unknown
8	✓	–	–	8	7	1	–	Unknown
9	✓	–	–	7	1	7[b]	–	Unknown
10	✓	–	–	16	13	3	–	Unknown
11	✓	–	–	10	9	1	–	Unknown
12	✓	–	–	9	6	3	–	Unknown
13	✓	–	–	3 program goals[a]	–	–	–	Unknown
14	✓	–	6	57	28	29[b]	–	Unknown
15	✓	–	6	15	14	1	–	Unknown
16	✓	–	–	8 program objectives	–	8[b]	–	Unknown
17	✓	–	4 courses	34	26	7	1	Unknown
18	✓	–	7	27	15	12	–	Unknown
19	✓	–	9	28	22	6	–	Unknown
20	✓	–	–	19 program objectives	12	7	–	Unknown
Total	20	3	–	458	357	96	5	—

[a] Excluded from analyses.
[b] ≥50% of competencies focused on knowledge transfer.
Data from Association of Schools of Public Health, Washington, DC.

specific competency behaviors. Only 5 (25%) specified actual competency domains of learning. Four other schools (20%) submitted nondomain-specific competencies by tracks of study or by specific courses. The remaining majority of the schools (N = 11; 55%) submitted listings of competencies with no overarching domain specifications or ties to specific tracks or courses.

Two (10%) submitted lists that outlined program objectives, rather than competency domains or competencies. Two other universities noted that their competency models were in development, including one which provided detailed information regarding their use of focus groups with 16 early and midcareerists working locally in multimillion dollar international health organizations. The other university did not specify the current development process. Also, no information was provided by the remaining 18 submitting organizations regarding the source or process for the selection of their specified program competencies (or objectives). Author experience finds that most early competency models are usually developed by faculty committees, or extracted from existing course-specific syllabi listing instructional goals and objectives, versus evidence-based competency identification, specification, and quantitative validation methodologies.[43,44]

Of note were the analyses of the taxonomic domains and level of expected outcomes for the specified competencies and objectives. Column E of **Table 2** provides the categorization for submitted competencies/objectives as well as the targeted level for student performance. The long-established and widely accepted Bloom's Taxonomy of Educational Outcomes was used for this review.[45,46] The two domains most applicable to the majority of general global health educational programs are the cognitive (thinking) and affective (feeling) domains, both of which are widely recognized in the literature as having equivalent impact on student learning outcomes, long-term retention, and professional development.[46–50] The third Bloom domain was not included in the review as it pertains more to the psychomotor skills most often unique to a particular profession or health specialist position. This psychomotor domain is more applicable to the development of health clinicians' physical and clinical skills.[51]

Of the 458 competencies, including the 27 objectives that were reported, only 5 (1%) addressed specific affective domain behaviors despite the impact that students values, appreciations, motivations, and views are universally known to have on their educational experiences and outcomes, as well as their long-term professional development.[50] However, more encouraging in relation to well-established adult and lifelong learning principles was the level at which 357 of the remaining 453 competencies/objectives were targeted. The outcome behaviors specifically stated for these competencies were found to match with the higher application (level 3.0) or above behaviors in Bloom's cognitive domain, including levels 4.0 analysis, 5.0 synthesis, and 6.0 evaluation.

In relation to individual program domain profiles, the majority reported having a higher proportion of their competencies in the higher cognitive domain taxonomic levels. For 4 of the programs, however, the specified competencies/objectives were dominated by lower-level cognitive learning behaviors, at the knowledge transfer levels of 1.0 knowledge or 2.0 comprehension. At these levels, expected learning outcomes were typically represented by verbs such as "identify", "discuss", "describe", and "explain", which are more appropriate to secondary or undergraduate education. By the time students have progressed to advanced coursework or specialization in graduate school, it is recognized that longer-term retention and higher-impact learning occurs at the higher taxonomic levels. These programs and their faculty would therefore best benefit their students by progressing beyond the stated emphasis on knowledge transfer and related lower-level performance learning outcomes. This would require the use of both learning and evaluation methods focused on application, analysis, extrapolation, and evaluation of concepts, principles, and theories–in contrast to short-term memorization of bodies of knowledge as their specified competencies denote.

Model development

Following the previous field survey, an ASPH Global Health Core Competency Development Consensus Conference was subsequently held in September of 2009. Nearly 50 national and international academic, practitioner, institute, and other organizational leaders participated in person or via video conferencing technologies. The aims for this conference were to establish the goal and charges for the development of the model outline, process guidelines and tenets, and to identify and specify the specific core competency domains for the model.

The project goal, charges, and targeted learner audience for the model are noted next.

Goal: To protect and promote population health, safety, and wellbeing at local and global levels, eliminating health and social disparities worldwide.

Charges: To identify key skills for the next generation of global health professional by

1. Defining what students at schools of public health should know and be able to do to improve health and eliminate disparities in populations around the world
2. Outlining other essential student attributes and characteristics for contributing to this goal.

Learner audience:
Master-level students majoring in global health programs

Seven core competency domains were also identified and further specified for more defined workgroup-specific development, including
Capacity-strengthening
Collaboration and partnering
Ethical reasoning and professional practice
Health equity and social justice
Program management
Socio-cultural and political awareness
Strategic analysis.

Expert panel workgroups, including more than 150 academic and field practitioner representatives, recently completed a series of structured protocol Delphi surveys for the identification and specification of the competencies for each domain. The completion of the model is slated for late 2011.[52] Subsequent efforts by ASPH include plans for an exploration of the common features and best practices for institutions aiming to globalize their entire curricula.

Future Imperatives for Graduate Health Profession Education

Graduate education, like primary, secondary, and postsecondary education, is under siege for its failings, and will need to evolve in line with educational best practices or be changed externally by mandate.[33] Oversight bodies are increasingly turning to reviewers from the disciplines of education and educational psychology for direction in the development of their standards, related review processes, and assessment methods.[37] Accordingly, leaders and faculty in graduate education will need to support the growing demand for transformation in pedagogy and learning and evaluation methods.[53–60]

As addressed in the Bridge to Quality report, faculty-focused, passive, lecture-based *teaching* needs to be replaced or supplemented with the student-centered, active, and experiential *learning* methodologies proven most effective for high-impact learning outcomes and long-term retention and performance.[54,59] A large body of knowledge exists regarding these methods and their related outcomes in the field of education and its associated behavioral disciplines. As well, the evolving recommended best practices, processes, and systems for optimal learning are firmly rooted in the plethora of investigative endeavors conducted throughout the past 6 to 7 decades of twentieth century educational research. Increasingly, graduate students will present with long histories of educational experiences that have been grounded in applied and integrative learning (AIL) principles and practices, as outlined below for global health educational program consideration:

1. AIL learning methods should be
   Action based
   Creative
   Engaging
   Entertaining
   Experiential
   Innovative
   Integrated with other classes
   Intrinsically reward based
   Used in a range of settings and contexts.

2. AIL learning methods should include
   Cognitive *and* affective outcomes
   Coaching and mentoring
   Evidence-based problem solving
   Higher-level educational taxonomic objectives (application, analysis, evaluation)
   Individualized performance planning
   Internalization of criteria for excellence and quality
   Multidisciplinary exchange
   Multicultural interaction
   Reflective learning and self-assessment
   Team-based problem solving.

As previously noted, a review of a recent accrediting body's adoption and transition to competency specifications revealed the establishment of accrediting standards similar to others across the health professions.[37] These organizations will increasingly expect evidence-based pedagogy, teaching and learning methods, and assessment practices aligned with the institution's and the program's missions and vision, their students' entry characteristics, and the roles they will be entering upon graduation (see **Fig. 2**). Instructional methods will therefore need to be examined in relation to stated behavioral performance expectations (competencies) as well as state-of-the-art practices. Investments in faculty pedagogical development will also be continually emphasized. And, the tracking of graduates' long-term performance and achievements will also be a core expectation.

Students as consumers faced with continued marketplace insecurity will increasingly expect more accountability for their tuition dollars. In line with workforce research and predictions, they will seek out those programs and educational experience that

closely simulate real-world and careerlike situations.[38,39] As has long been documented in the industrial and organizational psychology literature, knowledge alone
is not a discriminator in relation to long-term work achievement.[49] Such is the *tip* of
the performance iceberg with the real differentiators for recognized performance
excellence lying *below the surface of the water*: the behaviors, motivations, values,
and other characteristics that graduates bring to the workplace. These less obvious
learning outcomes are the critical affective domain attributes that are often left unad-
dressed in graduate education.[50]

DISCUSSION

In line with the Roger's innovation diffusion framework as a benchmark, it is evident
that the CBE journey in graduate health professions education has just begun. The
work of ASPH to date, other evolving research in health professions CBE efforts,
and this review support prior findings that there is little guidance in the current public
health literature for directing competency-based curriculum review and preparation
for new global health programs and curricula.[60]

Significant attention to the development of standards for both educational
outcomes and practices will need to be accomplished before a collaborative agenda
for global health workforce development will evolve across the health professions and
the many related specialty roles influencing the health of the world. In addition, these
initiatives will need to be widely shared and disseminated for the benefit of all working
toward the development of a competent global health workforce. Current indicators of
global collaborative success on these issues include: 1) the translation of the *Lancet*-
published Commission on the Education of Health Professionals for the 21st Century
report into multiple languages; 2) development of a commission website (at http://
www.healthprofessionals21.org/) to "provide news on progress, global networking
opportunities, and other ways to connect for all who share this [the Commission's]
global vision of reform;" and 3) future commission report follow-up meetings in Asia
and the Near East.

The colleges and universities currently conducting education and training programs
for global health are uniquely positioned to take a leadership role in building the body
of work required for the realization of the previously mentioned initiatives. Potential
opportunities include the development and showcasing of the following:

1. Model national demonstration projects for
   - Providing frameworks and educational system approaches for integrating and
     using competencies and competency-based practice in global health educa-
     tional programs
   - Developing student-centered curricula focused on individual, community, and
     population health
   - Elevating graduate curricula to higher taxonomic levels: analysis, synthesis, and
     evaluation
   - Incorporating the affective domain and related learning and assessment
     methods into global health curricula
   - Funding global health educational research related to the influence of CBE prin-
     ciples that support:
     1. Near and long-term global health leadership performance
     2. Interprofessional and multidisciplinary global health projects.
2. Educational development centers for sharing best practices and ongoing pedagogical innovation, development, and transfer

3. Forums for global exchange of experiences and lessons learned in identifying and specifying both competencies and compatible educational and training practices.

Leaders are clearly needed to advance the primary mission bequeathed to all universities and colleges: educating the next generation. Similar rigor, commitment to, and recognition of this graduate education imperative are unarguably overdue. Faculty would never consider not applying state-of-the-art best practices in their research endeavors, yet such is not currently required in educational practices across institutions of higher education today.

SUMMARY

As repeatedly outlined in the literature, global health success is dependent on workforce capacities, which are in turn integrally linked to the quality of educational practices provided for learner development of core competencies. Currently, the use of competencies and CBE has been significantly delayed despite the near century of educational research and advancement supporting the value of this educational methodology.

The rigor and applicability of the principles of strategic planning fit well for guiding future progress in diffusing the CBE movement globally. First an analysis of *current educational* methodologies *(the current state)* needs to be reconciled with emerging trends and requirements for education in the decades ahead *(the potential state)*. Upon completion of this review and analysis, advocates can then initiate the development of specific strategies and the required actions for the realization of *global health (the preferred state)*.

Findings from the deployment and research of educational innovation and evolving transformations, such as CBE and competency specification in graduate health professions education, will serve to inform and guide collaborative workforce capacity-building initiatives for the desired future: the development of an adaptable and productive workforce for global health and wellbeing.

ACKNOWLEDGMENTS

This paper is an outgrowth of work undertaken by the Association of Schools of Public Health (ASPH) to develop competencies for various public health arenas, in particular the initiative to create a competency model for students in master's-level global health programs. Special recognition is extended to the following for their ongoing championship and support of competency-based development in health professions education and research: 1) our ASPH colleagues—Elizabeth Weist and Jessica Petrush; 2) our University of Minnesota School of Public Health colleagues John Finnegan and Adrienne Voorhees; and 3) our research colleagues—Katie Droz, Natalia Maska, Krupa Patel, Susan Weidenbach, and Elizabeth Wurth.

REFERENCES

1. Shilton T. Health promotion competencies: providing a road map for health promotion to assume a prominent role in global health. Glob Health Promot 2009;16(2):42–6.
2. Hagopian A, Spigner C, Gorstein JL, et al. Developing competencies for a graduate school curriculum in international health. Public Health Rep 2008;12(3): 408–14.

3. Allegrante JP, Barry MM, Airhihenbuwa CO, et al. Domains of core competency, standards, and quality assurance for building global capacity in health promotion: the Galway consensus conference statement. Health Educ Behav 2009; 36(3):476–82.
4. Ehnfors M, Grobe SJ. Nursing curriculum and continuing education: future directions. Int J Med Inform 2004;73:591–8.
5. Institute of Medicine. Health professions education: a bridge to quality. Washington, DC: National Academies Press; 2003.
6. Institute of Medicine. To err is human: building a safer health system. Washington, DC: National Academies Press; 1999.
7. Institute of Medicine. Crossing the quality chasm: a new health system for the 21st century. Washington, DC: National Academies Press; 2001.
8. Bridging the skills gap. Alexandria (VA): American Society for Training & Development; 2006.
9. Calhoun JG, Wainio JA, Sinioris ME, et al. Outcomes-based health management education: baseline findings from a National curriculum development demonstration project. J Health Adm Educ 2009;36:171–92 Summer.
10. Calhoun JG, Vincent ET, Calhoun GL, et al. Why competencies in graduate health management and policy education. J Health Admin Educ 2008;25(1):17–36.
11. Health professions education for the future: schools in service to the nation. San Francisco (CA): Pew Health Professions Commission; 1993.
12. Committee on the Health Professions Education Summit. Health professions education: a bridge to quality. Washington, DC: Institute of Medicine; 2005.
13. The Joint Commission. Health care at the crossroads: strategies for improving health care profession education. Oakbrook Terrace (IL): The Joint Commission; 2005.
14. Barry MM, Allegrante JP, Lamarre MC, et al. The Galway Consensus Conference: international collaboration on the development of core competencies for health promotion and health education. Glob Health Promot 2009;16(2):5–11.
15. Fried L, Bentley ME, Buekens P, et al. Global health is public health. The Lancet 2010;375:535–7.
16. Frenk J, Chen L, Bhutta ZA, et al. Health professionals for a new century: transforming education to strengthen health systems in an interdependent world. Published online, 2010. DOI:10.1016/S0140-6736(10)61854-5. Available at: http://www.healthprofessionals21.org/. Accessed May 26, 2011.
17. Islam M, Yoshuda S. MDG: how close are we to success? BJOG 2009;116:2–5.
18. Rogers E. Diffusion of innovations. New York: Free Press; 1983. ISBN 0029266505.
19. Accreditation Council for Graduate Medical Education. Common program requirements: General competencies, 2007. Available at: http://www.acgme.org/outcome/comp/GeneralCompetenciesStandards21307.pdf. Accessed July 20, 2010.
20. Bruno A, Bates I, Brock T, et al. Towards a global competency framework. Am J Pharm Educ 2010;74(3):1–2.
21. Calhoun JG, Davidson PL, Sinioris ME, et al. Toward an understanding of competency identification and assessment in health care. Qual Manag Health Care 2002;11(1):14–39.
22. Dreachslin JL, Agho A. Domains and core competencies for effective evidence-based practice in diversity. J Health Admin Educ 2001;Spec No:131–47.
23. Garman AN, Johnson MP. Leadership competencies: an introduction. J Healthc Manag 2006;51(1):13–7.
24. Fitzpatrick JJ. Cultural competence in nursing education revisited. Nurs Educ Perspect 2007;28(1):5.

25. Hyndman B. Towards the development of skill-based health promotion competencies: the Canadian experience. Glob Health Promot 2009;16(2):51–5.
26. Morales ASM, Battel-Kirk B, Barry MM, et al. Perspectives on health promotion competencies and accreditation in Europe. Glob Health Promot 2009;16(2): 21–31.
27. Scheele F, Teunissen P, Van Luijk S, et al. Introducing competency based postgraduate medical education in the Netherlands. Med Teach 2010;30:248–53.
28. Speller V, Smith BJ, Lysoby L. Development and utilization of professional standards in health education and promotion: US and UK experiences. Glob Health Promot 2009;16(2):32–41.
29. Hiland J. Global health competencies. Centers for Disease Control and Prevention. Atlanta, GA; 2009. Unpublished Presentation.
30. Public health workforce study. Washington, DC: U.S. Department of Health and Human Services/Health Resources and Services Administration; 2005.
31. U.S. Department of Education (DOE). Secretary Spellings announces plans for more affordable, accessible, accountable and consumer-friendly U.S. higher education system. U.S. Department of education press release. 2006. Available at: http://www.ed.gov/news/pressreleases/2006/09/09262006.html. Accessed February 16 2008.
32. U.S. Department of Education (DOE). A test of leadership: charting the future of higher education. Washington, DC.U.S. Department of Education Press Release. 2006. Available at: http://www.ed.gov/news/pressreleases/2006/11/11292006. html. Accessed February 16, 2008.
33. U.S. Department of Education (DOE). Secretary spellings convenes accreditation forum in Washington, D.C. with key stakeholders. U.S. Department of education press release. 2006. Available at: http://www.ed.gov/news/pressreleases/2006/ 11/11292006.html. Accessed February 16, 2008.
34. Occupational programs and the use of skill competencies at the secondary and postsecondary levels. Washington, DC: U.S. Department of Education. National Center for Education Statistics; 1999.
35. Council on Education for Public Health (2005). Accreditation criteria for schools of public health. Available at: http://www.ceph.org. Accessed January 19, 2006.
36. Taub AT, Allegrante JP, Barry MM, et al. Perspectives on terminology and conceptual and professional issues in health education and health promotion credentialing. Health Educ Behav 2009;36:439–50.
37. Commission on Accreditation of Healthcare Management Education, "Criteria for Accreditation" 2011. Available at: http://cahme.org/Criteria.html. Accessed July 20, 2010.
38. Judy RW, D'Amico CD. Workforce 2020: work and workers in the 21st century. Indianapolis (IN): Hudson Institute; 1998. (Eric Document Reproduction Service No.ED409463).
39. Karoly LA, Panis CW. The 21st century at work: Forces shaping the future workforce and workplace in the United States. Santa Monica (CA): Rand Corporation; 2004.
40. Voorhees A, Finnegan JR, Calhoun JG. Schools of public health survey on implementation of competency-based education. Education Committee meeting presented at the annual meeting of the Association of Schools of Public Health. Philadelphia, November 7, 2009.
41. Association of Schools of Public Health (2009, April 24). ASPH Friday Letter #1566. Available at: http://fridayletter.asph.org/printing_press.cfm?fl_index=1566/. Accessed February 15, 2011.

42. Petrush J. Survey of competencies for global health programs. Washington, DC: Association of Schools of Public Health; 2008.
43. Linstone HA, Turoff M. The Delphi method: techniques and applications. Reading (MA): Addison-Wesley; 1975.
44. McClelland DC. Testing for competence rather than for intelligence. Am Psychol 1973;28:1–14.
45. Bloom BS, Engelhart MD, Furst EJ, et al. Taxonomy of educational objectives: handbook I: cognitive domain. New York: David McKay; 1956.
46. Krathwohl DR, Bloom BS, Masia BB, et al. The taxonomy of education objectives: the classification of educational goals, handbook ii: affective domain. New York: Longman; 1964.
47. Liff SB. Social and emotional intelligence: applications for developmental education. J Dev Educ 2003;26(3):28–34.
48. McClelland DC, Atkinson JW, Clark RA, et al. The achievement motive. New York (NY): Appleton; 1953.
49. McClelland DC. The achieving society. Princeton (NJ): D. Van Nostrand Co, Inc; 1961.
50. McClelland DC. Human motivation. 2nd edition. New York: Cambridge University Press; 1988.
51. Simpson E. The classification of educational objectives in the psychomotor domain: the psychomotor domain, vol. 3. Washington, DC: Gryphon House; 1972.
52. Buekens P. Global health competencies for master's students, Presentation, Annual Meeting of the American Public Health Association. Denver (CO), Fall 2010. November 6, 2010.
53. Koo D, Miner K. Outcome-based workforce development and education in public health. Annu Rev Public Health 2010;31:253–69.
54. Institute on High-Impact Practices and Student Success. Association of American Colleges and Universities. 2010. Available at: http://www.aacu.org/meetings/hips/index.cfm. Accessed September 6, 2010.
55. Abdelkhalek N, Hussein A, Gibbs T, et al. Using team-based learning to prepare medical students for future problem-based learning. Med Teach 2010;32:123–9.
56. Collins J. Education techniques for lifelong learning: Lifelong learning in the 21st century and beyond. Radiographics 2009;29:613–22.
57. Shortell SM, Weist EM, Mah-Sere KS, et al. Implementing the Institute of Medicine's recommended curriculum content in schools of public health: a baseline assessment. Am J Public Health 2004;94(10):1671–4.
58. Srinivasan M, Keenan C, Yager J. Visualizing the future: technology competency development in clinical medicine, and implications for medical education. Acad Psychiatry 2006;30:480–90.
59. Dale E. Audio-visual methods in teaching. 3rd edition. New York (NY): The Dryden Press; 1969.
60. Battel-Kirk B, Barry MM, Taub A, et al. A review of the international literature on health promotion competencies: identifying frameworks and core competencies. Glob Health Promot 2009;16(2):12–20.

Globalization and Infectious Diseases

Julio Frenk, MD, PhD[a], Octavio Gómez-Dantés, MD, MPH[b],*,
Felicia M. Knaul, PhD[c]

KEYWORDS

- Globalization • Infectious diseases • Security
- Global health challenges

In a report on global security developed by a high-level panel appointed by the Secretary General of the United Nations (UN), infectious diseases were included in a compact list of threats that the world must be concerned with now and in the decades to come.[1] According to the report, such threats recognize no national boundaries and need to be addressed at the global, regional, and national levels because no state, no matter how powerful, can, on its own, make itself invulnerable to them.

The purpose of this article is twofold: (1) to discuss the nature of the health challenges created by globalization and (2) to propose new forms of international cooperation to confront them. The discussion of global health challenges includes both the transfer of health risks, with an emphasis on infectious diseases, and the international dissemination of health opportunities, including the transfer of knowledge and technology. Consistent with the UN report on global security, we argue that the health-related challenges and opportunities of an increasingly interdependent world demand new forms of international cooperation. The authors suggest the promotion of 3 elements that, in their essence, contain the idea of collaboration: exchange, evidence, and empathy.

GLOBALIZATION AND HEALTH

Globalization is evolving at such speed and with such complexity that it challenges our ability to grasp its full extent. This dynamism is a good reason to constantly renew the discussion around the forces of globalization and their impact on everyday life.

Several processes illustrate the increasing degree of proximity in our world. The number of international travelers has reached 3 million people every day, telephone

Parts of this article are adapted from Frenk J, Gómez-Dantés O. Globalization and the challenges to health systems. Health Affairs 2002;21(3):160–5.
[a] Harvard School of Public Health, 677 Huntington Avenue, Boston, MA 02115, USA
[b] Center for Health Systems Research, National Institute of Public Health, Avenida Universidad 655, Santa María Ahuacatitlán, 62100 Cuernavaca, Morelos, México
[c] Department of Global Health and Social Medicine, Harvard School of Public Health, 677 Huntington Avenue, Boston, MA 02115, USA
* Corresponding author.
E-mail address: ocogomez@yahoo.com

Infect Dis Clin N Am 25 (2011) 593–599
doi:10.1016/j.idc.2011.05.003
id.theclinics.com

traffic amounts to 406 billion minutes a year, and there are more than 2 billion Internet users worldwide.[2] The antiglobalization movement itself went global in 2001 when activists gathered in Porto Alegre, Brazil in the first meeting of the World Social Forum.

These changes have profound implications for health. In all countries, the domestic health agenda has now been complicated by the international transfer of risks and opportunities.[3]

The transmission of communicable diseases is the best example of the increasing porosity of borders. To fully understand this phenomenon, we must first deal with 2 misconceptions that very often cloud the discussion on the role of infectious diseases in the global agenda.

The first misconception is that infections represent a sort of lower stage in the progression of disease patterns that has been characterized as the epidemiologic transition. Its original formulation by Omran[4] in the early 1970s viewed the epidemiologic transition as a linear movement from communicable to noncommunicable diseases.[4] Therefore, it was just a matter of time until societies got rid of the scourge of infection.

We know better now. We understand that the health transition is not a simple, linear, and unidirectional state, but rather a complex, contradictory, and dynamic process where several stages may overlap and where populations often experience veritable counter transitions with the reemergence of previously controlled infections.[5] This negative outcome reflects complex interactions among disease agents, hosts, and environments that often lead to the appearance of drug resistance. In addition, the world has witnessed the emergence of new communicable diseases, the most prominent of which is, of course, AIDS.

Furthermore, the separation between communicable and noncommunicable diseases is not as clear-cut as it was once thought. To begin with, diseases originally classified as noncommunicable have been found to have an infectious cause. According to the World Health Organization (WHO), one-fifth of all cancers worldwide are caused by chronic infections produced by agents, such as human immunodeficiency virus (HIV), human papillomavirus, and hepatitis B virus. On top of that, many of these diseases, or their treatments, weaken the immune system, giving rise to associated infections that are often the precipitating cause of death.

In sum, infectious diseases are not the exclusive domain of a primitive stage in the health transition, but rather a shifting component of every epidemiologic pattern. This conclusion also serves to counter the second misconception that infectious diseases are mostly a problem of underdeveloped countries. As we have seen, even in societies where noncommunicable diseases dominate the epidemiologic pictures, infection is a common companion of such diseases. Furthermore, the extent of integration in our world means that no country can be isolated from risks that emerge elsewhere.[6]

In fact, this is not a new phenomenon. The first documented case of a transnational epidemic was the Athenian plague of 430 BC.[7] Having probably originated in Ethiopia, it spread to Libya and Egypt and finally reached the heart of ancient Greece in grain boats.[8] According to Thucydides, this calamity was responsible for the defeat of Athens in the war against Sparta and the Peloponnesian League, which marked the decline of its golden age.[9]

The Black Death of 1347, which killed at least one-third of the European population, originated in Central Asia and spread through military conflicts and international trade. It was during this epidemic that Venetians invented quarantine, isolating arriving ships for 40 days.[10]

The conquest of the Aztec and Inca empires in the sixteenth century was an early example of involuntary microbiological warfare through the introduction of smallpox and measles into previously unexposed populations. The colonization of the Caribbean and Brazil almost led to the extermination of the indigenous populations, a situation that forced the importation of slaves from West Africa. This trade, in turn, brought malaria and yellow fever to the New World, creating additional disasters.[11] In this microbial exchange, Columbus probably took one dire disease from the Americas to Europe: great pox (syphilis).[12]

Another example in the uninterrupted history of the transnational transfer of infection is the 1829 cholera pandemic, which started in Asia, broke into Egypt and North Africa, entered Russia, and crossed Europe. Three years later it reached the eastern coast of the United States.[13]

In the twentieth century, the influenza pandemic of 1918, erroneously known as Spanish flu, accounted for an estimated 50 million deaths worldwide, 5 times more casualties than those produced in combat during World War I.[14]

As we can see, infectious diseases have an old record of cosmopolitan presence. What is new, however, is the scale of what has been called microbial traffic. The number of potentially infectious contacts has exploded as trade and travel bring persons and products closer than ever before. Today the longest intercontinental flight is briefer than the incubation period of any known human infectious disease, posing unprecedented challenges to disease surveillance and making classical quarantine measures obsolete. Even the existing therapeutic arsenal has lost a substantial part of its effectiveness in this context of growing health interdependence.[15]

Tuberculosis (TB) provides a dramatic example. In 2003, close to 9 million persons worldwide became infected with TB and more than 2 million died of it. Several reasons explain this unexpected comeback; one is the fragility of the immune suppressed. As we know, TB is often the first sign that a person harbors HIV. Other reasons include overcrowding, poor nutrition, and inadequate health care, which are common among the socially marginalized. Migrants are a particularly vulnerable population. Not surprisingly, morbidity and mortality rates for HIV and TB are several times higher among migrants and in the northern border states of Mexico than in this country as a whole. Likewise, more than 50% of TB cases in the United States are reported in the 4 states bordering Mexico.

The latest additions to the list of global epidemics are severe acute respiratory syndromes (SARS) and avian and swine flu. The 2003 SARS epidemic was the first serious warning of the potential health, social, economic, and security consequences of major disease outbreaks, and it confirmed the need for coordinated international action, timely reporting, and full transparency in handling epidemiologic information.[16] H1N5 avian influenza has remained a regional threat, but H1N1 swine influenza produced a second warning in 2009, when the outbreaks in Mexico and the United States eventually spread to the whole world in a matter of weeks. The fast and transparent response of the Mexican health authorities, and the immediate implementation of the national and global preparedness plans developed in the previous years were crucial in the contention of the health and economic consequences of this pandemic.

EXPORTING LIFE STYLES AND HEALTH PRODUCTS

The rise in the global spread of infectious disease is related to radical changes in our environment and lifestyles, which have led Arno Karlen to speak, in his book *Man and Microbes*, of a new bio-cultural era.[9] Such changes are also accounting for the global spread of noncommunicable diseases. Smoking and obesity are the exemplars of emerging health risks linked to globalization that are now placing a double burden on the health systems of developing countries, further compounding health inequities.

Indeed, *problems only of the poor*, like malaria, are no longer the *only problems of the poor*. Tobacco-related deaths are increasingly concentrated in developing countries that lack the legal and regulatory muscle to counter the power of multinational corporations.

Beyond diseases and risk factors, globalization is also affecting health products and services. This issue is particularly relevant for the Mexico-United States border. A recent study estimated that there are more than 17 million health-related crossings at this border every year.[17] Seventy-five percent of these crossings are from the United States into Mexico, most often to purchase pharmaceuticals without prescription, including antibiotics.

Thus, improper prescription practices are no longer a strictly national problem, but have acquired an added global dimension. Such practices are at least partly responsible for the emergence of new forms of microbial adaptation and mutation, which have, in turn, produced resistance to many antibiotics. This resistance has become one of the major hurdles in the fight against TB and malaria. Two thousand years after the first recorded treatment against malaria, we are still facing the challenge of devising an effective cure. Ironically, that ancient treatment came from the Chinese *quing hao* plant, the source of artemisinin, which today offers new hope in the fight against drug-resistant malaria.[18]

The mutagenicity of known infectious agents is of particular concern given their easy global transmission. It, therefore, places an added burden on surveillance systems and represents a major challenge to the scientific quest for new drugs.

Another recent development with potential implications for irrational prescription practices and the ensuing spread of antibiotic resistance is the growing commerce of services and drugs through the Internet. That this is no longer a marginal phenomenon is reflected in recent efforts by the WHO to curb it.[19]

All of these are contextual factors that constrain the final impact of efforts to develop new drugs and vaccines because, in the end, all technological innovations will have to be delivered through real-life health care systems. As we have seen in the acrimonious debates surrounding access to antiretrovirals, the development of life-saving drugs without generating the mechanisms to reach those in need can create very difficult ethical and political dilemmas.

Fortunately, this is an area where interdependence has opened up novel avenues for international collective action,[20] as expressed in compromises, such as the Doha declaration on public health and trade; new financial instruments, such as the Global Fund to Fight AIDS, Tuberculosis and Malaria; and successful negotiations to reduce the price of AIDS drugs.

KNOWLEDGE AND HEALTH IMPROVEMENT

The growing complexity of health systems has made international comparisons more valuable than ever. Given the enormous economic and social impact of policy decisions, countries can benefit from a process of shared learning. This was the significance of the effort by the WHO to assess the performance of all 191 health systems of the world.[21] Comparative analysis is likely to promote the international dissemination of good practice. Perfectible as it is, this exercise has nourished an intense and fruitful debate that, among other things, has improved the methodologies developed for the original assessment.

This type of knowledge-related global public goods[22] will be key for the design and implementation of solutions to global threats. In fact, we now know that most of the health gains achieved during the twentieth century can be attributed to the advancement of knowledge[23] through 3 main mechanisms. First, knowledge gets translated into new and better technologies, such as vaccines and drugs. This method is the best-understood mechanism through which it improves health. But knowledge is also internalized by individuals who use it to structure their everyday behavior in key domains, such as personal hygiene, feeding habits, sexuality, and child-rearing practices. Finally, knowledge becomes translated into evidence that provides a scientific foundation both for health care and for the formulation of public policies.[24]

Recent developments in our country illustrate this last point. Thanks to the cooperation among several academic and international organizations, the analytical armamentarium for health policy has been greatly enriched during the past few years to include such robust tools as the measurement of burden of disease, cost-effectiveness analysis, national health accounts, and standardized surveys. The rigorous application of these knowledge-related global public goods, coupled with excellent country-specific data, generated the evidence base to catalyze a major legislative reform in 2003 that will allow Mexico to offer publicly funded health insurance to the entire population.[25]

This development is a clear example of how globalization can turn knowledge into an international public good that can then be brought to the domestic policy agenda to address a local problem. Such application, in turn, feeds back into the global pool of experience, thus, generating a process of shared learning among countries. Everyone stands to benefit if we have the wisdom to move beyond the false dilemmas between research and action and between the global and the national levels.

More generally, false dilemmas have clouded the debate on the risks and opportunities of globalization. Progress requires that we avoid either of 2 extremes: on the one hand, a sort of unipolar globalization based on exclusionary trade, military might, or cultural uniformity, which would undermine global security by fostering marginalization and resentment; on the other hand, a sort of multipolar isolationism based on protectionist trade barriers, internal oppression of dissent or xenophobic nationalism, which would also undermine global security by fostering poverty and human rights violations.

NEW GLOBAL HEALTH

The only way of avoiding either of these extremes is to develop a new model of globalization. In fact, the current debates on globalization are reminiscent of those that surrounded structural adjustment policies in the late 1980s. Then, like now, positions were highly polarized. A virtuous middle course was at that time proposed by Cornia, Jolly, and Stewart from the United Nations Children's Fund as "adjustment with a human face."[26] What we now need is globalization with a human face.

Indeed, globalization is (and has been for a long time) an inescapable reality. But we can devise and implement a process of global integration that both minimizes ill effects and protects those who are vulnerable to them and, at the same time, maximizes benefits and produces a fair distribution of these benefits. "Global construction," writes the Nobel laureate Amartya Sen, "is the needed response to global doubts."[27]

Health may contribute to this pursuit because it has always been a key component of development. Thanks to economic research, we know that health is a contributing factor, at both the individual and population levels, for enhancing learning, increasing productivity, reducing inequity, promoting economic well-being and growth, preventing impoverishment, and reducing poverty, all of which strengthen national and global security.[28,29]

Equitable access to high-quality services has also become central to the global movement for human rights. In this way, health can contribute to humanizing globalization because it involves those domains that unite all persons. Health-related processes, such as birth, disease, suffering, recovery, and death, define the basis for our common humanity.

THE 3 E'S OF GLOBAL HEALTH

In the search for new ways of acting in global health the authors suggest the promotion of 3 key elements, the 3 e's, that, in their essence, contain the idea of collaboration: exchange, evidence, and empathy.

Health systems around the world are facing unprecedented challenges; many of them, as the authors have just discussed, are related to globalization. The communications revolution provides the opportunity to *exchange* experiences about the ways to deal with such challenges.

To be informative, such exchange should be based on sound *evidence* about alternatives, so that we may build a solid knowledge of what really works and what does not. This point is why global public goods, such as methodological tools, comparative analysis, and systematic evidence, are so important.

But there is another value, *empathy*, which is that human characteristic that allows us to emotionally participate in a foreign reality, understand it, relate to it, and, in the end, value the core elements that make us all members of the human race.

As we engage in this process of renewal, we would do well to remember the words of Dr Martin Luther King Jr, who, 4 decades ago, wrote the following:

"It really boils down to this: that all life is interrelated. We are all caught in an inescapable network of mutuality, tied into a single garment of destiny. Whatever affects one directly, affects all indirectly."[30]

In this rendition of interdependence lies the key to understanding and acting upon the complex realities that must be transformed if we are to realize the destiny of a more secure and prosperous world through better health for all.

REFERENCES

1. United Nations high level panel on treats, challenges and change. A more secure world: our shared responsibility. New York: United Nations; 2004.
2. Global Information Inc. International telephone traffic grew from 376 billion minutes in 2008 to an estimated 406 billion minutes in 2009. Available at: http://www.the-infoshop.com/press/tg34287.shtml. Accessed October 29, 2010.
3. Frenk J, Sepúlveda J, Gómez-Dantés O, et al. The new world order and international health. BMJ 1997;314:1404–7.
4. Omran AR. The epidemiologic transition: a theory of the epidemiology of population change. Milbank Mem Fund Q 1971;49:509–38.
5. Frenk J, Bobadilla JL, Sepúlveda J, et al. Health transition in middle-income countries: new challenges for health care. Health Pol Plann 1989;4:29–39.
6. Bloom B. Public health in transition. Sci Am 2005;(22):70–7.
7. Chen LC, Evans TG, Cash RA. Health as a global pubic good. In: Kaul Y, Grumberg Y, Stern MA, editors. Global public goods: international cooperation in the 21st century. New York: Oxford University Press for the United Nations Development Programme; 1999. p. 284–304.

8. Porter R. Illustrated history of modern medicine. Cambridge (UK): Cambridge University press; 1996. p. 25.
9. Karlen A. Man and microbes. Disease and plagues in history and modern times. New York: Simon & Schuster; 1995. p. 87–8.
10. The Encyclopaedia Britannica. Quarantine. London and New York: The Encyclopaedia Britannica Company 1926: vol. 21. p. 709–11.
11. Porter D. Health, civilization and the state. A history of public health from ancient to modern times. London and New York: Routledge, 1999. p. 47.
12. Porter R. Blood and guts. A short history of medicine. New York and London: WW Norton & Company, 2004. p. 13.
13. Porter R. The greatest benefit to mankind. A medical history of humanity. New York and London: WW Norton & Company, 1997. p. 402–3.
14. Kolata G. Flu: the story of the great influenza pandemic of 1918 and the search for the virus that caused it. New York: Farrar, Straus and Giroux; 1999. p. 9.
15. Chen L, Bell D, Bates L. World health and institutional change. In: Pocantico retreat: enhancing the performance of international health institutions. Cambridge (MA): Rockefeller Foundation, Social Science Research Council, Harvard School of Public Health; 1996. p. 9–21.
16. Kleinman A, Watson J, editors. SARS in China. Prelude to pandemic? Stanford (CA): Stanford University Press; 2006.
17. Sekri N, Gómez-Dantés O, MacDonald T. Cross-border health insurance: an overview. Oakland (CA): California HealthCare Foundation; 1999.
18. Specter M. What money can buy. New Yorker 2005;(24):57–71.
19. World Health Organization. Medical products and the Internet. Geneva (Switzerland): WHO; 1999.
20. Jamison D, Frenk J, Knaul F. International collective action in health: objectives, functions, and rationale. Lancet 1998;351:514–7.
21. World Health Organization. World health report. Health systems: improving performance. Geneva (Switzerland): WHO; 2000.
22. Kaul I, Grumberg Y, Stein MA, editors. Global public goods: international cooperation in the 21st century. New York: Oxford University Press for the United Nations Development Programme; 1999.
23. World Health Organization. World health report 1999. Making a difference. Geneva (Switzerland): WHO; 1999.
24. Frenk J. Bridging the divide: global lessons from evidence-based health policy in Mexico. Lancet 2006;368:954–61.
25. Knaul FM, Frenk J. Health insurance in Mexico: achieving universal coverage through structural reform. Health Aff (Millwood) 2005;24(6):1467–76.
26. Cornia GA, Jolly R, Stewart F. Adjustment with a human face. New York: Oxford University Press; 1987.
27. Sen A. Ten thesis on globalization. New Perspect Q 2002;18(4). Available at: http://www.youtube.com/watch?v=_il1m8NJbDY. Accessed June 20, 2011.
28. Commission on Macroeconomics and Health. Report of the Commission on Macroeconomics and Health. Geneva (Switzerland): WHO; 2001.
29. Comisión Mexicana sobre Macroeconomía y Salud. Invertir en salud para el desarrollo económico. Sinopsis del Informe de la Comisión Mexicana sobre Macroeconomía y Salud. México City (Mexico): Secretaría de Salud, Universidad de las Americas; 2004.
30. King ML Jr. The trumpet of conscience. New York: Harper; 1968.

Global Health Diplomacy and Peace

Ilona Kickbusch, PhD[a],*, Paulo Buss, MD, MPH[b]

KEYWORDS

• Global health • Diplomacy • Peace • Foreign policy

"The health of all peoples is fundamental to the attainment of peace and security"
—World Health Organization Constitution, Preamble.

Complex issues such as health, climate change, international financial stability, intellectual property rights, social and health inequalities between regions and countries, and human security are part of the overcrowded realm of today's global challenges, highlighting the need for better coordination among multiple actors at different levels for better global well-being. In this rapidly changing context, the term global health diplomacy has emerged to capture both the system and the method of the multilevel and multiactor negotiation processes that shape and manage the global policy environment for health.[1] But the World Report on Violence and Health[2] draws attention to another aspect of global health diplomacy that requires consideration: the 20th century was *"one of the most violent periods in human history: an estimated 191 million people lost their lives directly or indirectly as a result of conflict, and well over half of them were civilians."* If conducted successfully, global health diplomacy can move both health and peace agendas forward and respond to common structural challenges that they face. This article shows the complexity of this system and the opportunities for sustainable solutions that multistakeholder negotiations across national borders and disciplines can provide.

EVOLUTION OF GLOBAL HEALTH DIPLOMACY

The foundations of the complex multi-actor and multi-level system of international (multilateral) health efforts were set about 160 years ago with the First International Sanitary Conference in 1851 in Paris and the First International Sanitary Convention in 1892 (Hein W, Kickbusch I. Global health governance and the intersection of health and foreign policy. In: Schrecker T, editor. Research companion to the globalization of health. UK/USA: Ashgate; 2011. Submitted for publication.).[3–5] The beginning of the

[a] Global Health Programme, Graduate Institute of International and Development Studies, PO Box 136, 1211 Geneva 21, Switzerland
[b] FIOCRUZ Center for Global Health, FIOCRUZ National School of Public Health, Oswaldo Cruz Foundation (FIOCRUZ), Avenida Brasil, 4365 - Manguinhos, Rio de Janeiro 21040-900, Brazil
* Corresponding author.
E-mail address: kickbusch@bluewin.ch

Infect Dis Clin N Am 25 (2011) 601–610
doi:10.1016/j.idc.2011.05.006
0891-5520/11/$ – see front matter © 2011 Elsevier Inc. All rights reserved.

id.theclinics.com

twentieth century saw the creation of the first permanent international organizations: the Office International d'Hygiène Publique (OIHP) in Paris and the League of Nations Health Organization (LNHO) in Geneva, whereas the International Sanitary Bureau for the Americas (later the Pan American Sanitary Bureau) had existed since 1902. Even then, nonstate actors such as the Rockefeller Foundation and the International Committee of the Red Cross made significant contributions to transborder health.

In the wake of the destruction following 2 world wars, health was seen as fundamental to the achievement of peace and security, as the preamble of the WHO constitution expresses.[6] With great hope it was suggested that, for the first time, a single international organization with the broad mandate to coordinate international health efforts be created. Unanimous approval met the joint declaration by Brazil and China at the San Francisco Conference 1945 that called for its establishment.[4] This formative stage was filled with "trial and error with much improvisation because of the necessity of dealing with new problems promptly."[7]

The success of the WHO in fulfilling its directing and coordinating role in the first 30 years was reflected in many ways (Hein W, Kickbusch I. Global health governance and the intersection of health and foreign policy. In: Schrecker T, editor. Research companion to the globalization of health. UK/USA: Ashgate; 2011. Submitted for publication.): the eradication of small pox, a growing budget[7,8] or its function as an important diplomatic meeting place during the Cold War. The newly independent countries-several of them having emerged from violent conflicts that killed and continue killing millions of people, not only soldiers, but many civilians, especially women and children-were challenged to build and manage national health systems. This was made more difficult as the new infectious disease HIV/AIDS crossed the globe and contributed to a profound change of the global health landscape-a change described as a "political revolution"[9] or a Copernican shift.[10] The interface between health and peace still remains paramount 60 years after the creation of the WHO; in view of increasing global inequalities it has even gained renewed prominence. The health of all peoples is still fundamental to the attainment of peace and security, as the preamble of the WHO constitution emphasizes, but the context within which negotiations toward the two universal goals take place has changed.

CHANGING GEOPOLITICAL CONTEXT AND GROWING COOPERATION ON THE REGIONAL LEVEL

At a time when viruses can travel around the world in hours, without respect for any borders, and when disease threatens peace, economic growth, and development, countries have increasingly discovered the potential that global health diplomacy offers within the rapidly changing constellations of a geopolitical marketplace.[11] "[A] shift in power over global wealth has marked the beginning of a major change in governance from a G8 to G20 dominated world. The G20 currently represents approximately ninety percent of the world's wealth, eighty percent of the world's trade and two-thirds of the world population."[12] "A new geography of power is emerging and challenges prior alliances and divides among states and groupings." (Kickbusch I. 21st century health diplomacy: a new relationship between foreign policy and health. In: Kickbusch I, Novotny T, editors. 21st century global health diplomacy. UK: World Scientific. Imperial College Press. Submitted for publication.) In global health, there is a growing presence of countries such as Brazil, China, India, Kenya, Mexico, Thailand and South Africa.[13]

During the 128th session of the Executive Board (EB) of the WHO in Geneva, Switzerland, January 2011, the voice of a growing number of middle-income and low-income countries was clearly heard during the deliberations and drafting of texts. On some of the agenda items, such as health system strengthening, as much as 4 to 5 draft resolutions supported by various groups were proposed, – which shows the shifting alliances built in global health diplomacy. The rapid economic growth of such countries is changing their political position at the international level and has turned them into active members of the international community, including functions as aid providers and international investors.[14–16] With rising financial and discursive power, emerging economies also adopt new approaches to include health more systematically within their foreign policy, (Kickbusch I. 21st century health diplomacy: a new relationship between foreign policy and health. In: Kickbusch I, Novotny T, editors. 21st century global health diplomacy. UK: World Scientific. Imperial College Press. Submitted for publication.) while at the same time trying to promote unity and solidarity as a necessary condition to develop their negotiating capacity in international multilateral fora.[14,15]

A new understanding of the approach termed south-south cooperation (in health) is emerging and growing rapidly, and the donor nations organized in the G7/G8 continue to be pushed by both the United Nations (UN) system and the nongovernment organization (NGO) community, particularly as part of the Millennium Development Goals, to provide more support to health programs in low-income and middle-income countries through increased funding of north-south cooperation. In December 2009, the UN High Level Conference on South-South Cooperation, which took place in Nairobi, Kenya, highlighted this key trend on the international level. The importance of mutual assistance was emphasized also by a study published by the UN Development Programme (UNDP) in 2004 by the Special Unit for South-South Cooperation. Driven by the leadership of Brazil, China, Cuba, and India, south-south cooperation schemes have been examples of the principles referred to in the studies mentioned earlier.[14] For example, Brazil has been active in providing aid for development to other countries in public administration, health, education, agriculture, the environment, energy, and small companies. In 2010 Brazil hosted the I World Conference on the Development of Universal Social Security Systems and in 2011, Brazil hosts the Global Conference on Social Determinants of Health (whose organization has been decided by a WHO resolution approved by the World Health Assembly) working toward a comprehensive international political pact and a global strategy dedicated to fighting social inequalities in health.[14,15]

Leading for Brazil in health, the Oswaldo Cruz Foundation (a public institution belonging to the Ministry of Health) has been a prominent actor on the international stage since the 1980s, supporting the creation and development of the so-called "structuring institutions of the health systems", namely National Institutes of Health, Schools of Public Health and Health Governance and Schools of Health Technicians.

Other countries and regional organizations[17] also recognize the opportunities that global health diplomacy offers. For example, China and India have important technical training programs for nationals of developing countries, which in turn improves the institutional capacity of these countries.[14] Cuba has been supporting the establishment and the development of Schools of Health Sciences in many developing countries and sent medical personnel to about 70 countries,[18] in a process called by Cuban authors "internationalist solidarity" which is considered "a principle of the Cuban public health"[19] UNASUL health has defined its sub-regional specific South-American Health Agenda and its 2010–2015 Quadrennial Plan of Health. Even a Community of countries of four Continents, joined by the common idiom—the Community of Lusophonic Countries—has defined its Strategic Plan of Cooperation for Health. A 2008 to 2017 Health Agenda for the Americas,[20] launched among others by UN Secretary General Ban Ki-Moon and PAHO Director Dr Mirta Roses along with Organization of American States (OAS) Secretary General José Miguel Insulza, states in paragraph 1 of the Statement of Content:

> *The Governments of the Region of the Americas jointly establish this Health Agenda to guide collective action of national and international stakeholders who seek to improve the health of the peoples of this Region...*

The consequences are far-reaching: they create a habit of communication and a thickening of relations, highlighting the mutual benefits of peaceful negotiations, and can constitute a basis for building up alliances beyond health (Kickbusch I. 21st century health diplomacy: a new relationship between foreign policy and health. In: Kickbusch I, Novotny T, editors. 21st century global health diplomacy. UK: World Scientific. Imperial College Press. Submitted for publication.). The spill-over effects can offer opportunities to address the structural challenges of an increasingly interconnected world at a time when the power shift among nations is accompanied by a parallel power shift beyond the nation to other actors such as transnational companies and civil society.

AN INCREASINGLY DIVERSE GROUP OF (HEALTH) DIPLOMATS

One-hundred and eighty-two NGOs in official relations with the WHO in 2011,[21] more than 200 public private partnerships,[22] and innovative alliances such as the Global Fund or Global Alliance for Vaccines and Immunisation (GAVI) highlight a tremendous change in the system of global health diplomacy. Foreign policy and diplomacy no longer reside solely with the traditional diplomats but include today a wide range of other state and nonstate actors.[13,23-25] "Diplomacy" says Parag Khanna[26] "now takes place among anyone who is someone; its prerequisite is not sovereignty but authority." Health is again at the forefront of these changes.

At the health and peace interface, a clear example is provided by the Health as a Bridge for Peace initiative of the WHO. Building on the practice developed by the ministries of health in Central America with the support of the PAHO, it is defined as "the integration of peace-building concerns, concepts, principles, strategies, and practices into health relief and health sector development."[27] Although its achievements are multifaceted (and sometimes controversial) and range from a contribution to the integration of former enemies into the same national health system (Croatia, Bosnia Herzegovina, and Angola) or training initiatives (Sri Lanka, Indonesia) and at least 60 documented instances in 16 different countries of vaccination campaigns through Days of Tranquillity,[28] its illustration for the growing number and diversity of actors is straightforward. Together with the WHO and its regional offices, local and international NGOs, academia, local communities, regional entities, ministries of health and other government branches, national development agencies, as well as different international organizations, including the World Bank, have participated.

Non-state actors do not only exist alongside but also sometimes challenge the role of traditional actors such as the nation states and the WHO,[13,24,25] The ability of non-state actors to raise huge financial resources, their flexibility to act swiftly, and the active role in raising public attention have made them indispensable partners for global health diplomacy. The WHO Director General Report prepared for the 128th EB session in January 2011[29] took an important step forward:

> *Global health policy is shaped by a wide range of stakeholders from the public, private and voluntary sectors. It is of growing importance that these voices are*

also heard in WHO. Being more inclusive can contribute to a stronger leadership role for WHO by gathering broader-based support…

The diversification of actors in global health diplomacy and their changing roles have at the same time highlighted some key concerns about coherence, effectiveness and legitimacy. These debates are increasingly acknowledged in the UN. Article 21 of the third consecutive UN General Assembly (GA) Resolution on Health and Foreign Policy 65/95 from December 2010[30–32] requests the UN Secretary General, in close collaboration with the WHO, to prepare a report that:

1. Reflects on ways to improve the coordination, coherence, and effectiveness for global health
2. Discusses the role of the state and other stakeholders in improving the coordination, coherence, and effectiveness of governance for global health.

The same UN General Assembly Resolution already mentioned above[32] explicitly: *"Recognizes the leading role of the WHO as the primary specialized agency for health."* These words together with a growing number of co-sponsors of the UN GA Resolutions on health and foreign policy as well as the very important negotiations of the FCTC (2003), the revised IHR (2005) and the WHO Global Code of Practice on the International Recruitment of Health Personnel (2010) highlight that amidst the growing number and types of actors for global health diplomacy, the WHO, with its universal membership and equal member state representation in the World Health Association (WHA), is uniquely positioned to play a leading role in the increasingly complex and (overcrowded) global health landscape. It remains to be seen how this political support is translated into addressing the financial challenges faced by the organization.

THE DYNAMIC RELATIONSHIP BETWEEN HEALTH AND FOREIGN POLICY

In this rapidly changing environment with a growing number and diversity of the new health diplomats across the public, private, and civil society sectors on the national, regional, and international level, myriads of opportunities are open for health diplomacy, and this highlights the increasingly complex relationship between health and foreign policy as the UN GA Resolution on Global Health and Foreign Policy in Article 18[32] "urges Member States to continue to consider health issues in the formulation of foreign policy."

The evolving complexity (**Fig. 1**) can best be described as a continuum between a point where foreign policy neglects or even hinders health (A) to a situation where foreign policy is increasingly called to serve health (D). Along the whole continuum, national interests are served, but in a variety of ways and with different influences on health outcomes both at home and abroad. Although settings where diplomacy

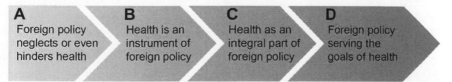

A Foreign policy neglects or even hinders health

B Health is an instrument of foreign policy

C Health as an integral part of foreign policy

D Foreign policy serving the goals of health

Fig. 1. The continuum of the relationship between health and foreign policy. (*Adapted from* Kickbusch I. Global health diplomacy: how foreign policy can influence health. BMJ 2011;345:1345–6.)

fails and military action take place, or where economic considerations have trumped health concerns, such as the TRIPS negotiations (A), continue to pose challenge, the points B and C on the continuum are of particular relevance for the regular practice of health diplomacy. The division between the 4 points along the continuum is fluid; from a public health perspective it seems that the goal is to move toward point D but also to be astute and practical in how to include health in points B and C and to advocate strongly against positions that endanger health at point A.

Today, health is used as an instrument of foreign policy (B) to serve a range of national interests within the geopolitical marketplace.[11] It can support political positioning, improve relations between states, and help build alliances for wider foreign policy goals; that is why the terms soft power or smart power are often used to describe global health initiatives.[33] Different countries are taking advantage of such approaches. The long-standing Cuban medical diplomacy and a significant part of development aid for health follow this pattern, as do China's health projects in Africa and US PEPFAR. It is hard to ignore their positive effect for health, but there are key problems with the politically framed conditionality, the selection of partners and recipients according to political factors not need, and with program sustainability should political intentions change.

The answer of the Secretary of State Hilary Clinton to the rhetorical question "What exactly does maternal health, or immunizations, or the fight against HIV and AIDS have to do with foreign policy? Well, my answer is everything"[34] highlights yet another important transition: health is becoming an integral part of foreign policy (C). The recent Japanese global health policy states at the beginning that "global health is an integral part of Japan's foreign policy strategy."[35] In an increasingly interconnected world, pandemics pose challenges not only to national and health security but also have significant economic implications. Other sectors have a strong interest in ensuring that global health security is managed well. Health is also one of the fastest growing industries worldwide and international health agreements can have significant impacts on national economies and multinational companies. Health becomes part of the system of diplomacy and therefore more diplomats are part of the health negotiations and health experts are increasingly pulled into the realm of foreign policy. It is critical that the public health perspective be part of the decision process on foreign policy goals related to health. There is also an increasing number of health attachés at the diplomatic representations to deal with the growing health portfolio, in particular in Geneva and Brussels, and many of these are now seconded by ministries of health. Health negotiations at the regional and global level can also create significant foreign policy spill-over effects including the possibility of alliances and deals in relation to other global issues at stake.

The global commitment to the Millennium Development Goals and the regular consideration of health in the context of the UN GA are indications of a further trend in which foreign policy serves to improve global health. Point D reflects the recognition of a double responsibility for health, serving the interest of the national and the global community simultaneously. Three UN resolutions on global health and foreign policy[30-32] have reinforced this understanding, based on an approach initially promoted by a group of Ministers of Foreign Affairs from Brazil, France, Indonesia, Norway, Senegal, South Africa, and Thailand a couple of years ago: health as a point of departure and a defining lens that countries will use to examine key elements of foreign policy.[36] Foreign policy can serve health; the cooperation between Thailand's strong national public health coalition and its diplomats made it possible to embark on a landmark General Agreement on Tariffs and Trade (GATT) case to contest the opening of its tobacco market to US companies on public health grounds.[37]

GLOBAL HEALTH DIPLOMACY AND PEACE: EXPANDING A MODEL FOR SYNERGIES

A higher political profile, more actors, and increasing attention from a growing number of nations create a cosmopolitan momentum. They highlight the diversity of possibilities to exert influence in the multilevel negotiations for global health diplomacy and peace, and invite exploration of additional opportunities to tackle, beyond concrete symptoms, the broader structural challenges. Searching for potential synergies, this article links the transitions in (global health) diplomacy along a broader understanding about the social determinants of health with analytical approaches in peace studies and action in conflict. It builds on the existing literature elaborating on the link between health and peace[38-44] and develops them further by highlighting the dynamic transitions in diplomacy and by putting emphasis on the importance of primary prevention acknowledging the need to address the determinants of health and peace.

The link between health and peace is most often established in the context of violent conflicts. The global disease burden of war, civil conflict, and violence measured in disability-adjusted life years is impressive and comparable with a significant part of the disease burden of HIV/AIDS. At the intersection of health and peace, efforts to mitigate the effects on health include humanitarian ceasefires, for example to allow immunization or other health interventions to take place. A good example was the joint efforts of UNICEF, PAHO, and the Roman Catholic Church, later also Rotary International and the International Committee of the Red Cross in El Salvador, to negotiate cease fires to allow the immunization of 300,000 children annually, before peace agreement was reached Immunization led to decreases in the incidence of measles and tetanus and polio and is even interpreted as supportive to the promotion of peace.

In postcrisis settings, health diplomacy can play an important role from individual health to contributing to the reconstruction of society infrastructure. The complexity of negotiations that might be required are illustrated by the efforts of the Red Cross or Medicins Sans Frontieres to reach an agreement with diverse parties (NATO, government, or donor/pharmaceutical companies). On the level of public health and society reconstruction, the PAHO experience since the 1980s or the WHO Health as a Bridge for Peace provide important lessons for global health diplomats through the facilitation of decentralized cooperation to create and/or consolidate long-term cultural, technical, and economic partnerships and confidence building (Bosnia and Herzegovina) as well as reintegrate health services (Croatia, Mozambique, and Angola).[28]

The transitions in the beginning of the twenty-first century highlight that global health diplomacy can do much more. UN GA Resolution 65/95, Article 3 encourages member states "to recognize that global health challenges require concerted and sustained efforts to further promote a global policy environment supportive of global health."[32] Within the WHO, prominent examples include the Code on Health Workers (2010), the FCTC, and the IHR. The importance of negotiations is also visible through the diversity of deliberations within the WHA and the executive bodies of the organization. The 128th WHO Executive Board (EB) session in 2011 provides a clear example: the topics cover pandemic influenza preparedness, health-related Millennium Development Goals, noncommunicable diseases, and health system strengthening. Not only is the number of topics growing but the debate is shifting toward more active participation of middle-income and low-income countries.

In 3 consecutive years, the UN GA has agreed on resolutions entitled Global Health and Foreign Policy, that show a diversity of topics that can be grouped along managing interdependence and development. It has previously deliberated on HIV/AIDS and, in 2011, set a special session on noncommunicable diseases. Even the

UN Security Council has devoted attention to HIV/AIDS. Other bodies such as the G8, the World Bank, UNICEF, UN AIDS and UN human rights bodies deliberate on health, as do many regional organizations,[17] and the effects for health can be huge: the 2010 G8 Muskoka Initiative will mobilize significantly more than $10 billion for health.

The importance of the deliberations of health in these many forums at different levels shows that, at a time when countries are challenged to manage complex issues from interstate and intrastate conflicts, conventional arms control, nuclear power use to climate change, economic cooperation, and human security, health has won a place on the already overcrowded world's urgent agenda.

A COSMOPOLITAN MOMENTUM CALLING FOR CAPACITY BUILDING AS EMPOWERMENT

At the beginning of the twenty-first century, global health diplomacy has gained unprecedented attention on the international level. Along with the diversification of actors for health and the reestablishment of the unique position of the WHO, it has a board agenda and hundreds of millions of dollars to implement it. But the cosmopolitan moment that has opened has highlighted the need for more comprehensive approaches to health, including the social determinants of health, better coordination among initiatives, and more active involvement of all members of the international community. These concerns were present at the deliberations of the 128th EB in 2011 and echoed in the UN GA resolutions, illustrating that although deliberations, negotiations and decisions made at these venues are likely to affect the interests of the middle and low income countries there are huge inequalities in countries' capacities to represent their own interests. Empowering them through capacity building to take initiatives in managing their own development and growth will be one of the key tasks, and this requires effective collaboration between the academic and policy worlds across national borders.

REFERENCES

1. Kickbusch I, Silberschmidt G, Buss P. Global health diplomacy: the need for new perspectives, strategic approaches and skills in global health. Bull World Health Organ 2007;85:230–2.
2. World report on violence and health, World Health Organization 2002. Available at: http://www.who.int/violence_injury_prevention/violence/world_report/en/index.html. Accessed March 4, 2011.
3. Lee K, World Health Organization (WHO). Global institutions series. London: Routledge; 2009. xx, p. 157.
4. WHO. The first ten years of the World Health Organization. Palais des Nations. Geneva (Switzerland): WHO; 1958.
5. Howard-Jones N. The scientific background of the International Sanitary Conferences 1851–1938. Geneva (Switzerland): World Health Organization; 1975.
6. Constitution of the World Health Organization, art. 2a. Available at: http://apps.who.int/gb/bd/PDF/bd47/EN/constitution-en.pdf. Accessed March 1, 2011.
7. WHO. The second ten years of the World Health Organization. Geneva (Switzerland): World Health Organization; 1968.
8. WHO, The third ten years of the World Health Organization. Geneva: World Health Organization; 2008. Available at: http://www.who.int/global_health_histories/who-3rd10years.pdf. Accessed March 4, 2011.
9. Fidler DP. Reflections on the revolution in health and foreign policy. Bull World Health Organ 2007;85:243–4.

10. Alcázar S. The Copernican shift in global health, Working Paper: Global Health Programme. Geneva (Switzerland): Graduate Institute of International and Development Studies; 2008.
11. Khanna P. The second world: empires and influence in the new global order. 1st edition. New York: Random House; 2008. p. xxvii, 466.
12. Garrett L, Alavian EH. Global health governance in a G-20 world. Global Health Governance 2010;IV(1):1–14.
13. Szlezak NA, Bloom BR, Jamison DT, et al. The global health system: actors, norms, and expectations in transition. PLoS Med 2010;7(1):e1000183.
14. Buss P, Roberto Ferreira J. Critical essay on international cooperation in health. RECIIS Rev Electron Comun Inf Inov Saude 2010;4(1):86–97.
15. Almeida C, de Campos RP, Buss P, et al. Brazil's conception of south-south "structural cooperation" in health. RECIIS Rev Electron Comun Inf Inov Saude 2010;4(1):23–32.
16. Almeida C. Global health and health diplomacy: an emerging dialogue between health and international relations. RECIIS Rev Electron Comun Inf Inov Saude 2010;IV(1):1–2.
17. United Nations. Global health and foreign policy: strategic opportunities and challenges. Note by the Secretary-General A/64/365. 2009.
18. Feinsilver JM. Cuban Medical Diplomacy. Council on Hemispheric Affairs, 2006. Available at: http://www.coha.org/cuban-medical-diplomacy-when-the-left-has-got-it-right/. Accessed January 17, 2011.
19. de la Torre Montejo E. La solidaridad en salud. In: Salud para todos: sí es posible. La Habana: Sociedad Cubana de Salud Pública; 2005. p. 239–89.
20. Health agenda for the Americas 2008–2017. Available at: http://www.paho.org/English/DD/PIN/Health_Agenda.pdf. Accessed March 1, 2011.
21. WHO, List of 182 NGOs in official relations with WHO reflecting decisions of EB 128 January 2011. Geneva (Switzerland). Available at: http://www.who.int/civilsociety/NGOs-in-Official-Relations-with-WHO-as-of-Jan-2011.pdf. Accessed March 1, 2011.
22. Kickbusch I, Hein W, Silberschmidt G. Addressing global health governance challenges through a new mechanism: the proposal for a Committee C of the World Health Assembly. J Law Med Ethics 2010;38(3):550–63.
23. Barston RP. Modern diplomacy. 3rd edition. Harlow (UK): Pearson/Longman; 2006. p. xx, 387.
24. Keusch GT, Kilama WL, Moon S, et al. The global health system: linking knowledge with action–learning from malaria. PLoS Med 2010;7(1):e1000179.
25. Moon S, Szlezak NA, Michaud CM, et al. The global health system: lessons for a stronger institutional framework. PLoS Med 2010;7(1):e1000193.
26. Khanna P. Future shock? Welcome to the new middle ages. Financial Times, December 28, 2010. Available at: http://www.ft.com/cms/s/0/02a84976-12ba-11e0-b4c8-00144feabdc0.html#axzz1QqIG5nlH. Accessed May 31, 2011.
27. WHO. What is health as a bridge for peace. Available at: http://www.who.int/hac/techguidance/hbp/about/en/index.html. Accessed March 1, 2011.
28. Department of emergency and humanitarian action, report on the Second World Health Organization Consultation on health as a bridge for peace. 2002. Available at: http://www.who.int/hac/techguidance/hbp/Versoix_consultation_report.pdf.   Accessed March 1, 2011.
29. The future financing for WHO. Report by the Director General, EB 128/21. Available at: http://apps.who.int/gb/ebwha/pdf_files/EB128/B128_21-en.pdf. Accessed March 1, 2011.

30. United Nations. Resolution adopted by the United Nations General Assembly on Global Health and Foreign Policy. A/Res/63/33. 2008.
31. United Nations. Resolution adopted by the United Nations General Assembly on Global Health and Foreign Policy. A/Res/64/108. 2009.
32. United Nations. Resolution adopted by the United Nations General Assembly on Global Health and Foreign Policy. A/Res/65/95. 2010.
33. Kickbusch I. Global health diplomacy: how foreign policy can influence health. BMJ 2011;345:1345–6.
34. Clinton H. The global health initiative: the next phase of American leadership in health around the world. Washington, DC: The School of Advanced International Studies; 2010.
35. Ministry of Foreign Affairs of Japan. Japan's global health policy 2011–2015. Available at: http://www.mofa.go.jp/policy/oda/mdg/pdfs/hea_pol_exe_en.pdf. Accessed January 13, 2011. 2010.
36. Oslo Ministerial Declaration–global health: a pressing foreign policy issue of our time. Lancet 2007;369(9570):1373–8.
37. Brandt AM. The cigarette century: the rise, fall, and deadly persistence of the product that defined America. New York: Basic Books; 2007. p. vii, 600.
38. Banatvala N, Zwi AB. Conflict and health - Public health and humanitarian interventions: developing the evidence base - part 1. BMJ 2000;321(7253):101–5.
39. MacQueen G, Santa-Barbara J. Peace building through health initiatives. BMJ 2000;321(7256):293–6.
40. Vass A. Peace through health - This new movement needs evidence, not just ideology. BMJ 2001;323(7320):1020.
41. Zwi AB, Garfield R, Sondorp E. Health and peace: an opportunity to join forces. Lancet 2001;358(9288):1183–4.
42. Arya N, Santa Barbara J. Peace through health: how health professionals can work for a less violent world. Sterling (VA): Kumarian Press; 2008. p. 340.
43. Khan AM, Janneck LM, Bhatt J, et al. Building a health-peace movement: academic medicine's role in generating solutions to global problems. Acad Med 2009;84(11):1486.
44. Kett M, Rushton S, Ingram A. Health, peace and conflict: roles for health professionals. Med Confl Surviv 2010;26(2):v–vii.

Poverty, Global Health, and Infectious Disease: Lessons from Haiti and Rwanda

Marcella M. Alsan, MD, MPH[a,b,*], Michael Westerhaus, MD, MA[b,c],
Michael Herce, MD, MPH[d,e], Koji Nakashima, MD, MHS[f,g],
Paul E. Farmer, MD, PhD[b,h]

KEYWORDS

- Poverty • Global health • Infectious disease • HIV/AIDS
- Malaria and inequality

The association between poverty and communicable disease is evident from a cursory exercise in cartography. The maps of those living on less than US $2 a day and the epidemiology of human immunodeficiency virus (HIV)/acquired immune deficiency syndrome (AIDS), malaria, tuberculosis (TB), and many other infectious diseases coincide nearly exactly (**Fig. 1**). Countries with higher incomes per capita tend to enjoy longer life expectancies (**Fig. 2**). Although notable exceptions exist in some low

Potential conflicts of interest: the authors have no conflicts of interest or financial support to disclose.

[a] Division of Infectious Diseases, Department of Economics, Brigham and Women's Hospital, Harvard University, 75 Francis Street, Boston, MA 02115, USA

[b] Partners In Health

[c] Division of Global Health Equity, Department of Global Health and Social Medicine, Brigham and Women's Hospital, Harvard Medical School, 75 Francis Street, Boston, MA 02115, USA

[d] Abwenzi Pa Za Umoyo, Partners In Health, Malawi

[e] Division of Global Health Equity, Department of Global Health and Social Medicine, Brigham and Women's Hospital, Harvard Medical School, FXB Building, 651 Huntington Avenue, 7th Floor, Boston, MA 02115, USA

[f] Zanmi Lasante, Partners In Health, Haiti

[g] Division of Global Health Equity, Brigham and Women's Hospital, Harvard Medical School, 888 Commonwealth Avenue, 3rd Floor, Boston, MA 02115, USA

[h] Division of Global Health Equity, Department of Global Health and Social Medicine, Brigham and Women's Hospital, Harvard Medical School, 641 Huntington Avenue, Boston, MA 02115, USA

* Corresponding author. Division of Infectious Diseases, Department of Economics, Brigham and Women's Hospital, Harvard University, 75 Francis Street, Boston, MA 02115.

E-mail address: malsan@fas.harvard.edu

Infect Dis Clin N Am 25 (2011) 611–622
doi:10.1016/j.idc.2011.05.004
0891-5520/11/$ – see front matter © 2011 Elsevier Inc. All rights reserved.

id.theclinics.com

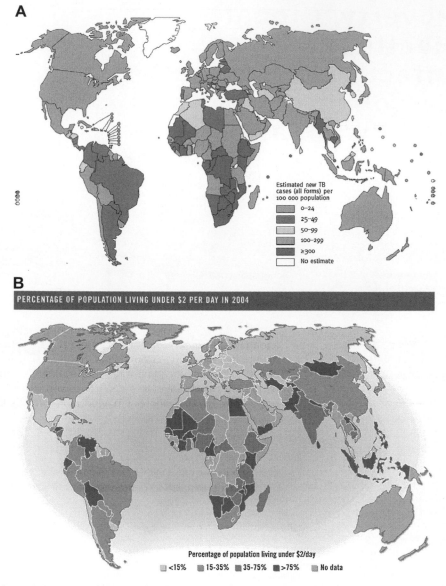

Fig. 1. (*A*) Estimated TB incidence by country, 2009. (*Adapted from* WHO Global Tuberculosis Control, 2010.) (*B*) Global poverty map. (*Reprinted from* The World Resources Institute; with permission.)

income settings, such as Cuba or Kerala State, where India has an excellent performance on population health measures, these instances represent important exceptions to the general rule. What are the linkages between poverty and ill health? How can the vicious cycle of destitution and sickness be broken?

Poverty is arguably the greatest risk factor for acquiring and succumbing to disease worldwide, but has historically received less attention from the medical community than genetic or environmental risk factors. Several factors likely contributed to this oversight: first, being poor is not considered a disruption of normal physiologic

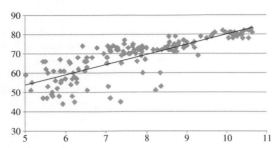

Fig. 2. Life expectancy at birth, total (years) versus log gross domestic product (GDP) per capita (constant US $2000). Data are from the most recent year of complete data, 2007, and include 146 countries with a population more than 1,000,000. (*Data from* The World Bank World Development Indicators.)

function. Physicians and basic scientists viewed themselves as ill-equipped to understand or manipulate an individual's socioeconomic status. Second, unlike the largesse dedicated to finding technical solutions for population health problems, funding for research dedicated to understanding and alleviating poverty was sparse. Third, although some acknowledged that poverty plays a pivotal role in determining disease vulnerability and outcomes, the resultant solutions intended to redress poverty were often wrongheaded. For example, structural adjustment programs (SAPs) intended to increase gross domestic product (GDP) growth often involved austerity measures, such as cuts in government spending, currency devaluation, and privatization. These macroeconomic shifts involved intertemporal trade-offs (temporary pain for long-term gains) and completely ignored the path-dependent nature of health care. If a child does not get vaccinated, a pregnant mother lacks antenatal care, or a TB clinic goes without drugs, the health consequences can reverberate for generations.

The tide in public health and medicine has started to shift. The global HIV/AIDS crisis brought into sharp relief the vulnerability of financially strapped health systems to epidemic disease and revealed disparities in health outcomes along economic fault lines. The protestations of injustice regarding the withholding of life-sustaining antiretroviral treatment from the developing world, made first by patient-activists, then students, and (more gradually) academics and politicians, have provided a template for addressing other diseases linked to poverty. This hope was echoed in the preface of Farmer's[1] *AIDS and Accusation*: "If AIDS care becomes a right rather than a commodity…we have no more excuses for ignoring the growing inequality that has left hundreds of millions of people without any hope of surviving preventable and treatable illnesses…Taking on AIDS forcefully would allow us to start a 'virtuous social cycle,' long overdue." And if a rights-based approach to controlling communicable disease falls on deaf ears, enlightened self-interest might still invoke concern. Severe acute respiratory syndrome (SARS), multidrug-resistant TB, and H1N1 remind the developed world of its porous borders. Many investors view the developing world as a potential market for their goods, and military strategists foresee the danger of allowing states to collapse from pandemic disease.

Economic thought regarding the link between poverty and disease has also evolved. Sen's[2] landmark treatise, *Development as Freedom*, exposed the false dichotomy between political and social and economic rights. Sen[2] posited that development was broader than income: an affluent, stable democracy could not be achieved without an educated and healthy populace. "There is a deep complementary between individual agency and social arrangements," Sen[2] wrote. And more pointedly: "Development requires the removal of major sources of unfreedom: poverty as well as tyranny, poor economic opportunities as well as systematic social deprivation, neglect of public facilities as well as intolerance or overactivity of the repressive states." Such insight paved the way for the creation of the Human Development Index (HDI) 20 years ago. The HDI is a composite measure of health, education, and income and was designed by Mahbub ul Haq to counter the inordinate reliance on income alone as a measure of well-being. Building on the conceptual framework created by Sen and parameterized (albeit imperfectly) by ul Haq, Jeff Sachs became the next economist to make a broader concept of development operational by promoting the Millennium Development Goals (MDGs). The 8 MDGs, endorsed by 189 countries, are time-limited commitments to reduce poverty, expand educational opportunities, promote gender equality, and safeguard population and environmental health.[3]

This article discusses the complex relationship between poverty and communicable disease, and draws on experience gleaned from working in solidarity with the destitute sick in Haiti, Peru, Rwanda, and elsewhere, as well as from anthropologic and economic theory and evidence. We conclude that the twin afflictions of poverty and disease cannot be treated in isolation and require a biosocial understanding to achieve lasting health gains.

POVERTY AND SUSCEPTIBILITY

One link between poverty and disease that is readily observable to most physicians is the increased vulnerability of the poor to communicable diseases, and the lack of medical care once infected. This link was eloquently documented by German pathologist Rudolf Carl Virchow, investigating an outbreak of typhus in the nineteenth century:

> The population had no idea that the mental and material impoverishment to which it had been allowed to sink, were largely the cause of its hunger and disease, and that the adverse climatic conditions which contributed to the failure of its crops and to the sickness of its bodies, would have not caused such terrible ravages, if it had been free, educated and well-to-do. For there can now no longer be any doubt that such an epidemic dissemination of typhus had only been possible under the wretched conditions of life that poverty and lack of culture had created in Upper Silesia. If these conditions were removed, I am sure that epidemic typhus would not recur. Whosoever wishes to learn from history will find many examples.[4]

To prevent typhus from recurring, Virchow announced a radical prescription: medicine must concern itself with the social condition of the population, and characterize efforts short of that as palliative. Although daunting, these words inspired the creation of social medicine, and the veracity of Virchow's observations are reflected in modern epidemics.

The recent cholera epidemic in Haiti provides a current example. In early December 2010, the US Centers for Disease Control and Prevention (CDC) *Morbidity Mortality and Weekly Report* announced that the outbreak had spread nationwide. At that time, the Haitian Ministry of Public Health and Population (MSPP) reported 91,770 cases of cholera, including 43,243 hospitalizations and 2071 deaths. Deaths occur "as rapidly as 2 hours after symptom onset and [identify] important gaps in access to life-saving treatments, including oral rehydration solution (ORS)."[5] Disentangling Haiti's dire health condition from historical, political, and economic concerns leads to the characterization of the epidemic as a medical disaster stemming from the twin natural disasters Haiti suffered in the last year: a 7.0 magnitude earthquake and subsequent flooding from Hurricane Tomas. However, a narrative that uses phrases such as medical and natural implies inevitability and general inculpability. A more careful reading of the context in which the cholera outbreak has occurred proves such ahistorical views misleading.

The Republic of Haiti is the only nation tracing its genesis to a successful slave revolt. After more than a decade of war that destroyed the country's infrastructure and cost tens of thousands of lives, the French relinquished military control in 1804. However, France maintained financial repression by demanding that the fledgling nation pay damages for property losses incurred during the revolution. These demands marked the birth of Haiti's longstanding debt burden. As historian von Tunzelmann[6] describes, Haiti was on the brink of humanitarian calamity even before the devastating earthquake of 2010:

> ... France gained the western third of the island of Hispaniola—the territory that is now Haiti—in 1697. It planted sugar and coffee, supported by an unprecedented increase in the importation of African slaves. Economically, the result was a success, but life as a slave was intolerable...After a dramatic slave uprising that shook the western world, and 12 years of war, Haiti finally defeated Napoleon's forces in 1804 and declared independence. But France demanded reparations: 150 [million] francs, in gold.
>
> For Haiti, this debt did not signify the beginning of freedom, but the end of hope... By 1900, it was spending 80% of its national budget on repayments. To manage the original reparations, further loans were taken out—mostly from the United States, Germany and France. Instead of developing its potential, this deformed state produced a parade of nefarious leaders, most of whom gave up the insurmountable task of trying to fix the country and looted it instead.

Staggering debt obligations hampered Haiti's ability to provide basic sanitation and public health interventions to its population. According to the United Nations Development Program (UNDP) Human Development Report, Haiti ranks 145th out of 169 countries.[7] It has occupied the unenviable position of poorest nation in the Western Hemisphere for decades. Income per capita is US $560, 54% of Haitians live on less than US $1 a day, and 78% live on less than US $2 a day. In 2005, total external debt owed was US $1.5 billion, more than one-quarter of total GDP,[8] whereas Haiti spent only 1.2% of GDP on health care.[7] Widespread lack of access to clean water has been a chronic threat to the health of the Haitian population.[9] In 2007, only 63% had access to an improved water source, and only 17% had access to sanitation.[10]

The earthquake on January 12, 2010 (which killed an estimated 250,000 people and displaced more than one-tenth of the Haitian population) turned the water situation in Haiti from bad to worse. It was in the context of hundreds of thousands of people living in refugee camps (1 million on the outskirts of Port-au-Prince alone) with intermittent access to drinking water and gross underprovision of sanitation facilities that cholera took hold.[11] Recent findings published in the New England Journal of Medicine and using third-generation single-molecule real-time DNA sequencing found that the clonal strain causing the Haiti outbreak was genetically similar to those previously isolated in Bangladesh. The study investigators concluded that, "Collectively, our data strongly suggest that the Haitian epidemic began with introduction of a V. cholerae strain into Haiti by human activity from a distant geographic source."[12] These results corroborated those from the CDC and the National Public Health Laboratory (NPHL) in Haiti.[13] The initial CDC findings were released in early November and sparked protests against the Nepali UN peacekeepers quartered near the river presumed to be the source of the outbreak. At least 3 Haitians were killed.[14] After a 100-year hiatus, cholera has now gripped Haiti and has started to spread to the Dominican Republic.[15] Given the increased virulence associated with this particular strain (the death rate in Haiti is 12 times higher than that of the 1991 Peruvian epidemic) there are calls from public health leaders to mass vaccinate the populations of the island and its closest neighbors.[16] Taking into account the long view of Haiti's history, from slavery to colonialism, debt, despotic leaders, and a woeful undersupply of public goods, the cholera outbreak seems less like an unforeseen catastrophe and more like an event that Virchow would have easily predicted.

Neglected tropical diseases (NTDs) provide another example of how economic position can interact with host susceptibility. According to the World Health Organization (WHO), NTDs are defined by their association with poverty: "though medically diverse, neglected tropical diseases form a group because all are associated with poverty."[17] Substandard housing, lack of access to safe water and sanitation, and inadequate vector control contribute to the efficient transmission of infection. Currently, of the world's 2.7 billion impoverished individuals, more than a billion people suffer from NTDs.[17] Thankfully, there is growing attention to this matter among the international community. The first annual report on NTDs was released by the WHO in 2010. Director-General Margaret Chan refers to the MDGs in her preface and provides several examples of how eliminating NTDs would foster economic development: "Onchocerciasis and trachoma cause blindness. Leprosy and lymphatic filariasis deform in ways that hinder economic productivity and cancel out chances for a normal social life. Buruli ulcer maims...Human African trypanosomiasis (sleeping sickness) severely debilitates before it kills. Chagas disease can cause young adults to develop heart conditions, so that they fill hospital beds instead of the labor force," and so on.[17] The emphasis on potential negative productivity implications associated with untreated NTDs is understandable. Like cancer and heart disease, NTDs do not travel widely. New justifications are needed to persuade the international community to intervene when the direct threat to the health of wealthy country inhabitants is muted. If the medical community is to be committed to global health equity and not simply to reducing morbidity or mortality from the cluster of diseases that most affect the wealthy world, a rights-based approach to health care must be adopted.

STRUCTURAL VIOLENCE AND RISK

As discussed earlier, poverty and associated disease rarely arise de novo. Heavy burdens of disease predictably strike those places, most often resource-poor communities, where structural violence weighs most heavily. Moreover, structural violence (institutionalized biases and inequalities including racism, elitism, gender inequality, militarism, and economic policy that fosters inequity) often emanates from global centers of power and privilege, and increases the risk of encounter with communicable disease.[18]

Rwanda's recent history makes these processes clear. The 1994 Rwandan genocide took an enormous toll on the population: at least 800,000 Rwandans massacred in 3 brutal months by approximately 15% of the population.[19] However, what commonly escapes our memories is that the Rwandan genocide was predicated on far more than physical violence alone. Structural violence played a significant role in setting the stage. Uvin[20] has argued that an uncritical development enterprise, dominated by foreigners, contributed to the creation of the processes that led toward genocide. In *Aiding Violence*, he summarizes:

[A]id financed much of the machinery of exclusion, inequality, and humiliation; provided it with legitimacy and support; and sometimes directly contributed to

it. To their credit, some aid agencies—some nongovernmental organizations (NGOs) foremost among them—may have had different impacts; they may have softened some parts of the crises faced by ordinary Rwandans. Yet, by and large, aid was an active and willing partner in the construction of structural violence in Rwanda, as it is elsewhere in Africa.

Many weapons used in the genocide did not originate in Rwanda, but in many of the political and economic powers of the world.[21]

The physical and structural violence of the Rwandan genocide directly affected the spread of communicable disease. Systematic rape during the genocide served as a vector for HIV transmission.[22] The exodus of Rwandans into refugee camps in the Democratic Republic of the Congo without adequate food, water, and sanitation gave rise to epidemics of infectious disease (such as cholera) that resulted in a crude mortality of 20 to 35 per 10,000 people each day.[23] Increased incidences of both malaria and tuberculosis have lasted far beyond the formal end of the genocide.[24]

Careful attention to Rwanda's and Haiti's places in global history, economics, and politics shows that the forces of structural violence increase risk of communicable disease for resource-poor populations in ways that are distinct from the behavioral and cultural explanations uncritically circulated in academic literature and the popular press.

DISEASE AND DEVELOPMENT

Conditions of poverty and structural violence facilitate disease acquisition. It is straightforward to extend this analysis to document the impact of poverty on access to care and health outcomes. Since the 2001 report by the WHO Commission on Macroeconomics and Health, chaired by Jeff Sachs, attention has shifted to exploring how investments in population health can spur economic growth.[25] Given that most of the developing world is engaged in physically demanding agricultural labor, health setbacks likely have a greater impact there than in the wealthy world. In economic terms, the marginal returns to good health in the labor force are higher in poorer countries. However, there are other, more nuanced channels by which ill health can affect economic prospects. These channels include the interactions among health and demography, cognition, and investment behavior.

Health and Demography

There is a strong association between child survival and fertility. Total fertility rate (TFR; the number of children that would be born to a woman if she were to live to the end of her childbearing years and bear children in accordance with current age-specific fertility rates) and mortality before 5 years of age (child mortality rate [CMR], the probability per 1,000 that a newborn baby will die before reaching the age of 5 years, if subject to current age-specific mortality) have a correlation coefficient of 0.876. **Table 1** shows the linear trend between these indicators.[10] Explanations

Table 1				
The association between fertility and mortality before 5 years of age				
Average mortality before 5 years of age	<50	50–100	100–150	>150
Average fertility rate	2.17	3.74	4.93	5.85

Data represent the average TFR and CMR of 187 countries for the 4 most recent complete years of data (2004–2008). Precise definitions of these measures are contained in the text.
Data from The World Bank World Development Indicators.

abound as to why the relationship between child survival and fertility are so robust. One view espoused by many demographers and economists is that families in societies where child survival is low tend to compensate for expected and actual child deaths by having more children. Nobel laureate and economist Gary Becker famously modeled this quality/quantity trade-off with respect to family size. Another explanation is that places with high child mortality also lack access to contraception, educational opportunities for women, and gender equality. Although desired family size is a difficult concept to define and measure, the World Bank does attempt to collect data on access to contraception and indices of gender inequality.[10] Although the correlation between the gender inequality index and child mortality in the World Bank's indicators database is negligible (0.01), perhaps at least in part because of the small sample size (75 countries) and imprecise measuring, contraceptive prevalence is negatively correlated with child mortality (−0.32). Although a major focus of academic inquiry is the direction of causality in the fertility-CMR relation, it seems safe to assume that the relationship is bidirectional. These data imply that efforts to improve public health through the provision of either culturally appropriate family planning or pediatric care would also pay dividends in the other health sector. From an economic standpoint, household resources are divided among fewer individuals as family size shrinks. This division allows parents to invest more in their children's education and nutrition, potentially interrupting the intergenerational transmission of poverty.

Health and Education

As with the relationship between child survival and fertility, the interplay between health and education is complex. As mentioned earlier, more-educated mothers tend to have fewer and healthier children. Moreover, the returns from education in terms of increased wages or agricultural output give heads of households the financial opportunity to promote their own health and that of their children. David Barker, a British physician who noted a correlation between low birth weight and cardiovascular health in midlife, put forward the fetal origins hypothesis that the in utero environment has important consequences for health and cognitive abilities later in life. Several epidemiologists have since confirmed this association.[26] Almond,[27] an economist at Columbia, used the natural experiment of the 1918 Spanish influenza epidemic to assess the impact of fetal health on educational and labor outcomes. Pairing data from the pandemic with those from the 1960 to 1980 decennial US censuses, Almond[27] found that cohorts in utero during the pandemic displayed reduced educational attainment, increased rates of physical disability, lower income, and lower socioeconomic status compared with other birth cohorts. Similarly, Miguel and Kremer[28] analyzed a randomized control trial of deworming in Kenyan schools at the facility level designed to capture the positive externalities associated with reducing the transmission of helminths. Miguel and Kremer[28] found that the program reduced absenteeism from school by one-quarter, although there was no significant effect on test scores. A series of follow-up studies have shown that those who received deworming for a longer period of time enjoy higher wages years later. Taken together, these results suggest that health investments, especially early in life, affect educational attainment.

Health, Savings, and Investment

There is perhaps an even more subtle way in which health affects education and economic outcomes: through the channel of savings and investment. Economic growth theory has repeatedly underscored that savings and investment are engines of development,[29] but what explains why some countries invest more than others?

This question was first posed by John Rae writing in the early nineteenth century. As Frederick and colleagues[30] explain, "Like [his contemporary] Adam Smith, Rae sought to determine why wealth differed among nations. Smith had argued that national wealth was determined by the amount of labor allocated to the production of capital, but Rae recognized that this account was incomplete because it failed to explain the determinants of this allocation. In Rae's view, the missing factor was 'the effective desire of accumulation,'" which determines the "rate of time preference." The rate of time preference is a mathematical representation of the tendency individuals have to weight the present more heavily than the future when making decisions. It summarizes how willing consumers are to delay immediate consumption and instead invest or save their income.[30] Thus, the relationship between the rate of time preference and savings behavior at the individual level can be linked to income growth and disparities at the aggregate level. Studies by psychologists and economists have shown that the poor discount the future more steeply than the wealthy.[31] This result has given rise to the view that the poor are impatient or, more pejoratively, lack self-control. However, this rationale fails to account for the uncertainty and risks associated with living in poverty. In particular, how do health status and expectation of longevity influence one's willingness to make trade-offs over time? Recent evidence from Sri Lanka sheds light on this question. Jayachandra and Lleras-Muney[32] examined how a sudden drop in maternal mortality between 1946 and 1953 sharply increased the life expectancy of girls. This increase in turn led to greater investment in their education: Jayachandra and Lleras-Muney[32] found that, for every extra year of life expectancy, literacy among girls increased by 0.7 percentage points (2%) and years of education increased by 0.11 years (3%). At Partners In Health, we often use the phrase antidote to despair to describe our work. Translating the language of social justice into the language of economics, the antidote is the extended time horizon afforded by longevity. Knowing that a healthy and well-fed tomorrow awaits may affect the psychology of those living in poverty. The impact of this health-led hope on investments in microenterprise, education, and complementary health inputs has yet to be fully measured.

APPLYING A BIOSOCIAL FRAMEWORK TO THE DESIGN OF HEALTH SYSTEMS

Having reviewed the ways in which poverty, structural violence, and infectious disease confine poor populations to vicious cycles of suffering and despair, we now examine the implications of these understandings on the design of health interventions. As shown by disease patterns in Haiti and Rwanda, social forces interact with human biology and affect who falls ill and who has access to care. Thus, use of a biosocial analytical framework provides a useful and effective tool for designing and implementing health interventions to address these inequalities. Failure to use a biosocial lens often gives rise to charity and development models of health intervention that replicate preexisting unequal structures. Such models localize blame for disease with the poor themselves. In contrast, a biosocial lens makes clear that disease among the poor results from the embodiment of structural violence and requires that any serious attempt to address disease in resource-poor settings incorporates efforts for social change. Through commitment to models built on the principles of social justice, we have found that advocacy and long-term partnerships with the public sector and the communities in which we work are indispensable to sustainable transformations in health that reduce suffering caused by infectious and chronic disease.

Biosocial understandings of disease in Haiti and Rwanda reveal that a sustainable response must not only make available the fruits of modern medicine (ie, diagnostic tools, pharmaceuticals, and trained clinicians) but must also address the consequences of deep poverty: limited transportation, poor housing, and food scarcity, among others. In Haiti, Rwanda, and numerous other settings, Partners In Health and local partners provide care that integrates social and economic programs. These programs include constructing homes and schools, establishing potable water systems, and providing food and transportation stipends. In addition, paid community health workers are used to deliver top-quality health care to patients in their homes, rather than requiring sick, impoverished individuals to confront innumerable barriers to reaching clinics and hospitals. Such solutions, which privilege a biosocial approach to identifying and breaking down barriers to care, have resulted in remarkable successes in addressing epidemics of HIV/AIDS, TB, malaria, and other communicable and chronic diseases in some of the most challenging domestic and global settings.[33]

SUMMARY

Poverty and infectious diseases interact in subtle and complex ways. Casting the problem of destitution as intractable, or epidemics that afflict the poor as accidental, erroneously exonerates us from responsibility for protecting and caring for those most in need. Our experience working in Haiti and Rwanda has shown that appropriately and adequately addressing the scourges of communicable diseases requires a biosocial appreciation of the structural forces that shape disease patterns. Although there is ample evidence that heath investments pay dividends in labor productivity, educational attainment, population control, and, potentially, capital investments, the idea that health is an instrument for development should complement, not supplant, a rights-based approach to health equity. It is plausible that most health interventions in resource-poor settings could garner support based on cost/benefit ratios with appropriately lengthy time horizons to capture the return on health investments and an adequate accounting of externalities; however, such a calculus masks the untold suffering of inaction and risks eroding the most powerful incentive to act: redressing inequality.

ACKNOWLEDGMENTS

The authors wish to thank Zoe Agoos, Burak Alsan, MD, Emily Bahnsen, and Cassia van der Hoof Holstein for their assistance in the preparation of this manuscript.

REFERENCES

1. Farmer P. AIDS and accusation: Haiti and the geography of blame. Berkley (CA): University of California Press; 2006.
2. Sen A. Development as freedom. New York: Alfred A. Knopf; 1999.
3. United Nations. United Nations millennium development goals. Available at: http://www.un.org/millenniumgoals/bkgd.shtml. Accessed December 12, 2010.
4. Brown TM, Fee E. Rudolf Carl Virchow: medical scientist, social reformer, role model. Am J Public Health 2006;96:2104–5.
5. Centers for Disease Control and Prevention. Update outbreak of cholera—Haiti 2010. MMWR Morb Mortal Wkly Rep 2010;59(48):1586–90. Available at: http://www.cdc.gov/mmwr/preview/mmwrhtml/mm5948a4.htm?s_cid=mm5948a4_w. Published December 8, 2010. Updated December 10, 2010. Accessed December 12, 2010.
6. Von Tunzelmann A. Haiti: the land where children eat mud. Available at: http://www.timesonline.co.uk/tol/news/world/us_and_americas/article6281614.ece. The Sunday Times; 2009. Accessed December 12, 2010.

7. United Nations Development Programme. Human Development Report 2010: the real wealth of nations - pathways to development. New York: United Nations Development Programme; 2010.
8. World Bank. Haiti at a glance 2005. Available at: http://siteresources.worldbank.org/INTHAITI/Resources/Haiti.AAG.pdf. Accessed December 12, 2010.
9. Varma MK, Satterthwaite ML, Klasing AM, et al. Woch nan Soley: the denial of the right to water in Haiti. Health Hum Rights 2008;10:67–89.
10. World Bank. World development indicators [database online]. Washington, DC: World Bank; 2010. Available at: http://data.worldbank.org/data-catalog/world-development-indicators/wdi-2010. Accessed December 12, 2010.
11. Beaubien J. Cholera cases spur containment efforts in Haiti. NPR.org. Available at: http://www.npr.org/templates/story/story.php?storyid=131181559. Published November 9, 2010. Accessed December 12, 2010.
12. Chin CS, Sorenson J, Harris JB, et al. The origin of the Haitian cholera outbreak strain. N Engl J Med 2011;364:33–42.
13. Laboratory test results of cholera outbreak strain in Haiti announced [news release]. Atlanta (GA): Center for Disease Control and Prevention; 2010. Available at: http://www.cdc.gov/media/pressrel/2010/r101101.html. Accessed February 13, 2011.
14. Katz J. Haiti cholera riots lessen, 3rd protester killed. Washington Times. Available at: http://www.washingtontimes.com/news/2010/nov/17/haiti-cholera-riots-lessen-3rd-protester-killed/. Published November 17, 2010. Accessed February 25, 2011.
15. Llorente E. More cholera cases reported in the Dominican Republic. Fox News Latino. Available at: http://latino.foxnews.com/latino/health/2010/12/11/cholera-cases-reported-dominican-republic/. Published December 11, 2010. Accessed December 12, 2010.
16. McNeil DG. WHO now sees cholera vaccine as viable. A18. Available at: http://www.nytimes.com/2010/12/11/world/americas/11cholera.html. New York Times; 2010. Accessed December 12, 2010.
17. World Health Organization. Working to overcome the global impact of neglected tropical diseases: first WHO report on neglected tropical diseases. Geneva (Switzerland): World Health Organization; 2010.
18. Farmer P. Partner to the poor. Berkeley (CA): University of California Press; 2010.
19. Gourevitch P. We wish to inform you that tomorrow we will be killed with our families: stories from Rwanda. New York: Farrar, Straus and Giroux; 1998.
20. Uvin P. Aiding violence: the development enterprise in Rwanda. West Hartford (CT): Kumarian Press; 1998.
21. International Campaign to Band Landmines. Landmine monitor report. New York: Human Rights Watch; 1999.
22. Mills EJ, Singh S, Nelson B, et al. The impact of conflict on HIV/AIDS in sub-Saharan Africa. Int J STD AIDS 2006;17:713–7.
23. Willis BM, Levy BS. Recognizing the public health impact of genocide. JAMA 2000;284:612–3.
24. Ghobarah HA, Huth P, Russett B. Civil wars kill and maim people—long after the shooting stops. Am Polit Sci Rev 2003;97:189–202.
25. World Health Organization. Commission on macroeconomics and health macroeconomics and health: investing in health for economic development. Geneva (Switzerland): World Health Organization; 2001.
26. Paul AM. Excerpt from origins: how the first nine months shape the rest of your life. Time Magazine. Available at: http://www.time.com/time/health/article/0,8599,2020815,00.html. Published September 22, 2010. Accessed December 12, 2010.

27. Almond D. Is the 1918 influenza pandemic over? Long term effect of in utero influenza exposure in the post-1940 U.S. population. J Polit Econ 2006;114:672–712.
28. Miguel E, Kremer M. Worms: identifying impacts on education and health in the presence of treatment externalities. Econometrica 2004;72:159–217.
29. Barro R, Sai-i-Martin X. Economic growth. 2nd edition. Cambridge (MA): MIT Press; 2003.
30. Frederick S, Loewenstein G, O'Donoghue T. Time discounting and time preference: a critical review. J Econ Lit 2002;40:351–401.
31. Lawrance E. Poverty and the rate of time preference: evidence from panel data. J Polit Econ 1991;99:54–77.
32. Jayachandra S, Lleras-Muney L. Life expectancy and human capital investments: evidence from maternal mortality declines. Q J Econ 2009;124:349–97.
33. Shin S, Furin J, Bayona J, et al. Community-based treatment of multidrug-resistant tuberculosis in Lima, Peru: seven years of experience. Soc Sci Med 2004;59:1529–39.

Global Health: Chronic Diseases and Other Emergent Issues in Global Health

Tracey Pérez Koehlmoos, PhD, MHA[a],*, Shahela Anwar, MPH[a],
Alejandro Cravioto, PhD, MD[b]

KEYWORDS

- Chronic disease • Injuries • Mental health
- Disaster risk reduction • Emergent issues

KEY MESSAGES

- The largest burden of noncommunicable diseases occurs in low-income and middle-income countries, making noncommunicable disease an urgent development issue
- The economic impact of noncommunicable diseases, such as cardiovascular disease and diabetes, places a significant burden on the development prospects for low-income and middle-income countries
- Approximately 1.3 million people die from road traffic injuries; 90% of these deaths occur in developing countries
- Rapid urbanization has a multiplier effect on many dimensions of existing disease and illness, and is introducing new health hazards
- Climate change is an emerging threat to global public health
- In the new millennium, global health decision makers and scientists must look beyond the traditional purview of public health regarding, for example, maternal and child health and communicable diseases.

Priority health issues are always a factor in country health policies that are shaped by global health discussions and initiatives, which in turn are influenced by existing risk factors and the interface with health systems. Priorities change quickly according to

No funding was received in the production of this article.

The authors report no conflicts of interest.

[a] Health & Family Planning Systems Programme, International Centre for Diarrhoeal Disease Research, Bangladesh (ICDDR,B), 68 Shahed Tajuddin Ahmed, Mohakhali, Dhaka 1212, Bangladesh

[b] International Centre for Diarrhoeal Disease Research, Bangladesh (ICDDR,B), Mohakhali, Dhaka, Bangladesh

* Corresponding author.

E-mail address: tracey@icddrb.org

Infect Dis Clin N Am 25 (2011) 623–638

doi:10.1016/j.idc.2011.05.008

id.theclinics.com

prevailing concerns and expected future trends, as seen clearly in the reemergence of tuberculosis and malaria as key health problems that have become global and individual country health priorities. Infectious diseases have always had a decisive and rapid impact on shaping and changing health policy with global pandemics such as severe acute respiratory syndrome (SARS) and H1N1, emerging without warning and challenging approved priorities within days if not hours.

However, it is important not to lose sight of other areas of health and to maintain a close and watchful eye on trends and developments in those diseases that do not generate the immediate impact that some infectious diseases have been able to do. Noncommunicable diseases fall into this group; they may not have garnered as much interest or importance over the past 10 or 20 years, but in fact have been affecting public health around the world in a very steady and critical way, becoming the leading cause of death in both developed and developing countries.[1]

This article discusses emergent issues in global health related to noncommunicable diseases and conditions. Trying to offer an in-depth discussion on such a wide range of issues in just one article is clearly not possible, and therefore focus and emphasis is given to defining the unique epidemiologic features and relevant programmatic, health systems, and policy responses concerning noncommunicable chronic diseases (NCDs), mental health, accidents and injuries, urbanization, climate change, and disaster preparedness.

NONCOMMUNICABLE CHRONIC DISEASES

In the shadow of global efforts to achieve the Millennium Development Goals (MDGs), by far the largest killer on the planet has continued to advance in low-income and middle-income countries. NCDs cause 60% of all global deaths but receive just 2.3% of international development assistance for health. Approximately 80% of deaths caused by NCDs occur in developing countries, generally in a younger population than those in high-income countries.[1,2] Over the next 10 years, the World Health Organization (WHO) predicts that NCD deaths will increase by 17% globally with the greatest increases in the African (27%) and the Eastern Mediterranean (25%) regions. In terms of the highest absolute number of deaths, the Western Pacific and South-East Asia are projected to lead the field.[3]

Noncommunicable diseases are a group of illnesses and include those conditions that have been identified as the leading causes of death around the world: heart disease, stroke, cancer, chronic respiratory diseases, and diabetes. These diseases are characterized by their long latency period often influenced by exposure to risk factors for extended periods over a patient's lifetime. The situation becomes more acute with the addition of the word "chronic," indicating that these diseases are mostly incurable and the duration of treatment may cover decades of a person's life.

Cardiovascular disease (mainly heart disease and stroke) is the biggest killer worldwide, contributing to 30% of global deaths each year.[1] The importance of such a high figure can be seen in the 47 countries that make up Latin America and the Caribbean, where cardiovascular disease alone accounts for 35% of the total mortality burden while AIDS, tuberculosis, malaria, and all other infectious diseases combined are responsible for only 10% of that burden.[4] Globally, chronic disease deaths have been predicted to increase by 17% between 2005 and 2015.[1] Although research on multimorbidity has been based primarily on high-income countries, experts estimate that around 50% of the population living with chronic disease may actually be living with multiple chronic conditions.[5]

Sometimes erroneously referred to as "lifestyle diseases," NCDs are affected by a variety of risk factors that are often outside the control of the individual. There is very little that can be done about some risk factors, such as age and genetic inheritance, and increasing evidence suggests that what happens before a person is born and during early childhood plays a key role in the onset of adult chronic disease, demonstrated by the proven association between low birth weight and increased rates of high blood pressure, heart disease, stroke, and diabetes.[6]

However, the most common chronic diseases share some of the same highly preventable or avoidable risk factors including physical inactivity, tobacco use, and obesity, leading researchers to study mortality for NCDs by risk factor. The WHO estimates that each year approximately 4.9 million people die from tobacco use, 2.6 million from being overweight or obese, 4.4 million as a result of raised cholesterol levels, and 7.1 million as a result of raised blood pressure.[1] Raised cholesterol and raised blood pressure (hypertension) are particularly dangerous risk factors because they can exist in an individual for a long time without presenting any obvious symptoms.

In its seminal book *Preventing Chronic Disease: A Vital Investment*, the WHO presents what it defines as effective and feasible interventions to reduce the threat of NCDs, with low-income and middle-income countries being specifically targeted.[1] The WHO seeks ideally to reduce the burden of NCD mortality by 2% per year through the implementation of the WHO Framework Convention on Tobacco Control (FCTC), which was the first global treaty negotiated by the WHO in 2003. As of 2010 it had been signed by 168 nations, although stages of ratification vary. The FCTC contains guidelines for implementing demand-reducing policies toward tobacco including health policies aimed at protecting the public with respect to commercial and other vested interests of the tobacco industry, protection from exposure to tobacco smoke, packaging and labeling of tobacco products; and limits or bans on tobacco advertising, promotion, and sponsorship.[7] Tax increases for tobacco control are considered to be clinically effective and very cost-effective relative to other health interventions,[8] while the implementation of smoking bans in public areas appears to reduce the risk of heart attacks significantly, particularly among younger individuals and nonsmokers, according to a study published in the *Journal of the American College of Cardiology* (September 29, 2009 issue). Researchers reported that smoking bans can reduce the number of heart attacks by as much as 26% per year.[9,10]

Policy level programs are also being discussed for reducing salt and sugared beverages[11,12] in the diet, consumer products, and food outlets. The WHO report also encourages screening for which there are clear public health benefits and cost benefit, and in situations in which the ability to treat the condition (such as raised blood pressure and cervical cancer) exists.[1] However, at present the quality and quantity of research investigating the actual benefits of different intervention programs to prevent noncommunicable diseases in developing countries is sparse and exists primarily as case studies.[1,11]

Low-income and middle-income countries have developed their health provision and policies according to a primary care or Alma Ata model, focused on meeting the needs of pregnant women and children younger than 5 years, and developing services for a variety of high-impact communicable diseases such as human immunodeficiency virus (HIV)/AIDS, tuberculosis, and malaria. The health systems in these countries are unprepared to deal with risk-factor education and behavior modification for the prevention, diagnosis, and treatment of NCDs, or the long-term management of these conditions. Despite growing interest among the population and health system leadership, one high-ranking health official pointed out that

> Currently, donor countries are operating a policy ban on funding NCDs, thereby starving low-income governments of the financial and technical assistance needed to turn around the NCD epidemic. This policy has to change, with overseas development assistance aligned to the priorities of recipient countries.[3]

This situation continues to be an issue for developing countries despite numerous calls for action in the area of NCDs and funding.[4,11,13–15] Furthermore, there is a clear inequity inherent in noncommunicable diseases, as the poor and less educated are more likely to be exposed to several preventable risk factors including tobacco use, high-fat and energy-dense food consumption, physical inactivity, and obesity.[16]

There is no denying that noncommunicable diseases are linked to economic loss, and the WHO highlighted this in 2005, predicting that national income loss due to heart disease, stroke, and diabetes for China, India, and the United Kingdom are expected to be $558 billion, $237 billion, and $33 billion, respectively, with part of the losses being the result of reduced economic productivity.[1]

The Global Burden of Disease (GBD) project began in 1990 and since then chronic diseases have exceeded the burden of infectious diseases.[17] Despite this, the international community has yet to display a sense of urgency toward reducing NCDs or supporting NCD-focused interventions in developing countries, even though they are threatening development and economic progress.[3] Perhaps the situation will change in the near future with the participation of United Nations (UN) member states in a high-level summit on noncommunicable diseases scheduled to take place in New York in September 2011.

Although nothing can be guaranteed, similar UN summits have provided the catalyst for change, as seen following the summit on HIV/AIDS in 2001 that resulted in significant funding and political commitment to a coordinated action plan.[3]

MENTAL HEALTH

Since 1946, the WHO has defined health as "a state of complete physical, mental and social well-being and not merely the absence of disease or infirmity."[18] However, mental illness and related conditions have never received the same importance or consideration as other areas of health despite their enormous burden on the population. This fact is exemplified by the routine exclusion of mental health services from Primary Health Care (PHC) and the absence of any mental health–related objectives in the MDGs.[19,20]

Mental illnesses, including behavioral, neurologic, and substance use disorders, affect a significant number of the world's population. In 2002, the WHO estimated that globally 154 million people suffered from depression, 25 million from schizophrenia, and 15 million from substance use disorders, with around 877,000 people committing suicide every year.[21] In the same year, unipolar depressive disorders were ranked as fourth in terms of burden of disease,[22] well on the way to prove the 1990 prediction of the GBD analysis that estimated mental illness, specifically unipolar major depression, would become the second leading cause of burden of disease by 2020, second only to ischemic heart disease.[17]

Studies in PHC settings in Turkey, the United Arab Emirates, France, Vietnam, and Zimbabwe revealed that the prevalence of mental illness ranges between 10% and 60% among adults,[23–30] with depression being the most common ranging from 5% to 20%, followed by generalized anxiety disorders (4%–15%) and dependency on addictive substances (5%–15%).[31–33]

Children are not immune to mental health problems, with those aged between 6 and 14 years exhibiting a prevalence of mental illness of between 20% and 30%,[34,35] the most common diagnoses being anxiety disorders, major depression, behavioral disorders, and attention-deficit/hyperactivity disorder.[28,35] Mental illness has an effect on other family members, which is seen clearly in a study looking at growth rates of children with mothers suffering from mental illness. The study showed that 20% of these children suffered from stunted growth, which could have been averted if interventions to treat the maternal depression had been performed.[28,35]

Individuals suffering from severe form of depression are at increased risk of attempting suicide,[36] as are women who experience abuse.[37] Meanwhile, the prevalence of mental health problems among elderly people is 33%, the majority of whom suffer from depression.[38,39]

Cost-effective treatment for most mental illnesses exists and, if correctly applied, most patients become functioning members of society, leading normal lives even in low-resource areas, and suicide risk is reduced.[40]

Of interest, poverty indicators are related to mental disorders[41–44] with low education level being the most influential determinant.[45] Extrapolating these data, it is feasible to suggest that developing countries with low education levels will tend to have a higher proportion of the population suffering from mental health problems. Despite this, however, most low-income and middle-income countries spend less than 1% of their health expenditure on mental health. Explicit mental health policy, legislation, mental health treatment facilities, and community care are all lacking.[21]

ACCIDENTS AND INJURIES

Injuries as a global health issue include many types that are routinely reported to and published by the WHO, such as poisoning, falls, drowning, burns, and intentional injuries including interpersonal violence such as elderly, partner, or child abuse, and collective violence such as war. However, two of the most important injuries that contribute to high global death rates are road traffic accidents and occupational injuries. In 2005, an estimated 9% of all global deaths were the result of an injury.[46] Injuries not only affect morbidity and mortality rates but also have a tremendous effect on the individual, the family, and the community. **Box 1** presents the scope of injuries and their importance as a national health issue.

Road Traffic Accidents

It is predicted that by 2030, road traffic injuries will be the fifth leading cause of death.[47] Already, approximately 1.3 million people die due to road traffic accidents each year, and an additional 20 to 50 million are injured or disabled.[47] Despite being home to fewer than 50% of the world's motor vehicles, low-income and middle-income countries have 90% of the mortality burden for road traffic accidents.[47] One

---

Box 1
Childhood injuries in Bangladesh

Injuries prove to be the largest killer of children between 1 and 17 years of age, accounting for 38% of all classifiable deaths. This means that 83 children per day die of injuries or 3 children per hour. The leading cause of injury-related deaths among children is drowning (59.3%) followed by road traffic accidents (12.3%), animal bites (9.3%), and suicide (8.0%). It is estimated that injuries permanently disable around 13,000 children per year in Bangladesh. Nonfatal injuries occur in approximately 1 million children per year or 2 per minute (Institute of Child and Mother Health, 2005). When injury-related deaths are broken down by type and by age group, children aged 1–4 and 5–9 years are most likely to die from drowning with a mortality rate of 86 per 100,000 and 26 per 100,000 child deaths, respectively. In the 10–14-year age group, road traffic accidents account for 8 per 100,000 child deaths, and in the 15–17-year age group, suicide accounts for 24 per 100,000 child deaths.

of the most important reasons for this apparent discrepancy is the high number of vulnerable road users in developing countries. Vulnerable road users include pedestrians, cyclists, and both the rider and passenger of motorcycles and scooters. Vulnerable road users account for 46% of deaths, and in low-income countries pedestrians account for nearly half of all road accident–related deaths.[48]

There are proven interventions that can lead to a reduction in the amount of road traffic deaths and injuries. Such measures include controlling or reducing the speed of traffic with speed bumps or low-speed zones in urban areas, establishing and enforcing blood alcohol concentration limits, enforcing the use of helmets for both riders and passengers on motorcycles, and enforcing the use of seat belts, infant seats, and child booster seats.[47] The wearing of seatbelts in automobiles can reduce front-seat passenger deaths by 40% to 65% and rear-seat passenger deaths by 25% to 75%; however, only 57% of countries require the wearing of seat belts by all passengers.[47] The problem is that because of the high numbers of both people and different types of vehicles in developing countries and the lack of resources to police traffic effectively, traffic laws are not easily enforced, despite evidence showing the benefit of specific interventions in the reduction of traffic-related morbidity and mortality.[49]

Occupational Injuries

Occupational injuries are a significant problem in global public health, contributing to between 312,000 and 334,000 deaths worldwide each year. With great shifts in industrialization from the developed to the developing countries, it is logical that the highest number of occupational injuries is shifting in the same way toward the developing world. However, it is very likely that published figures are underestimated, with numbers probably being 10% below the actual figure for the United States and as much as 85% for some locations such as rural Africa.[50,51] Although several factors come into play when analyzing the causes of underreporting in developing countries, one of the main reasons is the lack of adequate data.[52]

Determining the actual prevalence of occupational injury is critical for several reasons: (1) to provide accurate data to health providers, policy makers, nongovernmental organizations (NGOs), and the public; (2) to provide baseline data against which to measure interventions; (3) to aid priority setting and targeting for policy change and interventions; and (4) to estimate societal costs of rising occupational injuries. Tools to capture occupational injury have been designed and widely circulated by the UN's specialized agency, the International Labour Organization. However, field testing of the tools has been limited to small-scale surveys in diverse settings such as Vietnam, Ghana, and Bangladesh,[53–56] and larger, nationally representative studies are needed.

In many developing countries, there is a lack of policy for or enforcement of safe working environments, which naturally means that wood cutting, mining, agriculture, construction, and manufacturing are more hazardous than in developed countries. The developed world has accepted that poor working conditions and practices are unacceptable and has legislated against them, leading to a reduction in occupational injuries over the past century. However, it seems that globally the same care has not been forthcoming, and developing countries have taken on the burden of heavy industry and poor working conditions that generate increases in occupational injuries. This trend is perfectly exemplified by the phrase "export of hazard" to describe when an outdated and dangerous technology is relocated from a high-income country to a developing country, despite the knowledge that the risk of injury with this technology is high.[57]

Cost of production plays a key role in maintaining poor working conditions, and many industries in developing countries manage cost control through the use of manual labor, which is cheaper than the infrastructure and equipment needed to upgrade a process that produces the same amount of product at a much safer level. Manual labor is particularly exploited in the construction industry in developing countries, which have a disproportionate number of deaths from workers falling and injuries from falling objects. Working conditions at all levels of commerce are also full of risk factors to health, from the lack of ergonomically designed offices to avoid back injuries and repetitive stress disorders, to building materials used in construction, which may offer a long-term risk of health problems. The latter is of particular concern in many low-income and middle-income countries, with construction still making use of asbestos despite the documented links to lung cancer.[58,59]

URBANIZATION

Urbanization is a major public health challenge for the twenty-first century, with significant changes in our living standards, lifestyles, social behavior, and health. Previously more of a phenomenon in developed countries; it is now taking hold and being seen at a greater level in developing countries.[60] The United Nations Population Fund (UNFPA) predicts that over the next 2 to 3 decades, almost all the world's population growth will be in urban areas in developing countries.[61] WHO figures for the period 1995 to 2005 already show an alarming increase in urban population growth, with developing countries' urban areas growing at an average of 1.2 million people per week or around 165,000 people every day.[60]

While urban settings offer many opportunities including access to better health care, they can affect existing health risks and introduce new health hazards. The living and working conditions of those living in rapidly expanding and poorly planned urban areas often experience risks to health in some of the most basic areas such as unsafe drinking water, unsanitary conditions, poor housing, overcrowding, hazardous locations, and exposure to extremes of temperature. These increases in health risks are particularly critical for those most vulnerable: children younger than 5 years, infants, and the elderly.[60,62]

The rapid growth of urban settlements is often due to poor economic performance of the area in question and lack of urban planning and regulation, which has resulted in an increase in the number and size of informal settlements or slums in many cities. It is estimated that in the developing regions, more than 70% of urban residents live in slums.[61]

The Urban Health Situation

The current pattern of urban growth is expected to have a multiplier effect on many dimensions of illness and disease. Child mortality is already high in the urban areas of developing regions. In Nairobi, where 60% of the city's population lives in slums, child mortality in these slums is 2.5 times greater than in other areas of the city.[63] Evidence from various surveys and studies points to a heavier burden of diseases such as diarrheal diseases, acute respiratory diseases, malnutrition among children, HIV/AIDS, tuberculosis, malaria, diabetes, and obesity on the urban poor.[60,61,64]

Migration, increased mobility, changes in the ecology of urban environment, high population density, poor housing, and poor provision of basic services all act as pathways for emerging and reemerging communicable diseases.[61,62] The consequence of these changes is evident in the spread of multidrug-resistant strains of tuberculosis that is placing the urban poor of India, Indonesia, Myanmar, and Nepal at a higher risk. Vector-borne diseases such as dengue and malaria are also increasing in many urban areas, due to migration, climate change, stagnant water, insufficient drainage, flooding, and improper disposal of solid waste.[61,62]

Unhealthy lifestyles characterized by unhealthy nutrition, reduced physical activity, and tobacco consumption due to rapid and unplanned urbanization are associated with common modifiable risk factors for chronic diseases such as hypertension, diabetes mellitus, and obesity.[60] Urban environments tend to discourage physical activity and promote unhealthy food consumption. Overcrowding, heavy use of motorized transport, poor air quality, and lack of safe public spaces are some urban factors that restrict participation in physical activities. In the larger populated cities of Asia obesity is becoming a significant problem, and the rapid transition of diets in developing countries is typified by the coexistence of child malnutrition and maternal obesity in the same household. One of the main factors identified as causing an increase in diabetes worldwide is the change in traditional diets caused by urbanization.[65]

Urbanization is exacerbating the health risks in terms of traffic accidents, injuries on the street or in the home, and mental health problems. The changes in climate and rising sea levels work toward increasing urbanization, with 600 million people living in the low-elevation coastal zones being at heightened risk of flooding, which will lead to migration to higher elevations and larger cities.[61]

Adopting preventive measures to control communicable diseases, upgrading the infrastructure of existing health facilities, increasing human resource capacity, and taking appropriate measures for providing equitable health services to all, especially the most vulnerable groups, are vital for improving urban health. Recently, the WHO identified 5 key areas of action for improving urban health:

1. Promote urban planning for healthy behaviors and safety
2. Improve urban living conditions, including access to adequate shelter and sanitation for all
3. Involve communities in local decision making
4. Ensure cities are accessible and age-friendly
5. Make urban areas resilient to emergencies and disasters.[60]

However, these actions will only be effective if there is strong collaboration between health authorities, urban planning agencies, environmental agencies, energy providers, and the transportation systems.

CLIMATE CHANGE

Climate change is an emerging threat to global public health. It is now widely accepted that climate change is occurring as a result of emission of greenhouse gases, especially from fossil-fuel combustion.[66] Climate change is predicted to affect many natural systems and habitats, for example, increasing the frequency and intensity of heat waves, increasing the number of floods and droughts, altering the geographic range and seasonality of certain infectious diseases, and disturbing food-producing ecosystems,[67] which in turn will affect human health both directly and indirectly. Direct health effects include changes in mortality and morbidity, and changes in respiratory diseases from heat waves. In terms of indirect health effects, these are much more extensive and include changes in the distribution of vector-borne diseases, the nutritional and health consequences of regional changes in agricultural productivity, and the various consequences of rising sea levels, flooding, and droughts.[66–68]

Climate change is highly inequitable, and the paradox is that those at greatest risk are the poorest populations in developing countries who have contributed least to greenhouse gas emissions. However, the rapid economic development and concurrent pollution means that developing countries are now vulnerable to adverse health effects from climate change and, simultaneously, are becoming an increasing contributor to the problem.[67,69]

Although the effects of climate change affect all levels and ages of any single population, the elderly and those with preexisting medical conditions are seen as being the most vulnerable. Conversely, major diseases that are most sensitive to climate change such as diarrhea, malaria, and infection associated with malnutrition are most serious in children living in poverty, making them highly vulnerable to the resulting disease burden.[67]

Heat waves are expected to increase the occurrence of heat-related illnesses such as heat exhaustion and heat stroke, and aggravate existing conditions related to circulatory, respiratory, and nervous system problems, especially among the elderly.[67,68] In 2003, a major heat wave affected most of Western Europe and caused 2000 additional deaths in England and Wales.[68] Another consequence of high temperatures is that they raise the levels of ozone and other air pollutants, which in turn aggravate respiratory diseases such as asthma.

Meanwhile, health impacts due to natural disasters, such as floods, droughts, and storms, range from immediate effects that include physical injury, mortality and morbidity, and communicable diseases, to possible long-term effects such as malnutrition and mental health disorders. From 1992 to 2001, flooding was the most frequent natural disaster (43%), killing almost 100,000 people and affecting over 1.2 billion people worldwide.[70] Droughts increase the risk of food shortages and malnutrition, and increase the risk of diseases spread by contaminated food and water, because viral load increases in water sources when levels drop dramatically.

Rising temperatures, irregular rainfall patterns, and increasing humidity affect the transmission of many vector-borne and water-borne diseases such as malaria, dengue, cholera, and other diarrheal diseases. Vector-borne diseases currently kill approximately 1.1 million people each year while 2.2 million die from diarrheal diseases.[71] Studies suggest that by 2030, climate change may put 170 million people in Africa at risk of malaria,[67,72] and by the 2080s the global population at risk of dengue is likely to increase to 2 billion.[67,73] Recent published data provides evidence of an association between the El Niño and La Niña phenomena, which are major determinants of global weather patterns, and some infectious diseases. Evidence shows that there is an association between El Niño and malaria epidemics in parts of South Asia and South America, and with cholera in coastal areas of Bangladesh.[68,74] Studies of malaria have already revealed the health impacts of climate variability associated with El Niño, including large epidemics on the Indian subcontinent, Colombia, Venezuela, and Uganda.[75]

One of the most immediate problems related to changes in climate and climate patterns is that on food production and availability. Each year approximately 3.5 million people, mostly children from developing countries, die from malnutrition and related diseases. It is projected that climate change will decrease agricultural production in many tropical developing regions, thus putting tens of millions more people at risk of food insecurity and adverse health consequences of malnutrition.[67] Disasters in certain areas of high food production will also affect global prices, thereby affecting not only those people living in the affected region but others around the world who depend on food produced from that region.

The WHO GBD study in 1990 indicated that the climatic changes that have occurred since the mid-1970s would be having an effect by the year 2000, with 150,000 deaths (0.3% deaths globally each year) and 5.5 million lost disability-adjusted life years

(DALYs) per year (0.4% global DALYs lost per year). The estimated effects are predicted to be most severe in those regions that already have the greatest disease burden of climate-sensitive health outcomes, such as malnutrition, diarrhea, and malaria.[17,67,71]

Many of the projected impacts on health are avoidable, and public health policy makers need to act to reduce or negate the impact caused by climate change through a combination of short-term public health interventions that aim to adapt measures in health-related sectors, such as agriculture and water management, and long-term strategy. The most effective responses are likely to be strengthening of the key functions of environmental management, surveillance and response to protect health from natural disasters and changes in infectious disease patterns, and strengthening of the existing public health systems.[67,68] However, countries need to assess their main health vulnerabilities and prioritize adoptive action accordingly, keeping in mind the costs involved.

COMPLEX DISASTER PREPAREDNESS AND RESPONSE

Natural disasters know no boundaries, and any nation or population can be subject to a catastrophic disaster at any time. However, some nations and populations are more at risk of disasters than others due to geographic location, poverty, and several sociopolitical factors. This issue of disaster risk reduction (DRR) rose to global prominence in the aftermath of the tsunami in the Indian Ocean in December 2004.

Following a disaster, some populations suffer more acutely than others. It is worth considering the complex issues of how societies organize themselves in terms of risk and actual prevention and care, for access to clean water and sanitation, and how they communicate and initiate behavioral change among the displaced or fragile populations. At the forefront of most discussions when planning post-disaster management and action is the priority placed on certain elements of disaster relief, such as the building of embankments, the distance to clean water, or the time from incident to response. Recent examples of varying responses and outcomes were seen following the two cyclones in South Asia. There was a relative success in Bangladesh in terms of lives saved and response coordination after Cyclone Sidr in November 2007, compared with the devastating loss of more than 100,000 lives after Cyclone Nargis in Myanmar in May 2008, not to mention the loss of draft animals and dykes, and the flooding of fields during planting season.[76] Bangladesh reverted to its well-developed program for DRR that includes national-level coordination, whereas in Myanmar there was no national platform for disaster preparedness, and delays occurred in the coordination of international response to the disaster. In addition to the immediate and obvious impact of natural disasters, conditions often worsen in poorly coordinated settings, as evidenced in 2010 when *Vibrio cholerae* emerged in post-flood Pakistan, and for the first time since the 1960s in post-earthquake Haiti.[77]

In general, there are 7 factors that can turn a natural disaster into a complex disaster regardless of the severity or magnitude of the initiating event such as a hurricane, earthquake, or tsunami. According to the UN Department of Humanitarian Affairs, the 7 factors are: poverty, ungoverned population growth, rapid urbanization and migration, transitional cultural practices, environmental degradation, lack of awareness and information, and war and civil strife.[78]

Poverty is by far the single greatest factor that contributes to the vulnerability of a population to complex disasters. In addition to lacking financial resources to prepare for or recover from a disaster, impoverished people are also more likely to have low levels of education and low amounts of political influence to properly deal with a disaster situation. In addition to increases in birth rates, rapid population growth can be the consequence of urbanization or migration. Population growth without limits produces a population that is more likely to settle in areas that are unsuitable or at risk for natural disasters, meaning that more people are at risk of disease and, most importantly, are more likely to undergo civil strife while competing for scarce resources.

As mentioned previously, rapid urbanization and migration lead to impoverishment. Former rural populations make themselves more vulnerable to disaster by settling in less developed or high-risk city environs, often leading to homelessness or living in urban slums that have circumvented any planning controls or regulations. Such populations therefore are made more vulnerable to floods, landslides, and the destruction of their dwelling during a hurricane or earthquake.

Transition of cultural, economic, or government practices such as the increase in migration from rural to urban areas, economic advancements, families moving away from traditional support networks and to unfamiliar surroundings, and the shift from an agrarian to an industrialized society leave certain societies vulnerable to natural disasters.

Environmental degradation can play a role by either causing or exacerbating a disaster. For example, deforestation can work in two ways: firstly enabling runoff or secondly, making landscapes vulnerable to storms, due to lack of natural wind breaks. Everyone is aware of the natural conditions that provoke droughts, but through the construction of dams, unchecked urbanization, implementation of poor cropping patterns, and the depletion of water supplies, man-made droughts are becoming more widespread.

It is clearly of upmost importance to ensure that populations are informed about what to do to prepare in advance of a natural disaster such as a hurricane, and also are able to fend for themselves following the event. A lack of awareness and the dissemination of accurate information is a major factor that can turn one disaster into a multiple or complex disaster involving, for example, subsequent outbreaks of cholera, malnutrition, and physical injury.

War and civil strife are extreme events that can both produce disasters or be caused by disasters, normally as a result of the preceding 6 factors.[78] The phrase for disasters that specifically strike war-torn populations is Complex Humanitarian Emergencies.[79]

Global efforts to address and capture the importance of disaster risk and poverty have been hampered by a lack of data, especially from Asia, Latin America, and the Caribbean. Empirical evidence linking disaster risk to poverty tends to come from microstudies within one community, making it impossible to generate generalized findings across regions or entire countries.[80]

Prompted by the devastation that followed the tsunami on 26 December, 2004, there was widespread acceptance that an early-warning system should be installed and other actions taken to prevent loss of life where possible. The World Conference on Disaster Reduction was held in Japan in January 2005, and resulted in the creation of the Hyogo Framework for Action 2005-2015 (HFA), which was endorsed by 168 UN member states and urges all countries to make major efforts to reduce their disaster risk by 2015. The HFA outlines the need to increase awareness and understanding about DRR, the importance of knowing the real and potential risks, and taking action against them. Specific recommendations included the need to create or enhance early-warning systems, build DRR into education, and reduce risk factors such as deforestation, unstable housing, and the location of communities in risk-prone areas.

Although different areas of the planet experience different risks, the one common factor is that DRR "concerns everyone, from villagers to heads of state, from bankers and lawyers to farmers and foresters, from meteorologists to media chiefs."[81] To support common needs within regions, associations and networks have been established to support DRR, such as the South Asian SAARC Disaster Management Center and the Caribbean Disaster Emergency Response Agency.

Types of activities that can feature in a national or regional DRR program can include: establishing early-warning systems; using local knowledge of events; building an awareness of risk and risk preparedness through community activities; building flood-resistant buildings and safe homes; developing contingency plans; helping communities and individuals develop alternative sources of income; and establishing insurance or microfinance programs to help transfer the risk of loss and provide additional resources to the community.[82]

SUMMARY

In addition to chronic diseases, mental health problems, injuries, and complex disasters, communities should consider increasing risks from more than 30 new or reemerging diseases that have appeared since the 1970s: liver disease due to the hepatitis C virus; Lyme disease; food-borne illnesses caused by *Escherichia coli* O157:H7; *Cyclospora*, a water-borne disease caused by *Cryptosporidium*; hantavirus pulmonary syndrome; and human disease caused by the avian H5N1 influenza virus.[83] The increasing number of new and reemerging diseases is not the only risk factor that should be added to the planning processes for developing a DRR program. Drug resistance in treating many diseases and illnesses is a major concern, as witnessed in malaria and tuberculosis, and with a highly mobile world population, global pandemics such as SARS, H5N1, and H1N1, for which treatments either are not available or levels of suitable drug are clearly not sufficient for a worldwide epidemic, are proving to be very challenging. This clear inability to predict and maintain sufficient levels of treatment for potential threats makes health risk reduction extremely difficult, and in developing countries where resources are already stretched to cope with existing health issues, creating effective programs will require intervention from social partners, global support organizations, and aid from the developed world. An ever quickening pace of globalization means that public health–related problems in one area of the world will have an impact on those living in another area and therefore, it is in everyone's interest to ensure that all countries, irrespective of their economic development and available resources, are sufficiently supported to maintain and review strategies that will effectively reduce morbidity and mortality rates in all spheres of public health.

REFERENCES

1. World Health Organization [WHO]. Preventing chronic diseases: a vital investment. Geneva (Switzerland): WHO; 2005.
2. Leeder S, Raymond S, Greenberg H, et al. A race against time: the challenge of cardiovascular disease in developing economies. New York: Columbia University; 2004.
3. Non-communicable Disease Alliance. Non-communicable diseases: time to pay attention to the silent killer. Press release. 2010 6 December, Available at: http://www.ncdalliance.org/node/3231. Accessed December 10, 2010.
4. Anderson G. Missing in action: international aid agencies in poor countries to fight chronic disease. Health Aff (Millwood) 2009;28(1):202–5.
5. Jadad A, Cabrera A, Lyons R, et al. When people live with multiple chronic diseases: a collaborative approach to an emerging global challenge. Granada (Spain): Andalusian School of Public Health; 2010.

6. Barker DJ. The developmental origins of chronic adult disease. Acta Paediatr Suppl 2004;93:26–33.
7. World Health Organization Framework Convention on Tobacco Control [WHO FCTC]. Guidelines for implementation. Geneva (Switzerland). 2009. Available at: http://www.who.int/fctc/guidelines/en/. Accessed December 10, 2010.
8. Ranson MK, Jha P, Chaloupka C, et al. Global and regional estimates of the effectiveness and cost-effectiveness of price increases and other tobacco control policies. Nicotine Tob Res 2002;4:311–9.
9. Meyers DG, Neuberger JS, He J. Cardiovascular effect of bans on smoking in public places: a systematic review and meta-analysis. J Am Coll Cardiol 2009; 54(14):1249–55.
10. Schroeder SA. Public smoking bans are good for the heart. J Am Coll Cardiol 2009;54(14):1256–7.
11. Ebrahim S. Chronic diseases and calls to action. Int J Epidemiol 2008;37:225–30.
12. Brownell K, Frieden T. Ounces of prevention—the public policy case for taxes on sugared beverages. N Engl J Med 2009;360(18):1805–8.
13. Horton R. The neglected epidemic of chronic disease. Lancet 2005;366:1514.
14. Horton R. Chronic diseases: the case for urgent global action. Lancet 2007;370: 1881–2.
15. Daar AS, Singer PA, Persad DL, et al. Grand challenges in chronic noncommunicable diseases. Nature 2007;450:494–6.
16. Bartley M, Fitzpatrick R, Firth D, et al. Social distribution of cardiovascular disease risk factors: change among men in England 1984–1993. J Epidemiol Community Health 2000;54:806–14.
17. Murray C, Lopez A, editors. The global burden of disease: a comprehensive assessment of mortality and disability from disease, injuries, and risk factors in 1990 and projected to 2020. Cambridge (MA): Harvard University Press; 1996.
18. World Health Organization. Preamble to the Constitution of the World Health Organization as adopted by the International Health Conference. New York, June 19–22, 1946. (Official Records of the World Health Organization, no. 2. p. 100).
19. Prince PM, Patel PV, Saxena S, et al. No health without mental health. Lancet 2007;370(9590):859–77.
20. UNDP. The millennium development goals report 2009. UNDP; 2010 [updated 2010; cited 2010 01/01/2010]; Available at: http://www.un.org/millenniumgoals/pdf/MDG_Report_2009_ENG.pdf. Accessed December 12, 2010.
21. WHO. Mental health. World Health Organization; 2010 [updated 2010; cited 2009 12/12/2009]; Available at: http://www.who.int/mental_health/en/. Accessed December 12, 2010.
22. Mathers CD, Loncar D. Projections of global mortality and burden of disease from 2002 to 2030. PLoS Med 2006;3(11):2011–30.
23. Danaci AE, Dinç G, Deveci A, et al. Postnatal depression in Turkey: epidemiological and cultural aspects. Soc Psychiatry Psychiatr Epidemiol 2002;37(3):125–9.
24. Patel V, Todd C, Winston M, et al. Outcome of common mental disorders in Harare, Zimbabwe. Br J Psychiatry 1998;172(1):53–7.
25. Birchall H, Brandon S, Taub N. Panic in a general practice population: prevalence, psychiatric comorbidity and associated disability. Soc Psychiatry Psychiatr Epidemiol 2000;35(6):235–41.
26. Araya R. Trastornos mentales en la práctica médica general [Mental disorders in general medical practice]. Santiago (Chile): Saval; 1995.
27. Norton J, Roquefeuil GD, Benjamins A, et al. Psychiatric morbidity, disability and service use amongst primary care attenders in France. Eur Psychiatry 2004;19(3):164–7.

28. Eapen V, Al-Sabosy M, Saeed M, et al. Child psychiatric disorders in a primary care Arab population. Int J Psychiatry Med 2004;34(1):51–60.
29. Eapen VM, Al-Gazali LF, Bin-Othman SM, et al. Mental health problems among schoolchildren in United Arab Emirates: prevalence and risk factors. J Am Acad Child Adolesc Psychiatry 1998;37(8):880–6.
30. Giang KB, Dzung TV, Kullgren G, et al. Prevalence of mental distress and use of health services in a rural district in Vietnam. Global Health Action. 3: 2025. DOI: 10.3402/gha.v3i0.2025. Available at: http://www.globalhealthaction.net/index.php/gha/article/viewArticle/2025. Accessed December 14, 2010.
31. Rucci P, Gherardi S, Tansella M, et al. Subthreshold psychiatric disorders in primary care: prevalence and associated characteristics. J Affect Disord 2003; 76(1–3):171–81.
32. Aragonès E, Piñol J, Labad A, et al. Prevalence and determinants of depressive disorders in primary care practice in Spain. Int J Psychiatry Med 2004;34(1):21–35.
33. Olfson M, Shea S, Feder A, et al. Prevalence of anxiety, depression, and substance use disorders in an urban general medicine practice. Arch Fam Med 2000;9(9):876–83.
34. Pedreira MJ, Sardinero GE. Prevalence of mental disorders in childhood in pediatric primary care. Actas Luso Esp Neurol Psiquiatr Cienc Afines 1996;24(4): 173–90.
35. Gureje O, Omigbodun OO, Gater R, et al. Psychiatric disorders in a paediatric primary care clinic. Br J Psychiatry 1994;165(4):527–30.
36. Mullick M, Karim M, Khanam M. Depression in deliberate self harm patients. Bangladesh Med Res Counc Bull 1994;20(3):128.
37. Naved R, Rimi N, Jahan S, et al. Paramedic conducted mental health counselling for abused women in rural Bangladesh: an evaluation from the perspective of participants. J Health Popul Nutr 2009;27:477–91.
38. Olafsdóttir M, Marcusson J, Skoog I. Mental disorders among elderly people in primary care: the Linköping study. Acta Psychiatr Scand 2001;104(1):12–8.
39. Almeida O, Forlenza O, Lima N, et al. Psychiatric morbidity among the elderly in a primary care setting—report from a survey in São Paulo, Brazil. Int J Geriatr Psychiatry 1997;12(7):728–36.
40. Hamid M, Munib A, Ahmed S. Psychiatric morbidity in cancer patients. Bangladesh Med Res Counc Bull 1993;19(1):15–20.
41. Wilton RD. Poverty and mental health: a qualitative study of residential care facility tenants. Community Ment Health J 2004;39(2):139–56.
42. Laughame J. Poverty and mental health in Aboriginal Australia. Psychiatr Bull 1999;23:364–6.
43. Ludermir AB, Lewis G. Links between social class and common mental disorders in Northeast Brazil. Soc Psychiatry Psychiatr Epidemiol 2001;36(3):101–7.
44. Ssanyu R. Mental illness and exclusion: putting mental health on the development agenda in Uganda. Journal [serial on the Internet]. 2007 Date: Available at: http://www.chronicpoverty.org/pubfiles/CPRC-UG_PolicyBrief2(2007).pdf. Accessed December 12, 2010.
45. Patel V, Kleinman A. Poverty and common mental disorders in developing countries. Bull World Health Organ 2003;81:609–15.
46. Strong K, Mathers C, Leeder S, et al. Preventing chronic disease: how many lives can we save? Lancet 2005;366:1578–82.
47. World Health Organization [WHO]. Ten facts on global road safety. Fact File 2009. Available at: http://www.who.int/features/factfiles/roadsafety/facts/en/index.html. Accessed December 14, 2010.

48. Naci H, Chisholm D, Baker TD. Distribution of road traffic deaths by road user group: a global comparison. Inj Prev 2009;15(1):55–9.
49. Sharma BR. Road traffic injuries: a major global public health crisis. Public Health 2008;122(12):1399–406.
50. Concha-Barrientos M, Nelson DI, Fingerhut M, et al. The global burden due to occupational injury. Am J Ind Med 2005;48:470–81.
51. Takala J. Introductory Report: decent work—safe work. XVIIth World Congress on Safety and Health at Work, 2005. Geneva (Switzerland): International Labour Organization; 2005.
52. Eijkemans GJ, Takala J. Moving knowledge of global burden into preventive action. Am J Ind Med 2005;48:395–9.
53. Taswell K, Wingfield-Digby P. Occupational injuries statistics from household and establishment surveys: an ILO manual. Geneva (Switzerland): International Labour Organization; 2008.
54. Mock C, Adjei S, Acheampong F, et al. Occupational injuries in Ghana. Int J Occup Environ Health 2005;11(3):238–45.
55. Phung DT, Nguyen HT, Mock C, et al. Occupational injuries reported in a population-based injury survey in Vietnam. Int J Occup Environ Health 2008;14(1):35–44. Prevention Web. Myanmar, Available at: http://www.preventionweb.net/english/countries/asia/mmr/?x=14&y=10. Accessed January 3, 2010.
56. Davies HW, Koehlmoos T, Courtice M, et al. Occupational Injury in Rural Bangladesh: Data Gathering using Household Survey. Int J Occup Environ Health 2011;17(3):214–22.
57. LaDou J, Jeyaratnam J. Transfer of hazardous industries: issue and solutions. In: Jeyaratnam J, Chia KS, editors. Occupational health in national development. Singapore: World Scientific Publishing Co Pte Ltd; 1994. p. 227–44.
58. Feachem R, Kjellstrom T, Murray CJ, et al. The health of adults in the developing world. Oxford (England): Oxford University Press; 1992.
59. Kazan-Allen L. The asbestos war. Int J Occup Environ Health 2003;9:173–93.
60. World Health Organization. Urbanization and health. Bull World Health Organ 2010;88:245–6.
61. World Health Organization. Our cities, our health, our future: Acting on social determinants for health equity in urban settings. Kobe (Japan): WHO Centre for Health Development; 2008.
62. Godfrey R, Julien M. Urbanization and health. Clin Med 2005;5(2):137–41.
63. McMichael AJ, McKee M, Shkolnikov V, et al. Mortality trends and setbacks: global convergence or divergence? Lancet 2004;363:1155–9.
64. Campbell T, Campbell A. Emerging disease burdens and the poor in cities of the developing world. J Urban Health 2007;84(1):i54–63.
65. World Health Organization. Diet, nutrition and the prevention of chronic diseases. Report of a joint WHO/FAO expert consultation. WHO Technical Report Series, No. 916. Geneva (Switzerland): World Health Organization; 2003.
66. McMichael AJ, Haines A. Global climate change: the potential effects on health. BMJ 1997;315:805.
67. World Health Organization [WHO]. Protecting health from climate change: connecting science, policy and people. Geneva (Switzerland): World Health Organization; 2009.
68. Haines A, Kovatsa RS, Campbell-Lendrumb D, et al. Climate change and human health: impacts, vulnerability and public health. Public Health 2006;120:585–96.
69. Campbell-Lendrum D, Corvalàn C. Climate change and developing-country cities: implications for environmental health and equity. J Urban Health 2007;84(1):i109–17.

70. McMichael AJ, Woodruff RE, Hales S. Climate change and human health: present and future risks. Lancet 2006;367:859–69.
71. World Health Organization [WHO]. The global burden of disease: 2004 update. Geneva (Switzerland): World Health Organization; 2008.
72. Hay SI, Tatem AJ, Guerra CA, et al. Foresight on population at malaria risk in Africa: 2005, 2015 and 2030. Scenario review paper prepared for the Detection and Identification of Infectious Diseases Project (DIID), Foresight Project, Office of Science and Innovation, London, UK, 2006. Available at: http://www.foresight.gov.uk/Detection_and_Identification_of_Infectious_Diseases/Reports_and_Publications/Final_Reports/T/T8_2.pdf). Accessed January 5, 2011.
73. Hales S, de Wet N, Maindonald J, et al. Potential effect of population and climate changes on global distribution of dengue fever: an empirical model. Lancet 2002; 360:830–4.
74. Kovats S, Bouma MJ, Hajat S, et al. El Nino and health. Lancet 2003;361:1481–9.
75. Patz JA, Campbell-Lendrum D, Holloway T, et al. Impact of regional climate change on human health. Nature 2005;438:310–7.
76. BBC News 2010. Burma death toll jumps to 78,000. Available at: http://news.bbc.co.uk/1/hi/world/asia-pacific/7405260.stm. Accessed November 4, 2010.
77. Rottman S 2010. Haiti cholera outbreak causes not clear, experts say. Available at: http://www.bbc.co.uk/news/world-latin-america-11618352. Accessed October 25, 2010.
78. United Nations, Department of Humanitarian Affairs [UN-DHA] The use of military and civil defence assets in relief operations. MCDA Reference Manual. 1995. Available at: www.Reliefweb.int. Accessed December1, 2010.
79. Burkholder B, Toole M. Evolution of complex disasters. Lancet 1995;346:1012–5.
80. United Nations-International Strategy for Disaster Reduction [UN-ISDR]. Global assessment report on disaster risk reduction. Geneva (Switzerland): United Nations; 2009.
81. United Nations- International Strategy for Disaster Reduction [UN-ISDR] Living with Risk. A global review of disaster reduction initiatives 2004. Geneva (Switzerland): UN/ISDR; 2004.
82. Development Research Network. Disaster risk management and climate change adaptation in South Asia. Dhaka: Portfolion; 2010. Issue 3.
83. Fauci A. New and reemerging diseases: the importance of biomedical research. Emerg Infect Dis 1998;4(3):374–8. Available at: http://www.cdc.gov/ncidod/EID/vol4no3/fauci.htm. Accessed November 30, 2010.

Global Health: Neglected Diseases and Access to Medicines

Nisha Jain Garg, PhD[a]

KEYWORDS

• Neglected diseases • Public health • Therapeutics • Vaccines

Neglected tropical diseases (NTDs) share several common features, the most profound being that the affected population is ravaged by poverty. These ancient diseases are endemic in Africa, Asia, and the Americas,[1] and are believed to cause the death of a million people annually. The major impact of NTDs on public health stems from chronic conditions that result in disfigurement, and lifelong disability and morbidity, afflicting the lives of more than a billion people worldwide.[2,3] Despite NTDs being coendemic with AIDS and malaria, and morbidity resulting from NTDs being additive to morbidity inflicted by human immunodeficiency virus (HIV), malaria, and tuberculosis,[2] and impeding the realization of the Millennium Development Goals,[4,5] NTDs, are recognized as other diseases by the developed economies. This recognition is shown by NTDs receiving less than 1% of the more than 7.7 billion US dollars spent by the G8 summit, Bill & Melinda Gates Foundation, Global Funds, and PEPFAR and PMI initiatives on HIV/AIDS, malaria, and tuberculosis.[6]

No safe, single-dose, or approved vaccines are available for control of NTDs.[7] The World Health Organization (WHO) recommends a 5-prong approach against NTDs, including preventive chemotherapy; intensified case management; vector control; the provision of safe water, sanitation, and hygiene; and veterinary public health.[8] This 5-prong strategy is based on scientific evidence and targets control and prevention of NTDs and even elimination of several NTDs. Evidence suggests that effective

The work in NJG's laboratory has been supported in part by grants from the American Heart Association, John Sealy Memorial Endowment Fund for Biomedical Research, American Health Assistance Foundation, and the National Institutes of Health.
Conflict of interest: The author has nothing to disclose.
[a] Department of Microbiology & Immunology, Center for Tropical Diseases, Sealy Center for Vaccine Development, Institute for Human Infections and Immunity, The University of Texas Medical Branch, Galveston, 3.142C Medical Research Building, 301 University Boulevard, Galveston, TX 77555-1070, USA
E-mail address: nigarg@utmb.edu

Infect Dis Clin N Am 25 (2011) 639–651
doi:10.1016/j.idc.2011.05.007
0891-5520/11/$ – see front matter © 2011 Elsevier Inc. All rights reserved.

id.theclinics.com

control is achieved when all 5 components are combined and delivered locally by intersectoral collaboration involving mass drug administration (MDA), education, nutrition, and agriculture.[9,10] However, most efforts to date have focused on preventive chemotherapy, partly because partnerships with the pharmaceutical industry and subsequent donations made to support control of NTDs have increased access, free of charge, to high-quality medicines. For example, unlimited supplies have been made available of albendazole from GlaxoSmithKline for control of lymphatic filariasis (LF),[11] ivermectin from Merck for control of LF and onchocerciasis,[11,12] and azithromycin from Pfizer for control of trachoma.[13] Likewise, available or soon to be provided are multidrug therapy (rifampicin, clofazimine, and dapsone) and clofazimine (all from Novartis) for control of leprosy,[14] and melarsoprol, pentamidine eflornithine (all from Sanofi-Aventis),[15] and suramin (Bayer) for control of Trypanosoma brucei–mediated sleeping sickness.[1] Large commitments have also been made by other pharmaceutical companies to provide drugs free of charge to the WHO.[1] For example, a donation of 50 million tablets per year of mebendazole by Johnson & Johnson for control of soil-transmitted helminthes (STH) in children will be increased to 200 million tablets annually from 2011. Bayer has committed 0.9 million tablets of nifurtimox per year by 2014 for treatment of Trypanosoma cruzi infection and Chagas disease, and Merck has committed to provide 200 million tablets of praziquantel during 2008 to 2017 for control of schistosomiasis. Triclabendazole has been made available by Novartis for control of fascioliasis. Thus, overall access to medicine for distribution to those affected by NTDs has significantly increased.[1]

CONTROL EFFORTS AGAINST HELMINTHES INFECTION

The concept of integrated preventive chemotherapy (ie, coordinated use of anthelminthic medicines, against 4 of the NTDs (LF, onchocerciasis, schistosomiasis, and STH) has gained support from several public health sectors. Fundamental to the development of integrated drug delivery programs was the geographic overlap of the helminthes infections that allowed targeting of multiple diseases by the existing mechanisms, (eg, delivery of vitamins to babies at the time of immunization), thus having a public health approach.[16,17] The broad-spectrum anthelminthic medicines include albendazole, diethylcarbamazine, ivermectin, levamisole, mebendazole, praziquantel, and pyrantel.[18] These medicines require once (or twice) a year treatment to control morbidity, have an impressive safety record, and exhibit no pharmacokinetic interactions or increased adverse effects when delivered in combination,[19] thus making it feasible for them to be delivered by nonmedical volunteers.[20–22] Depending on the choice of medicine(s), this intervention also relieves strongyloidiasis, scabies, and lice. Further, pilot research projects have provided a degree of confidence in the concept that, if the prevalence of helminthes infection in patients can be reduced to less than a threshold level, then transmission will remain sufficiently low to prevent the reemergence of infection as a public health problem.[23–25] Accordingly, numerous partnerships of local governments; donors; the pharmaceutical industry and other agencies, including nongovernmental organizations (NGOs); and volunteer distributors and coordinators have worked out economies of scale in delivering chemotherapeutic interventions. Community participation and mobilization that have given people greater control of their health have been essential components of an integrated approach to NTD control and prevention, and the results achieved by this approach for the delivery of medicines are commendable.[26,27]

STH (large roundworms, whipworm, and hookworms) collectively parasitize more than 1 billion people worldwide. Humans are the only definitive host, and transmission of STHs, and persistence and prevalence of the resultant disease, continues primarily because of a lack of access to safe water and proper sanitation (reviewed in Refs.[28,29]). The main consequence of infection with STHs is malnutrition and impaired development in infected children, and symptoms of reduced physical fitness and cognitive capacity in adulthood. It is estimated that up to 300 million people suffer from severe morbidity caused by STH infection.[29,30] There is no vaccine available; however, albendazole and mebendazole, administered as a single dose, are highly effective against hookworms and roundworms; and efficacy of albendazole in combination with ivermectin is significantly enhanced against whipworm.[31] Numerous studies involving hundreds of millions of patient exposures in a 20-year period have also repeatedly documented a remarkable safety record of albendazole.[19,22,28,31] A call for treatment of more than 75% of school-aged children to attain control of STH was made at the World Health Assembly (WHA; WHA54.19) in 2001, and it was recommended that treatment for 3 consecutive years would suffice to attain STH control. However, several studies indicate that infections return to pretreatment levels within 3 years after the termination of the program,[32,33] and sustained yearly treatment would be required to effectively maintain nematode removal. The data reported to WHO for treatment coverage indicate that ~16% of infected children were treated worldwide in 2008, and one-third of these children received treatment through LF control programs.[1] It is anticipated that the percentage of coverage of STH treatment will decline significantly once LF control programs are terminated, and reinfection and reemergence of disease will occur unless significant steps are taken to integrate STH control with other existing or newly developed public health programs. Resistance to albendazole is frequently noted in farm animals as a result of frequent drug use[34] and may be a cause for concern in humans. Integration of education and community participation in environmental hygiene and sanitation (access and use of closed-pit toilets, availability of decontaminated water at the point of use, and elimination of the practice of defecation in open fields), along with therapeutic treatment, will have a major impact on control of STH.[30]

Before the Global Program to Eliminate Lymphatic Filariasis, launched by WHO in 2000, there were an estimated 115 million people infected with *Wuchereria bancrofti* and 13 million with *Brugia* spp.[35] Chronic complications caused by the presence of adult worms in the lymphatic system include lymphedema or elephantiasis of the limbs, testicular hydrocele in males, and potential damage of the kidneys and lymphatic system.[35] The microfilariae released by female worms in circulation are taken up during blood meals by the mosquito (*Culex* spp), which is the most important vector for *W bancrofti* transmission worldwide.[36] The existing epidemiologic data suggest that ivermectin/albendazole combinatorial therapy is more effective than a diethylcarbamazine/albendazole combination (100% vs 83%) in reducing microfilariae levels, whereas the reverse is true in decreasing female fertility and microfilariae production (96% vs 100%).[37] Efforts to prevent infection or control morbidity by intervention therapy, along with hydrocele case management, have been successful in several countries, including China, Egypt, and countries in the African continent.[38] According to the WHO, all countries in Asia and most on the African continent have initiated LF treatment programs, and the number of people treated every year has increased from 10 million in 2000 to 546 million in 2007, reaching 32% to 42% of the at-risk population. Moreover, there are some areas where treatment coverage has reached more than 65%.[38,39] A major increase in efforts in 2008 to 2009 resulted in delivery of more than 2. 5 billion drug treatments per year to populations in endemic countries.[1] The modeling of the available data predicts that a coverage of more than 80% of the at-risk population for at least 6 consecutive years would be required to achieve elimination of transmission,[24,40] and coverage at 65% (or less) would not yield desirable results. Therefore, the drug treatment of a sufficiently high percentage of the population would remain of prime importance for the LF control programs. Preventive chemotherapy is cost-effective to control the morbidity caused by LF, but it does not remove the worms that can live for more than 15 years in the human host, and the potential for transmission to vector remains for long periods of time. The experiences from low-prevalence areas, and high-endemicity countries (China and India) have led to the suggestion that vector control efforts alongside drug treatment would be most effective in the interruption of filarial transmission and reemergence.[41,42] The integrated strategy of drug treatment with vector control is also favored, because it reduces the time needed for the interruption of filarial transmission and the risk of development of drug resistance against albendazole. Thus, a major impact on the reduction of LF (similar to that noted earlier for STH) would occur after controlling the vectors of *Wuchereria* and *Brugia* by appropriate management of water resources through country-specific health system strengthening and integration with other economic development programs.

Onchocerciasis (river blindness) is caused by the nematode filarial *Onchocerca volvulus*, transmitted by black fly vectors that live in fast-running streams.[43,44] The chronic form of the disease can result in severe visual impairment, when the adult female worm starts to produce microfilariae resulting in lesions of the eye and skin and general debilitation.[44] The earliest onchocerciasis control program, started in West Africa in 1974, was based on vector control.[43,45] With the established safety and efficacy record of ivermectin against *O volvulus*,[46] the African Program for Onchocerciasis Control (APOC) was launched in 1995 with the objective of controlling onchocerciasis by self-sustaining community-directed treatment with ivermectin.[47] The current strategy is to treat the entire population with a greater than 40% prevalence of positive skin snips or greater than 20% prevalence of palpable nodules with 1 dose of ivermectin. According to the WHO, 56.7 million people were treated with ivermectin for onchocerciasis control in Africa by 2008, and the disease has been eliminated as a public health program in 11 West African countries by joint vector control and drug treatment efforts.[1,48] The network of onchocerciasis control programs spans 30 African countries, and encompasses more than 107 projects to create a comprehensive approach to eliminating the disease as a public health problem.[45] However, there is a need for the expansion of ivermectin delivery in sub-Saharan Africa where more than 99% of the population at risk resides.[49] The strategy of the Onchocerciasis Elimination Program in Americas (OEPA) is to sustain ivermectin treatment every 6 months and to reach at least 85% of the 500,000 people at risk of the disease. By the end of 2007, all 6 endemic countries (Brazil, Colombia, Ecuador, Guatemala, Mexico, and Venezuela) had established effective national programs in the 13 foci and had treatment coverage of at least 85% twice a year.[23] The program has been highly effective, perhaps also aided by low virulence of the circulating pathogen, and has reported cessation of transmission in 7 of the 13 foci in the Americas and is on track to eliminate onchocerciasis in the region by 2015.[23] No new cases of blindness attributable to onchocerciasis have been reported in the Americas, and eye lesions caused by onchocerciasis have been eliminated in 9 of the 13 foci.[50]

Future efforts to overcome the public health threat of onchocerciasis will depend on maintaining high treatment coverage through country ownership. As is the case with albendazole efficacy against LF, ivermectin also acts on microfilariae and reduces the productivity of female worms but does not kill adult worms, which are estimated to live longer than 14 years in a human host. A recent study in Ghana showed that, after 17 years of treatment, microfilariae repopulation levels reached ~54% of the pretreatment level within 3 months after stopping the treatment.[51] It is considered that the proposed treatment with ivermectin for 6 years may not be sufficient, and, accordingly, treatment may need to be extended for longer than 20 years (range 25–35 years, depending on the coverage rate) to successfully interrupt the transmission.[52] Alternative strategies to kill or sterilize the female worm to shorten the length of ivermectin treatment will have a major impact on improving the cost-effectiveness and efficacy of the onchocerciasis control programs. One such strategy has been considered through tetracycline treatment that kills the *Wolbachia* symbiont of *O volvulus* and sterilizes the female worm.[53] Several randomized drug trials with doxycycline or rifampicin treatment for a 3-week to 8-week course have shown the effectiveness of antibiotic approach of targeting *Wolbachia* endobacteria for control of *O volvulus* and lymphatic filarial nematode.[53] However, the use of doxycycline with ivermectin is not feasible because of the long courses needed and contraindication in children and pregnant women. Increased understanding of the host-symbiont relationship would aid the identification of new targets and the development of new drugs for targeting *Wolbachia* endobacteria for control of onchocerciasis.

Schistosoma spp (intestinal disease) and *Schistosoma haematobium* (urinary schistosomiasis) are largely spread on contact with contaminated freshwater sources (intermediate host: freshwater snails), with the exception of *S japonicum* for which amphibians are an intermediate host.[9] Blood loss in stool, iron deficiency caused by blood loss, and liver enlargement are the major causes of morbidity, although if left untreated, severe disorders of the bladder, urethra, and liver may emerge.[54] The use of praziquantel has proved effective,[55] and, despite many years of use, significant incidences of drug resistance have not been widespread.[56,57] The experience in China suggests the reemergence of prevalence of infection after termination of successful control programs targeting treatment of people with praziquantel and molluscicide treatment of water sources.[10,54] However, because of the safety of the drug even for pregnant lactating women, and the efficacy of a single treatment with praziquantel in providing a greater than 80% reduction in the prevalence of *Schistosoma mansoni* and greater than 90% reduction in egg burden, at least in high-endemicity areas, the use of praziquantel for targeting *Schistosoma* control is an attractive strategy.[58] Schistosomiasis is largely confined to sub-Saharan Africa now, where ~200 million people suffer from this morbid disease. The reports from WHO indicate that 17.5 million people were treated with praziquantel worldwide in 2008, and, of these, 11.7 million treatments were delivered in sub-Saharan Africa.[1,58] There is an immense need to increase the scale of programs for praziquantel distribution, especially in sub-Saharan Africa. However, the limited supply of praziquantel and the availability of only 10% of the needed drug as a donation from pharmaceutical companies pose an enormous hindrance to scaling efforts up.[59] Besides consistent efforts to enhance praziquantel availability and distribution, improved water management and hygiene and sanitation practices, thereby preventing reentry of eggs into the human environment, would be required to have a long-term health impact on the control of schistosomiasis as a public health problem.[10]

CONTROL EFFORTS AGAINST OTHER NTDs

Excluding trachoma, no single-dose, safe vaccine or drugs are available for other protozoan and bacterial neglected diseases such as Chagas disease, human African trypanosomiasis (HAT), leishmaniasis, Buruli ulcer, leprosy, and yaws.

Trachoma (chronic follicular keratoconjunctivitis) is caused by *Chlamydia trachomatis* spread from eye to eye by flies (*Musca sorbens*), contaminated fingers, and human secretions. Active trachoma affects an estimated 84 million people worldwide, of whom 7.6 million have end-stage disease, and ~1.3 million are blind.[60] The WHO-supported Global Elimination of Trachoma Initiative was launched in 1998, to achieve anticipated elimination of trachoma by 2020. The program suggests preventive chemotherapy using azithromycin (or tetracycline) eye ointment to control morbidity from trachoma among populations at risk, which forms an effective component of the SAFE (surgery, antibiotic treatment, facial cleanliness, and environmental improvement by sanitation and hygiene) strategy.[61] Surgery for trichiasis (inward turning of the eyelids) prevents progression to blindness.[60] SAFE is recommended for all individuals in communities with a greater than 10% prevalence of clinical signs of trachoma. Several studies indicate that SAFE may not be effective in preventing the onset of active trachoma and blindness among those already infected.[62] However, SAFE is highly effective in preventing the spread of pathogens, and, thereby, in reducing new cases of infection.[60] Accordingly, implementation of SAFE strategy for fewer than 6 years has been shown to result in the reduction of active trachoma by more than 99% in Morocco.[63] Trachoma was estimated to contribute a decade ago to 15% of cases of blindness worldwide (~7 million people).[64] A striking reduction in recorded trachomatous blindness to less than 4% is attributable in part to an improvement in socioeconomic conditions, and possibly to more accurate data, but might also be because of widespread implementation of the SAFE strategy.[60] A switch to annual administration of 1 oral dose of azithromycin, compared with self-use of eye ointment, may be desirable, because it is more effective in reducing the prevalence of infection to a low level, likely because of a higher rate of compliance.[65]

The currently available medicines against parasitic protozoans include nifurtimox and benznidazole for control of T cruzi infection and Chagas disease; pentamidine, suramin, melarsoprol, eflornithine, and nifurtimox for control of T brucei, the causative agent of HAT; and pentavalent antimonials (sodium stibogluconate and meglumine antimoniate), amphotericin B, paromomycin, and miltefosine for control of visceral leishmaniasis. Mycobacterium leprae infection causes leprosy, and multidrug therapy (ie, a combination of rifampicin and dapsone, with or without clofazimine) is recommended depending on the presence of multibacillary or paucibacillary leprosy. A combination of rifampicin and streptomycin or amikacin is effective for control of Buruli ulcers, as is benzathine penicillin for yaws. Most of these medicines are donated to the WHO in limited quantities, facilitating their delivery free of charge to targeted populations in endemic areas. Most of these pathogens result in asymptomatic conditions for long periods, and chronic evolution of disease occurs several years after exposure.

The available drugs for treatment of Chagas disease, HAT, and visceral leishmaniasis are effective mainly during the early phase of infection and exhibit variable efficacy in different regions of high endemicity.[66–68] The efficacy of drugs against Chagas, HAT, and leishmaniasis during the chronic phase is debatable and, because of pronounced toxicity of drugs in adults, monitoring by the medical practitioners or hospitalization are generally required, resulting in low compliance.[66,68] Further, highly sensitive and specific diagnostic tests are not available, and multiple tests are needed for confirmed diagnosis of infection by trypanosomes and Leishmania.[69–71] The complexity of the life cycle and pathologic mechanisms involved have made it difficult to tackle these diseases, and significant commitment of academia, governments, nongovernment organizations, and for-profit organizations is required to promote the development of simpler-to-use diagnostic methods and safer medicines for administration in shorter treatment regimens.[72] Until then, to prevent mortality and reduce morbidity by these diseases, innovative public health approaches or integration in existing public health services are required to improve case detection so that treatments are delivered immediately after exposure.[1]

Country-owned programs exist for control of some of the neglected diseases. For example, India has recently eliminated yaws through the effective distribution of penicillin to those afflicted, and no new cases have been reported since 2004.[5] The control of dracunculiasis (guinea worm disease), for which no effective drug or vaccine is available, shows that well-designed public health programs are capable of delivering the needed services.[73,74] Dracunculiasis was estimated to afflict 3.5 million people annually in 1986. By the end of 2007, dracunculiasis transmission had been eliminated from 15 of the 20 countries where the disease was endemic in 1986, and only 9585 cases were reported worldwide.[75,76] During 2009 to 2010, the annual incidence was reduced to 3185 cases (ie, greater than 99% reduction in cases since 1989), and Ethiopia, Sudan, Ghana, and Mali, the remaining endemic countries, were addressing their final challenges to interrupting all remaining transmission.

KEY CHALLENGES AND OPPORTUNITIES

A scale-up of intervention with preventive therapies is required to meet the targets for coverage set by the WHA to achieve control or elimination of LF, *Schistosoma*, STH, and trachoma as public health problems, especially in African and the south-east Asia regions, otherwise disease may persist or reemerge. Most intervention programs based on preventive therapy seem to be less effective than originally planned and, depending on the initial disease prevalence, would need to continue for longer periods. Thus, sustained support, at least at current levels, from donor countries and public and private partners, who participated in building up the NTD control programs, along with additional support from others, are needed to expand the program for overcoming NTDs. Pharmaceutical companies may not be willing to upscale their facilities to produce drugs that are to be given away free of cost. However, considering that the commitment to providing unlimited drugs for the treatment of helminthes infection is increased, the logistics of making, shipping, storing, distributing, and delivering to ensure that drugs reach the people who need it most can be an impinging factor.[77,78] Countries need to have access to immense resources to strengthen the health systems and to train and support staff in technical and management expertise for the implementation of expanded prevention and control activities.[77]

Despite these challenges, the enormous global health impact and low cost of poverty reduction efforts makes NTD reduction a best buy in public health.[4,6] The political will and policies that support mass drug/vaccine delivery have worked in controlling the debilitating infectious diseases of the poor in Japan and Korea after World War II, in China beginning in the 1990s, and in southern North America in the 1930s after the New Deal Program, which brought agricultural industrialization. In developing countries, country-owned deworming programs against *Schistosoma* and STH covered 100% of children in Cambodia[79–81] and more than 90% in Burkina Faso,[82–84] which rank 175/177 on the Human Development Index. The exemplary success of these programs shows that national and international commitment to make drugs accessible, and the innovative use of community-based drug distribution approaches, are still valid to target control or elimination of NTDs.

A research strategy is required to develop and implement new medicines, notably for leishmaniasis and trypanosomiasis; new methods for vector control; vaccines for dengue; and new diagnostics that will be accessible to all who need them.[78] However, private industries have not been interested in investing in research, development, and advancement of products for the diseases of the poor. However, NIH and the US Centers for Disease Control, the United Nations Development Program, the World Bank, as well as private foundations such as the Bill & Melinda Gates Foundation, and the Global Fund continue to have a strong commitment to strengthening capacity in developing countries, aiming at identification of technologies and development of new products, and large new initiatives have began to take shape.[72,77] These initiatives also focus on the education and training of in-country scientists, provision of technical assistance, and infrastructure development. Thus, public-private partnerships will continue to be the driving forces for research and development of new drugs and vaccines against NTDs. In addition, the alliances within developing countries for drug and vaccine development and production locally have great potential for the advancement of products against NTDs.[85]

Lessons learned from efforts to control helminthes infections by intervention therapy only and Chagas disease by vector control only make it clear that sanitation alongside integrated efforts for vector control and therapeutic treatment of infected individuals must be addressed to prevent reemergence of the infection. The NTD control programs have an opportunity to integrate educational campaigns on the role of vectors in disease transmission, to use appropriate tools to prevent exposure to infectious agents, and to measure process indicators based on health and education improvements and a decline in new cases and vector-mediated transmission to facilitate a reduction in NTD prevalence and maximize the achievements made.

Many of the NTDs, once widespread in the United States and other developed countries, disappeared with economic development, and sustained control efforts alongside improved sanitation, hygiene, and lifestyle changes. Therefore, it can be argued that resource-poor communities can achieve NTD control by increased awareness and public health education programs targeting hygiene as an important component of lifestyle. Social marketing (ie, ownership of victory over diseases that have treatment available and accessible) can invigorate public involvement. Thus, it is important that policies be integrated in drug delivery programs to support local campaigns to educate people against specific, targeted diseases, and enhance efforts to provide free treatment distribution via mobilization of resources within the countries. The decline in guinea worm disease worldwide by more than 99% is an exemplary success model, achieved by health education and improved access to safe drinking water. Thus, empowering the neglected population to take charge of their own health would promote healthier nations and economic productivity, the most potent forces in eliminating NTDs.

SUMMARY

The benefits of integrating NTDs in the donor and recipient country policies will be numerous. These benefits include eradication of NTDs for which high-quality treatments are available (eg, leprosy, soil-borne helminthes); increased community-based surveillance and case management of NTDs for which no treatment is currently available (eg, Buruli ulcer); and better control of sleeping sickness, Chagas disease, and other diseases that require continuous efforts for greater coverage and additional treatments administrable without skilled health workers. Operational issues, compliance, pharmacologic vigilance, multidrug toxicity, and the emergence of drug resistance would remain the burning issues in mass drug delivery efforts. However, if the specter of resistance is carefully considered, an integrated NTD plan continued, and new drug development supported, there is every reason to believe that control and elimination of NTDs can be achieved, leading to extreme poverty reduction and economic productivity in developing nations.

REFERENCES

1. World Health Organization. Working to overcome the global impact of neglected tropical diseases, in First WHO report on neglected tropical diseases. Geneva (Switzerland): World Health Organization; 2010. p. 1.
2. Hotez PJ, Fenwick A, Savioli L, et al. Rescuing the bottom billion through control of neglected tropical diseases. Lancet 2009;373:1570.
3. Hotez PJ, Molyneux DH, Fenwick A, et al. Control of neglected tropical diseases. N Engl J Med 2007;357:1018.
4. Boutayeb A. Developing countries and neglected diseases: challenges and perspectives. Int J Equity Health 2007;6:20.
5. Narain JP, Dash AP, Parnell B, et al. Elimination of neglected tropical diseases in the South-East Asia Region of the World Health Organization. Bull World Health Organ 2010;88:206.
6. Moran M, Guzman J, Ropars AL, et al. Neglected disease research and development: how much are we really spending? PLoS Med 2009;6:e30.
7. Bethony JM, Cole RN, Guo X, et al. Vaccines to combat the neglected tropical diseases. Immunol Rev 2010;239:237.
8. World Health Organization. Global plan to combat neglected tropical diseases. Geneva (Switzerland): World Health Organization; 2007. p. 1.
9. Utzinger J, Raso G, Brooker S, et al. Schistosomiasis and neglected tropical diseases: towards integrated and sustainable control and a word of caution. Parasitology 2009;136:1859.
10. Wang LD, Guo JG, Wu XH, et al. China's new strategy to block *Schistosoma japonicum* transmission: experiences and impact beyond schistosomiasis. Trop Med Int Health 2009;14:1475.
11. Gustavsen KM, Bradley MH, Wright AL. GlaxoSmithKline and Merck: private-sector collaboration for the elimination of lymphatic filariasis. Ann Trop Med Parasitol 2009;103(Suppl 1):S11.
12. Colatrella B. The Mectizan Donation Program: 20 years of successful collaboration - a retrospective. Ann Trop Med Parasitol 2008;102(Suppl 1):7.
13. Burton MJ, Frick KD, Bailey RL, et al. Azithromycin for the treatment and control of trachoma. Expert Opin Pharmacother 2002;3:113.
14. Sunderkotter CH, Lan Ma H. Clofazimine. Current status of therapy with clofazimine (Lampren) for leprosy, erythema leprosum, and other dermatoses after donation of the medicine to the WHO by Novartis. Hautarzt 2005;56:478 [in German].
15. Sebbag R. Drug access in poor countries. Bull Acad Natl Med 2007;191:1601 [in French].
16. Gyapong JO, Gyapong M, Yellu N, et al. Integration of control of neglected tropical diseases into health-care systems: challenges and opportunities. Lancet 2010;375:160.
17. Kabatereine NB, Malecela M, Lado M, et al. How to (or not to) integrate vertical programmes for the control of major neglected tropical diseases in sub-Saharan Africa. PLoS Negl Trop Dis 2010;4:e755.
18. Keiser J, Utzinger J. The drugs we have and the drugs we need against major helminth infections. Adv Parasitol 2010;73:197.
19. Olsen A. Efficacy and safety of drug combinations in the treatment of schistosomiasis, soil-transmitted helminthiasis, lymphatic filariasis and onchocerciasis. Trans R Soc Trop Med Hyg 2007;101:747.

20. Ali BH. A short review of some pharmacological, therapeutic and toxicological properties of praziquantel in man and animals. Pak J Pharm Sci 2006;19:170.
21. Brown KR, Ricci FM, Ottesen EA. Ivermectin: effectiveness in lymphatic filariasis. Parasitology 2000;121(Suppl):S133.
22. Horton J. Albendazole: a review of anthelmintic efficacy and safety in humans. Parasitology 2000;121(Suppl):S113.
23. Cupp EW, Sauerbrey M, Richards F. Elimination of human onchocerciasis: history of progress and current feasibility using ivermectin (Mectizan (R)) monotherapy. Acta Trop 2010. [Epub ahead of print].
24. Michael E, Malecela-Lazaro MN, Simonsen PE, et al. Mathematical modelling and the control of lymphatic filariasis. Lancet Infect Dis 2004;4:223.
25. Ray KJ, Lietman TM, Porco TC, et al. When can antibiotic treatments for trachoma be discontinued? Graduating communities in three African countries. PLoS Negl Trop Dis 2009;3:e458.
26. Babu BV, Behera DK, Kerketta AS, et al. Use of an inclusive-partnership strategy in urban areas of Orissa, India, to increase compliance in a mass drug administration for the control of lymphatic filariasis. Ann Trop Med Parasitol 2006;100:621.
27. Smits HL. Prospects for the control of neglected tropical diseases by mass drug administration. Expert Rev Anti Infect Ther 2009;7:37.
28. Bethony J, Brooker S, Albonico M, et al. Soil-transmitted helminth infections: ascariasis, trichuriasis, and hookworm. Lancet 2006;367:1521.
29. Brooker S, Clements AC, Bundy DA. Global epidemiology, ecology and control of soil-transmitted helminth infections. Adv Parasitol 2006;62:221.
30. Brooker S, Hotez PJ, Bundy DA. The global atlas of helminth infection: mapping the way forward in neglected tropical disease control. PLoS Negl Trop Dis 2010;4:e779.
31. Keiser J, Utzinger J. Efficacy of current drugs against soil-transmitted helminth infections: systematic review and meta-analysis. JAMA 2008;299:1937.
32. Haswell-Elkins MR, Elkins DB, Manjula K, et al. An investigation of hookworm infection and reinfection following mass anthelmintic treatment in the south Indian fishing community of Vairavankuppam. Parasitology 1988;96(Pt 3):565.
33. Quinnell RJ, Slater AF, Tighe P, et al. Reinfection with hookworm after chemotherapy in Papua New Guinea. Parasitology 1993;106(Pt 4):379.
34. Harfoush MA, Abd el AA, El-Seify MA. Resistance of gastrointestinal nematodes of sheep to some anthelmintics. J Egypt Soc Parasitol 2010;40:377.
35. Hooper PJ, Bradley MH, Biswas G, et al. The global programme to eliminate lymphatic filariasis: health impact during its first 8 years (2000–2007). Ann Trop Med Parasitol 2009;103(Suppl 1):S17.
36. Ottesen EA. Lymphatic filariasis: treatment, control and elimination. Adv Parasitol 2006;61:395.
37. de Kraker ME, Stolk WA, van Oortmarssen GJ, et al. Model-based analysis of trial data: microfilaria and worm-productivity loss after diethylcarbamazine-albendazole or ivermectin-albendazole combination therapy against *Wuchereria bancrofti*. Trop Med Int Health 2006;11:718.
38. Ottesen EA, Hooper PJ, Bradley M, et al. The global programme to eliminate lymphatic filariasis: health impact after 8 years. PLoS Negl Trop Dis 2008;2:e317.
39. Addiss D. The 6th Meeting of the Global Alliance to Eliminate Lymphatic Filariasis: a half-time review of lymphatic filariasis elimination and its integration with the control of other neglected tropical diseases. Parasit Vectors 2010;3:100.
40. Michael E, Gambhir M. Transmission models and management of lymphatic filariasis elimination. Adv Exp Med Biol 2010;673:157.

41. El-Setouhy M, Abd Elaziz KM, Helmy H, et al. The effect of compliance on the impact of mass drug administration for elimination of lymphatic filariasis in Egypt. Am J Trop Med Hyg 2007;77:1069.
42. Sunish IP, Rajendran R, Mani TR, et al. Vector control complements mass drug administration against bancroftian filariasis in Tirukoilur, India. Bull World Health Organ 2007;85:138.
43. Boatin BA, Richards FO Jr. Control of onchocerciasis. Adv Parasitol 2006;61:349.
44. Thylefors B, Alleman M. Towards the elimination of onchocerciasis. Ann Trop Med Parasitol 2006;100:733.
45. Amazigo UV, Noma M, Bump J, et al. Onchocerciasis. In: Jamison DT, Feachem RG, Makgoba MW, editors. Disease and mortality in sub-Saharan Africa. Washington, DC: World Bank; 2006.
46. Basanez MG, Pion SD, Boakes E, et al. Effect of single-dose ivermectin on *Onchocerca volvulus*: a systematic review and meta-analysis. Lancet Infect Dis 2008;8:310.
47. Seketeli A, Adeoye G, Eyamba A, et al. The achievements and challenges of the African Programme for Onchocerciasis Control (APOC). Ann Trop Med Parasitol 2002;96(Suppl 1):S15.
48. Boatin B. The Onchocerciasis Control Programme in West Africa (OCP). Ann Trop Med Parasitol 2008;102(Suppl 1):13.
49. Ogoussan KT, Hopkins A. Mectizan (R) procurement and delivery for onchocerciasis mass drug administration programmes. Acta Trop 2010. [Epub ahead of print].
50. Report from the 2009 Inter-American Conference on Onchocerciasis: progress towards eliminating river blindness in the region of the Americas. Wkly Epidemiol Rec 2010;85:321 [in English, French].
51. Osei-Atweneboana MY, Eng JK, Boakye DA, et al. Prevalence and intensity of *Onchocerca volvulus* infection and efficacy of ivermectin in endemic communities in Ghana: a two-phase epidemiological study. Lancet 2007;369:2021.
52. Winnen M, Plaisier AP, Alley ES, et al. Can ivermectin mass treatments eliminate onchocerciasis in Africa? Bull World Health Organ 2002;80:384.
53. Slatko BE, Taylor MJ, Foster JM. The *Wolbachia* endosymbiont as an anti-filarial nematode target. Symbiosis 2010;51:55.
54. Zhou XN, Bergquist R, Leonardo L, et al. Schistosomiasis japonica control and research needs. Adv Parasitol 2010;72:145.
55. Botros S, El-Lakkany N, Seif El-Din SH, et al. Comparative efficacy and bioavailability of different praziquantel brands. Exp Parasitol 2011;127(2):515–21.
56. Gryseels B, Stelma FF, Talla I, et al. Epidemiology, immunology and chemotherapy of *Schistosoma mansoni* infections in a recently exposed community in Senegal. Trop Geogr Med 1994;46:209.
57. Ismail M, Botros S, Metwally A, et al. Resistance to praziquantel: direct evidence from *Schistosoma mansoni* isolated from Egyptian villagers. Am J Trop Med Hyg 1999;60:932.
58. Uneke CJ. Soil transmitted helminth infections and schistosomiasis in school age children in sub-Saharan Africa: efficacy of chemotherapeutic intervention since World Health Assembly Resolution 2001. Tanzan J Health Res 2010;12:86.
59. Hotez PJ, Engels D, Fenwick A, et al. Africa is desperate for praziquantel. Lancet 2010;376:496.
60. Wright HR, Turner A, Taylor HR. Trachoma. Lancet 2008;371:1945.
61. Burton MJ. Trachoma: an overview. Br Med Bull 2007;84:99.
62. Yorston D, Mabey D, Hatt S, et al. Interventions for trachoma trichiasis. Cochrane Database Syst Rev 2006;3:CD004008.

63. Ferriman A. Blinding trachoma almost eliminated from Morocco. BMJ 2001;323: 1387.
64. Thylefors B, Negrel AD, Pararajasegaram R, et al. Available data on blindness (update 1994). Ophthalmic Epidemiol 1995;2:5.
65. Melese M, Alemayehu W, Lakew T, et al. Comparison of annual and biannual mass antibiotic administration for elimination of infectious trachoma. JAMA 2008;299:778.
66. Barrett MP, Gilbert IH. Perspectives for new drugs against trypanosomiasis and leishmaniasis. Curr Top Med Chem 2002;2:471.
67. Boscardin SB, Torrecilhas AC, Manarin R, et al. Chagas' disease: an update on immune mechanisms and therapeutic strategies. J Cell Mol Med 2010;14:1373.
68. Paulino M, Iribarne F, Dubin M, et al. The chemotherapy of Chagas' disease: an overview. Mini Rev Med Chem 2005;5:499.
69. Adams ER, Hamilton PB. New molecular tools for the identification of trypanosome species. Future Microbiol 2008;3:167.
70. Desquesnes M, Davila AM. Applications of PCR-based tools for detection and identification of animal trypanosomes: a review and perspectives. Vet Parasitol 2002;109:213.
71. Rodgers J. Human African trypanosomiasis, chemotherapy and CNS disease. J Neuroimmunol 2009;211:16.
72. Hotez PJ, Pecoul B. "Manifesto" for advancing the control and elimination of neglected tropical diseases. PLoS Negl Trop Dis 2010;4:e718.
73. CDC. Progress toward global eradication of dracunculiasis, January 2009-June 2010. MMWR Morb Mortal Wkly Rep 2010;59:1239.
74. Rinaldi A. Free, at last! The progress of new disease eradication campaigns for guinea worm disease and polio, and the prospect of tackling other diseases. EMBO Rep 2009;10:215.
75. Dracunculiasis eradication - global surveillance summary, 2009. Wkly Epidemiol Rec 2010;85:166.
76. Hopkins DR, Ruiz-Tiben E, Downs P, et al. Dracunculiasis eradication: neglected no longer. Am J Trop Med Hyg 2008;79:474.
77. Cohen J, Dibner MS, Wilson A. Development of and access to products for neglected diseases. PLoS One 2010;5:e10610.
78. Trouiller P, Torreele E, Olliaro P, et al. Drugs for neglected diseases: a failure of the market and a public health failure? Trop Med Int Health 2001;6:945.
79. Chigusa Y, Ohmae H, Otake H, et al. Effects of repeated praziquantel treatment on schistosomiasis mekongi morbidity as detected by ultrasonography. Parasitol Int 2006;55:261.
80. Hisakane N, Kirinoki M, Chigusa Y, et al. The evaluation of control measures against Schistosoma mekongi in Cambodia by a mathematical model. Parasitol Int 2008;57:379.
81. Sinuon M, Tsuyuoka R, Socheat D, et al. Financial costs of deworming children in all primary schools in Cambodia. Trans R Soc Trop Med Hyg 2005;99:664.
82. Gabrielli AF, Toure S, Sellin B, et al. A combined school- and community-based campaign targeting all school-age children of Burkina Faso against schistosomiasis and soil-transmitted helminthiasis: performance, financial costs and implications for sustainability. Acta Trop 2006;99:234.
83. Koukounari A, Gabrielli AF, Toure S, et al. Schistosoma haematobium infection and morbidity before and after large-scale administration of praziquantel in Burkina Faso. J Infect Dis 2007;196:659.

84. Toure S, Zhang Y, Bosque-Oliva E, et al. Two-year impact of single praziquantel treatment on infection in the national control programme on schistosomiasis in Burkina Faso. Bull World Health Organ 2008;86:780.
85. Mrazek MF, Mossialos E. Stimulating pharmaceutical research and development for neglected diseases. Health Policy 2003;64:75.

Global Health: Injuries and Violence

Hadley K. Herbert, MD[a], Adnan A. Hyder, MD, MPH, PhD[a],*,
Alexander Butchart, MA, PhD[b], Robyn Norton, MPH, PhD[c]

KEYWORDS

- Injury • Violence • Burden of injury • Trauma
- Accidents • Global health

Injury and violence rank among the 10 leading causes of death worldwide. In 2004, more than 5 million deaths resulted from injuries, representing 12% of the global burden of disease, as measured by disability-adjusted life years (DALYs).[1] Injuries accounted for 1 in 7 healthy life-years lost worldwide in 2004, which is projected to increase to 1 in 5 by 2020. Nearly a quarter of injury-related deaths in 2004 were caused by road traffic injuries (RTIs) and each year, more than 1.5 million people die from acts of violence including 800,000 suicides and 500,000 homicides.[1]

Approximately 90% of injury-related fatalities occur in low-income and middle-income countries (LMICs), illustrating one of many global inequalities in health. Injuries contribute approximately 15 times as many total DALYs in LMICs as in high-income countries (HICs). When adjusted for population, injury-related DALYs are 4 times greater in LMICs than in HICs: 4198 DALYs per 100,000 people, compared with 1403 DALYs per 100,000 people, respectively.[1]

Injury has traditionally been defined as physical damage that results from exposure to an excessive form of energy or from a lack of essential agents. Energy is defined as chemical, thermal, electrical, radiation, or kinetic, such as that transmitted by a crash, fall, or bullet. Essential agents include oxygen or toxins and as such, drowning and poisoning are also categorized as injuries. In 2002 the World Health Organization (WHO) proposed this definition to be too narrow and has since reframed injury to include psychological harm, maldevelopment, and deprivation.[2] Through this approach, injury can be also described according to the presumed underlying intent

Disclosures/Funding support: The authors have nothing to disclose.
[a] International Injury Research Unit, Department of International Health, Bloomberg School of Public, Johns Hopkins University, 615 North Wolfe Street, Baltimore, MD 21205, USA
[b] Department of Violence and Injury Prevention and Disability, World Health Organization, Avenue Appia 20, 1211 Geneva 27, Switzerland
[c] The George Institute for Global Health, The University of Sydney, Level 7, 341 George Street, Sydney NSW 2000, Australia
* Corresponding author. International Injury Research Unit, Department of International Health, Bloomberg School of Public, Johns Hopkins University, 615 North Wolfe Street, Suite E-8132, Baltimore, MD 21205.
E-mail address: ahyder@jhsph.edu

Infect Dis Clin N Am 25 (2011) 653–668
doi:10.1016/j.idc.2011.06.004
0891-5520/11/$ – see front matter © 2011 Elsevier Inc. All rights reserved.

as unintentional or intentional. This formal effort to categorize injury emphasizes that injuries are not "accidents" and that violence does not occur per se.[2]

Unintentional injuries occur in the absence of predetermined intent, resulting from causes such as road traffic crashes, falls, burns, drowning, and poisoning. *Intentional injuries* result from violence, defined as "the intentional use of physical force of power, threatened or actual, against oneself, another person, or against a group or community, that either results in or has a high likelihood of resulting in injury, death, psychological harm, mal-development, or deprivation."[2] *Violence* is categorized into 3 groups: *self-directed violence*, in which a person inflicts the violent act on themselves; *interpersonal violence*, in which violence is inflicted by another individual or a small group of individuals; and *collective violence*, in which violence is inflicted by larger groups such as a state, organized political groups, religious groups, militia groups, and terrorist organizations.[2]

This article considers how injury and violence relate to global health, using the most recent global burden of disease data and selected reviews of key articles and databases in the field.[1–11] By highlighting cause-specific injuries, this article describes the burden of injury in terms of mortality and DALYs, and summarizes the evidence and global recommendations regarding risk factors and prevention initiatives. In doing so, the article serves as a call to action to increase injury research and prevention efforts at national and global levels.

BURDEN OF UNINTENTIONAL INJURY AND VIOLENCE
Unintentional Injuries

The WHO estimates that more than 3.9 million unintentional injury deaths occurred in 2004, accounting for 61 unintentional injuries per 100,000 population or 6.6% of the global mortality burden. More than 90% unintentional injury deaths occurred in LMICs (**Table 1**). The rate of unintentional injuries was highest in Southeast Asia with 80 injuries per 100,000, and lowest in the Americas with 39 injuries per 100,000. Unintentional injuries were responsible for more than 138 million DALYs in 2004, of which 94% occurred in LMICs (**Fig. 1**).[1] The overall DALY burden of highest in the South-East Asian and Western Pacific regions of the WHO. Of these injuries, nearly two-thirds afflicted men (**Fig. 2**). While **Fig. 2** illustrates that majority of injury occurs among men, the data may also suggest an underreporting of injuries that occur among women.

RTIs are the ninth leading cause of death worldwide, responsible for more than 1.2 million deaths in 2004 or 2.2% of the global mortality. While RTI mortality varies across regions, from fewer than 130,000 in Europe to almost 350,000 in the Western Pacific, the burden is disproportionately high in LMICs.[1,3] Approximately 1 million RTIs in 2004 occurred in LMICs, corresponding to 20 deaths per 100,000 population.

Falls caused more than 424,000 deaths worldwide in 2004 with a reported mortality rate of 7 per 100,000 and a loss of 3 DALYs per 1000 population. Falls were the second leading cause of death by unintentional injury globally, of which Europe and the Western Pacific region accounted for nearly 60%. Globally, adults older than 70 years had significantly higher mortality rates than younger individuals. While fatality rates for men exceeded those for women in all age groups, women were more likely to experience nonfatal falls. In the United States, the total direct cost of fall injuries for people 65 years and older exceeded $19 billion; this was expected to increase to approximately $54.9 billion by 2010.[12] Falls rank 12th among the leading causes of death among children 5 to 9 years old and 15 to 19 years old.[9] Falls in children younger than 15 years contribute to significant morbidity, comprising almost 50% of the total global DALYs lost to falls.[9]

Table 1
Global number of injury-related deaths (in thousands) by income and regions, 2004

	Income Level		WHO Regions						Total
	Low- and Middle-Income Countries	High-Income Countries	Africa	South East Asia	Eastern Mediterranean	The Americas	Europe	Western Pacific	
Population (millions)	5454	971	738	1672	520	874	883	1738	6437
All injury	5269	506	769	1949	485	586	789	1196	2629
Unintentional injury	3558	341	496	1331	321	342	564	846	2569
RTI	1158	30	205	306	146	152	129	336	1274
Fall	348	76	19	126	24	41	79	134	423
Fires	302	9	48	186	29	8	23	16	310
Drowning	371	114	62	100	30	22	34	139	387
Poisoning	316	17	42	96	17	25	107	59	346
Other	1068	94	121	517	76	93	191	163	1161
Intentional injury[a]	1474	165	273	392	163	238	226	348	1640
Self-directed violence	707	137	50	252	36	69	151	286	844
Interpersonal violence	573	26	182	115	25	155	65	37	579
War and conflict	180	1	40	20	99	11	10	2	182

[a] For the purposes of this article, the WHO definition of intentional injury in synonymous with violence.
Data from WHO. Global burden of disease. Available at: http://www.who.int/healthinfo/global_burden_disease/GBD_report_2004update_full.pdf. Accessed July 4, 2011.

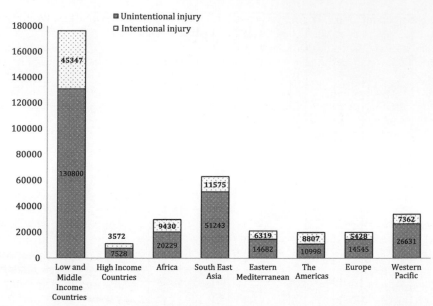

Fig. 1. Injury-related total DALYs (in thousands) by income level and regions, 2004. (*Data from* WHO. Global burden of disease. Available at: http://www.who.int/healthinfo/global_burden_disease/GBD_report_2004update_full.pdf. Accessed July 4, 2011.)

Fires were responsible for more than 310,000 deaths in 2004, resulting in more than 2 DALYs per 1000 population.[1] More than 90% of fatal fire-related burns occurred in LMICs. South-East Asia alone accounted for more than half of the total number of fire-related deaths worldwide.[1,13,14] Children younger than 5 and those older than 70 years had the highest fire-related burn mortality rates. In addition to fires, there are many more burn-related deaths from scalds, electrical burns, and other types of burns for which global data are not available. Although few data exist on the medical costs of burns in LMICs, the costs of burn injury in HICs are staggering. In Spain, for example, the mean cost of one burn injury, including social and labor costs, was US$95,551, of which health care comprised only 10%.[15]

In 2004 an estimated 387,000 people drowned, making drowning the third leading cause of unintentional death globally. These estimates exclude drowning that results from floods, boating, water transport, and intentional injury. Approximately 97% of all drowning deaths occur in LMICs.[16] Of this, the Western Pacific and South-East Asia

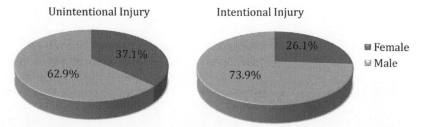

Fig. 2. Percentage of injury-related deaths by gender, 2004. (*Data from* WHO. Global burden of disease. Available at: http://www.who.int/healthinfo/global_burden_disease/GBD_report_2004update_full.pdf. Accessed July 4, 2011.)

regions account for 60% of mortality and DALYs.[1] Over half of the mortality worldwide and 60% of the total number of DALYs lost due to drowning occur among children younger than 14 years. Children younger than 5 years have the highest drowning mortality rates, of which the highest rates occur in China, followed by Sub-Saharan Africa.[16,17]

The WHO estimates that 346,000 deaths were caused from poisoning in 2004. While more than 90% of poison-related deaths occurred in LMICs, poisoning is the fourth leading cause of death and DALYs in HICs.

Violence

Violence is an emerging field in public health, having only been declared in 1996 by the WHO World Health Assembly as a major public health issue; despite this, global, regional, and country-based data remain scarce. However, the widespread nature of violence is evident: in 2004 the WHO estimated that 1.6 million people died as a result of violence, accounting for more than 2.5% of the world's deaths.[1] Almost half of these deaths were suicides, nearly one-third were homicides, and one-fifth were war-related. Nearly three-quarters of those injured through violence were men. To understand the true burden of violence-related injury, research shows the repercussions of violence to be much broader than mortality and morbidity statistics: violence affects psychological and behavioral factors, including depression, alcohol abuse, anxiety, and suicidal behaviors. These factors are also root causes of violence, and thus further fuel the vicious circle of violence.[2,18]

Self-directed violence resulted in more than 840,000 deaths globally in 2004, making suicide the 13th leading cause of death worldwide and responsible for more than 19 million DALYs lost. Among individuals aged 15 to 44 years, it is the fourth leading cause of death and sixth leading cause of disability.[2] Deaths are only a portion of self-directed violence, as many individuals survive following suicide attempts, often resulting in serious medical harm, self-destructive behaviors, and self-mutilation (this form of violence includes repeated and intentional self-infliction of injuries, including cutting, burning, head banging, and nonlethal overdose).[19] These injuries are difficult to recognize, and obtaining data on self-directed injuries remains challenging.

Interpersonal violence, which includes child maltreatment, youth violence, intimate partner violence, sexual violence, and abuse of the elderly, accounted for 600,000 deaths in 2004, of which more than 90% occurred in LMICs. The estimated rate of violent deaths per 100,000 was nearly 4 times higher in LMICs than HICs (10.41 vs 2.68 per 100,000 respectively).[4]

Violence against children is the least reported, studied, and understood area of childhood injuries.[20] The WHO estimates that 25% to 50% of children younger than 18 years reported suffering from physical abuse.[7] In addition, 20% of girls and 5% to 10% of boys reported having experienced sexual abuse.[7] The United Nations International Labor Organization estimated that in 2000, 5.7 million children were in forced labor, 1.8 million were in prostitution or pornography, and 1.2 million were victims of trafficking.[21] Estimates of the economic costs in the United States for child maltreatment are more than $250 billion per year.[22,23] While studies show that violence against children occurs in all countries, rates are higher in LMICs.[4]

In 2004 youth violence, defined as violence by or against an individual 10 to 29 years old, resulted in more than 247,000 youth homicides or an average of 677 youth deaths each day. Youth homicide rates vary by region, ranging from 3.95 per 100,000 in HICs to 11.51 per 100,000 in LMICs, of which the highest rates occur in Africa and Latin America.[1] For each youth homicide, it is estimated that 20 to 40 youths sustain injuries that require medical management.[24]

Intimate partner violence is "any behavior within an intimate relationship that causes physical, psychological or sexual harm to those in the relationship," and includes acts of physical aggression, psychological abuse, and forced intercourse.[4] Sexual violence includes rape, attempted rape, gang rape, and other forms of forced sexual acts. A WHO multicountry study of domestic violence against women found that among 24,000 women 15 to 49 years old, physical abuse by a partner was reported by 13% to 61% of women, sexual violence by a partner was reported by 6% to 59% of women, and sexual violence by a nonpartner older than 15 years was reported by 0.3% to 11.5% of women.[25] Estimates regarding the global prevalence of intimate partner and sexual violence remain limited, however; data are difficult to obtain and relatively few studies have measured intimate partner and sexual violence outside North America.[26–29]

Elderly abuse incorporates physical, sexual, emotional, and psychological acts or neglect directed toward older people. A systematic review of the prevalence of elder abuse and neglect found 1 in 4 vulnerable elders to be at risk, but only a small proportion are identified by health care providers.[30] The barriers to research in elder abuse and neglect are substantial. Even in HICs, such as the United States, where there are mandatory elderly abuse reporting laws, challenges to research include appropriate diagnosis, assessment, recruitment, and attrition of the elderly.[31]

RISK FACTORS FOR INJURIES AND VIOLENCE

Causes and risk factors associated with injury and violence are complex and multifactorial. The Haddon matrix and the WHO ecological model provide frameworks to describe the causes of unintentional injury and violence, respectively, and highlight interrelated risk factors. Through the application of the Haddon matrix, the traditional epidemiologic triangle of host, vector, and environment has been used to describe injury-causing events in terms of pre-event, event, and post-event phases (**Table 2**).[32] This matrix allows analysis of potential interventions from primary prevention to treatment.

To describe violence-related causes, the WHO adopted a 4-level ecological model to represent the interplay between individual, relationship, community, and societal factors (**Table 3**). The first level identifies biological and personal factors that influence how individuals behave, including demographic characteristics, personality disorders, and history of experiencing violent behavior. The second level focuses on close relationships. The third level explores the community context, including schools, workplaces, and neighborhoods. The fourth level takes into account societal factors that propagate or dissuade violence.[2] This section applies these models to summarize known and potential risk factors for the leading cause-specific injures.

Unintentional Injuries

RTI risks are factors that affect or influence exposure to risk, crash involvement, and crash and post-crash injury severity. Factors that influence crash involvement include economic development, social inequality, demographic factors, land use planning, the ratio of motorized traffic to vulnerable road users, and lack of awareness regarding the design of road functions. Risk factors that influence crash involvement include speeding, use of alcohol, fatigue, inexperienced and young drivers, defects in the road design, and vehicle factors such as braking and maintenance. Factors that influence crash severity include speeding, lack of safety restraints and crash helmets, insufficient vehicle crash protection, and the presence of alcohol. Risk factors that

Table 2
The Haddon matrix, as it applies to road traffic injury

Phase		Host	Vehicles and Equipment	Environment
Pre event	Crash prevention	Information Attitudes Impairment Police enforcement	Roadworthiness Lighting Braking Handling Speed management	Road design and layout Speed limits Pedestrian facility
Event	Injury prevention during the crash	Use of restraints Impairment	Occupant restraints Other safety devices Crash-protective design	Crash-protective roadside objectives
Post event	Life sustaining	First aid skill Access to medics	Ease of access Fire risk	Rescue facilities Congestion

Data from WHO. World report on road traffic injury prevention. Available at: http://whqlibdoc. who.int/publications/2004/9241562609.pdf. Accessed July 4, 2011.

affect post-crash outcomes include lack of appropriate pre-hospital and hospital care, as well as inappropriate extrication of the injured.[8]

Risk factors for falls in the elderly are categorized into 4 dimensions: biological, behavioral, environmental, and socioeconomic.[5] Biological factors include demographics and changes that result from aging, such as a decline in physical and occupational abilities. Behavioral risk factors include actions and choices, such as excess alcohol use. Environmental risk factors include individuals' physical conditions, such as hazards in the home. Socioeconomic factors include low income and education levels, inadequate housing, and limited access to health care. Among children, risk factors for falls include development stages, gender, poverty, underlying disabilities, physical and social environments, and agents such as consumer products and playground equipment. Incidence and severity of fall injuries are influenced by the height of the fall, type of surface, mechanism, and setting.[9]

Burn injuries are coded differently throughout the world, often making it difficult to study variable coding systems.[9] Risk factors for burn injuries differ according to geographic regions, but generally include alcohol, smoking, use of open fires for space heating, use of ground-level stoves for cooking, high-set water heater temperatures, and substandard electrical wiring.[33] Gender differences play a significant role in the risk of burn injuries, with a predominance of women injured in fires from cooking and heating fuels in LMICs, whereas industrial events primarily affect men in HICs.[34] Burn research in LMICs identified childhood risk factors that include poverty, use of kerosene, cooking in open spaces, overcrowding, and lack of parental supervision.[34–37]

Drowning in HICs is often associated with recreational swimming, such as in swimming pools, whereas drowning in LMICs often occurs with everyday activities near bodies of water.[38] Few studies, however, have formally researched risk factors associated with drowning; those that are available found a correlation between alcohol and drowning among adults.[39,40] A systematic review of pediatric injuries found drowning to be considered in only 3 studies: 2 studies found poverty to be associated with drowning in children younger than 5 years, while the third study found no evidence to suggest income level was a risk factor for drowning.[41–44]

Table 3
WHO ecological model for intentional violence analysis

	Individual	Relationship	Community	Societal
Self-Directed Violence	• Psychiatric factors • Psychological factors • Family history of suicide	• Personal loss • Interpersonal conflict • Broken or disturbed relationship • Legal or work-related problems	• Poverty • Lack of employment • Immigration status • Place of residence	• Role of cultural values • Religious affiliation • Economic conditions • Availability of means of suicide
Interpersonal Violence				
Child maltreatment	• Age • Gender • Special characteristics (prematurity, twins, handicapped) • Personality and behavioral characteristics • Prior history of abuse	• Caregiver's and family's behavioral characteristics • Family structure and resources • Family size • Violence in the home • Stress and social isolation	• Poverty • Preventive health care for infants and children	• Role of cultural values and economic forces • Inequalities related to sex and income • Cultural norms surrounding gender roles, parent-child relationships, and privacy of the family • Child and family policies • Strength of social welfare system • Nature and extent of social protection
Youth violence	• Biologic, psychological, and behavioral characteristics	• Family influence or lack of cohesion • Parental conflict or poor attachment • Family size • Young/teenage parents • Peer influence	• Poverty • Presence of gangs, guns, or drugs • Limited social integration within a community	• Cultural norms • Demographic or social change • Political structures • Law enforcement

Intimate partner and sexual violence: *factors that influence the perpetrator*	• Alcohol and drug use • Attitudes supportive of sexual violence • Impulsive and antisocial tendencies • Preference for impersonal sex • Prior history of sexual abuse and family violence	• Family environment characterized by physical violence and few resources • Strongly patriarchal relationship • Emotionally unsupportive family environment • Peer influence	• Poverty, mediated through forms of crisis of male identity • Lack of employment opportunities • Lack of institutional support • General tolerance of sexual assault within the community • Weak sanctions against perpetrators	• Societal norms supportive of sexual violence, male superiority, and sexual entitlement • Weak laws and policies regarding sexual violence and gender equality • High levels of crime and other forms of violence
Abuse of the elderly	• Mental health disorders • Alcohol	• Career and care recipient relationship • Care recipient's disruptive behavior • Caregiver's depression or stress • Overcrowded living arrangements • Lack of privacy	• Poverty • Social isolation	• Cultural norms regarding ageism and sexism • Societal lack of stability and social security • High unemployment
War and Conflict Violence			• Inequality between groups • Readily available small arms or other weapons	• Lack of democratic processes • Unequal access to power • Unequal distribution of and access to resources • Control over key resource production or trading • Group fanaticism • Rapid demographic change

Data from WHO. World report on violence and health. Available at: http://whqlibdoc.who.int/publications/2002/9241545615_eng.pdf. Accessed July 4, 2011.

Risk factors for poisoning almost exclusively relate to poisoning in children, although the majority of poisoning occurs in adults. In HICs, product accessibility, such as safe packaging and storage, is a key risk factor.[45] Storage and availability of poisons are also risk factors in LMICs, as several studies showed that kerosene and pesticides are commonly ingested by children.[46–49] Sociodemographic risk factors include poverty, low education levels, young parental age, residential mobility, and lack of adult supervision.[9,47]

Violence

Many root causes of particular forms of violence are similar, such as poverty, social isolation, alcohol, and access to firearms, placing individuals at an increased risk of experiencing more than one type of violence. By emphasizing the need to explore links between different types and causes of violence, this section highlights how risks are framed within the WHO ecological model of violence (see **Table 3**).

Factors that place individuals at risk for self-directed violence include psychiatric, biological, social, and environmental factors. Many studies of suicide research are derived from "psychological autopsies," in which surviving family members are interviewed regarding the presence of these factors.[50] Biological markers, such as a family history of suicide, may suggest a genetic predisposition.[51] Life events, such as personal loss, interpersonal conflict, or legal difficulties, may also be precipitating factors for suicide. Social and environmental factors that increase the risk of suicidal behaviors include social isolation, lack of employment, immigration status, religious affiliation, and poverty.[2,52]

Age is the greatest risk factor among children who suffer maltreatment, as children younger than 4 years are at the highest risk of abuse. However, when describing child abuse it is important to place this and other risk factors within the context of the children and their relationships with their family, the perpetrator, their community, and their economic and cultural environment.[2] The ecological model can be applied to youth violence to understand how adolescence influences and propagates violent behaviors. Over the last decade, emerging research has linked intimate partner and sexual violence to individual, community, and societal risk factors as well.[2,53–55] Research regarding the risks of elder abuse is scarce, limited to HICs settings, and is often being revised. For example, early theoretical models identified caregiver's stress as a risk factor, but current research suggests stress may be a contributing factor and not an independent risk factor.[56,57] Nevertheless research efforts are beginning to place risk factors for elderly abuse within the ecological model, of which depression, social network, and social engagement are at the forefront.[58]

Ethnic conflict, political violence, and war have deep-seated structural causes. The Carnegie Commission on Preventing Deadly Conflict proposed that community, societal, demographic, political, and economic factors play important roles.[59] However, research regarding the immediate and long-term impact of societies affected by conflict violence remains scarce. Studies on the collective suffering and trauma-related disorders among survivors are only now emerging in the scientific literature.[60,61]

INTERVENTIONS FOR UNINTENTIONAL INJURIES AND VIOLENCE

Evidence-based and cost-effective interventions are available for injury prevention and control, yet their coverage is dismally low in LMICs. This section highlights proven interventions or prevention initiatives covering both unintentional injuries (RTIs, child injuries) and violence; some of these have received widespread global acknowledgments from experts through the publication of WHO World Reports in the past decade (**Table 4**).

Unintentional Injuries

In 2004, the WHO proposed the motto "safer systems, safer roads, safer vehicles, and safer people" to implement strategies to reduce motor vehicle traffic, encourage safer modes of traffic, and minimize exposure to high-risk scenarios.[8] Effective interventions to improve road-user safety include the introduction of relevant legislation, combined with strict enforcement and supportive education. The WHO and the World Bank jointly proposed a set of 6 recommendations to member states in 2004, which encouraged countries to both assess their burden of RTI and respond to it systematically (see **Table 4**). Despite this focus, however, only 48% of countries have national

Table 4
WHO recommended interventions for specific injuries

Road Traffic Injury[75]	Child Injury[76]	Violence[77]
1. Identify a lead agency in government to guide the national road traffic safety effort	1. Integrate child injury into a comprehensive approach to child health and development	1. Create, implement, and monitor a national action plan for violence prevention
2. Assess the problems, policies, and institutional settings related to road traffic injury and the capacity for road traffic injury prevention in each country	2. Develop and implement a child injury prevention policy and a plan of action	2. Enhance capacity for collecting data on violence
3. Prepare a national road safety strategy and plan of action	3. Implement specific actions to prevent and control child injuries	3. Define priorities for and support research on the causes, consequences, costs, and prevention of violence
4. Allocate financial and human resources to address the problem	4. Strengthen health systems to address child injuries	4. Promote primary prevention responses
5. Implement specific actions to prevent road traffic crashes, minimize injuries and their consequences, and evaluate the impact of these actions	5. Enhance the quality and quantity of data for child injury prevention	5. Strengthen responses for victims of violence
6. Support the development of national capacity and international cooperation	6. Define priorities for research and support research on the causes, consequences, costs, and prevention of child injuries	6. Integrate violence prevention into social and educational policies, and thereby promote gender and social equality
	7. Raise awareness of and target investments toward child injury prevention	7. Increase collaboration and exchange of information on violence prevention
		8. Promote and monitor adherence to international treaties, laws, and other mechanisms to protect human rights
		9. Seek practical, internationally agreed responses to the global drugs trade and the global arms trade

and subnational laws regarding all risk factors as of 2009; and even when legislation exists enforcement is limited, especially in LMICs.[3]

Multifactorial interventions have shown a reduction in the rate of falls but not the risk of falling among the elderly. Exercise interventions, however, such as Tai Chi, have shown the greatest promise in reducing both the risk and rate of falls.[62] Interventions to prevent falls among children emphasize strengthening relationships, such as parental awareness, and community support, including the provision of safer playground equipment.[9]

There is limited evidence regarding the effectiveness of interventions related to burns. Interventions that have been proposed, but have yet to be shown to be effective, include separating the cooking area from the living area, reducing the amount of flammable substances available in the household, and enhancing child supervision— all in LMICs.[9,13,63,64]

Evidence regarding the effectiveness of drowning prevention interventions in both HICs and LMICs is relatively nonexistent. The only available data are from case-controlled studies, which suggest that fencing around domestic swimming pools reduces the risk of drowning in HIC.[65] Field trials are needed in LMICs to establish the effectiveness of such interventions.[66] Interventions to prevent drowning linked to water-related transport include providing well-maintained and functional flotation devices; however, evidence regarding the effectiveness of these interventions is currently not available.[16]

Suggested interventions to reduce exposure to poisoning include appropriate storage of poisons in terms of position and vessels, warning labels, and first aid education.[9,67] In addition, home safety education and behavioral change efforts may be potentially effective interventions.[68] Many of these child injury interventions were proposed as part of a comprehensive approach addressing this burden in the youngest ages by the WHO and UNICEF in 2008 (see **Table 4**).

Violence

The WHO ecological model serves as a framework for violence prevention interventions, addressing multiple levels of risk factors. Prevention efforts that focus on individual behaviors encourage positive attitudes and behavioral change models. Relationship approaches can influence interactions with family and negative peer pressure. Community-based efforts can stimulate community action and support victims. Societal approaches focus on economic conditions, cultural norms, and social influences.[2] This multisector approach to prevent violence was promoted by the WHO a decade ago and calls on public health, criminal justice, social services, and education sectors to invest in national surveillance, intervention research, and effective legislation, furthering partnerships and collaboration (see **Table 4**).[69]

Post-Injury and Violence

In addition to preventing injury and violence, the burden and economic loss associated with injury can be decreased by improving the care of the injured in the pre-hospital and hospital settings.[70] Improvements in pre-hospital care include strengthening existing emergency medical services (EMS), instituting new formal EMS systems, and strengthening existing informal systems.[71] Hospital care can be strengthened by investing in human resources, such as staffing and training regarding appropriate injury-specific care and timely referrals; physical resources, such as airway equipment, chest tubes, and trauma-specific medications; and administration resources.[71,72] The WHO and the International Association for Trauma Surgery recently set forth Essential Trauma Care Guidelines to promote the availability of universal core essential trauma care services and to serve as the first steps in prioritizing trauma care worldwide.[73,74]

SUMMARY

This article serves as a call to action to expand our understanding of the growing burden of injury and violence in LMICs and to prioritize epidemiologic and intervention injury prevention research initiatives. The public health community must play a leadership role in galvanizing a multisector response to injury and violence, to advocate for investments at national and international levels, and to catalyze sharing of knowledge and lessons learned across communities and nations. The increasing impact of injury and violence on global health makes it imperative that the international public health community invest in research and prevention of injury and violence.

REFERENCES

1. World Health Organization. Global burden of disease: 2004 update. Geneva (Switzerland): World Health Organization; 2008.
2. Krug EG, Mercy JA, Dahlberg LL, et al. The world report on violence and health. Geneva (Switzerland): World Health Organization; 2002.
3. World Health Organization. Global status report on road safety: time for action. Geneva (Switzerland): World Health Organization; 2009.
4. World Health Organization. Violence prevention: the evidence overview. Geneva (Switzerland): World Health Organization; 2009.
5. World Health Organization. WHO global report on falls prevention in older age. Geneva (Switzerland): World Health Organization; 2007.
6. World Health Organization/London School of Hygiene and Tropical Medicine. Preventing intimate partner and sexual violence against women: taking action and generating evidence. Geneva (Switzerland): World Health Organization; 2010.
7. World Health Organization, ISPCAN. Preventing child maltreatment: a guide to taking action and generating evidence. Geneva (Switzerland): World Health Organization; 2006.
8. Peden M, Scurfield R, Sleet D, et al. World report on road traffic injury prevention. Geneva (Switzerland): World Health Organization; 2004.
9. Peden M, Oyegbite K, Ozanne-Smith J, et al. World report on child injury prevention. Geneva (Switzerland): World Health Organization; 2008.
10. International road and traffic accident database. Available at: www.internationaltransportforum.org/irtad/coverage.html. Accessed December 28, 2010.
11. World Bank. Available at: www.data.worldbank.org/data-catalog. Accessed December 28, 2010.
12. Centers for Disease Control and Prevention (CDC). Fatalities and injuries from falls among older adults—United States, 1993-2003 and 2001-2005. MMWR Morb Mortal Wkly Rep 2006;55(45):1221-4.
13. Atiyeh BS, Costagliola M, Hayek SN. Burn prevention mechanisms and outcomes: pitfalls, failures and successes. Burns 2009;35(2):181-93.
14. Ahuja RB, Bhattacharya S. Burns in the developing world and burn disasters. BMJ 2004;329(7463):447-9.
15. Sanchez JL, Pereperez SB, Bastida JL, et al. Cost-utility analysis applied to the treatment of burn patients in a specialized center. Arch Surg 2007;142(1):50-7 [discussion: 57].

16. Peden MM, McGee K. The epidemiology of drowning worldwide. Inj Control Saf Promot 2003;10(4):195–9.
17. Perrement M. China development brief. Beijing: WHO, UNICEF, the China Centre for Disease Control, Beijing (China); 2006.
18. Tegegne A. The primary solution of global poor health and poverty. Med Confl Surviv 2008;24(2):107–14.
19. Haswell DE, Graham M. Self-inflicted injuries. Challenging knowledge, skill, and compassion. Can Fam Physician 1996;42:1756–8, 1761–4.
20. Newton AW, Vandeven AM. Child abuse and neglect: a worldwide concern. Curr Opin Pediatr 2010;22(2):226–33.
21. ILO. A future without child labour. Geneva (Switzerland): International Labour Office; 2002.
22. Miller TR, Fisher DA, Cohen MA. Costs of juvenile violence: policy implications. Pediatrics 2001;107(1):E3.
23. Waters HR, Hyder AA, Rajkotia Y, et al. The costs of interpersonal violence—an international review. Health Policy 2005;73(3):303–15.
24. Mercy JA, Butchart A, Rosenberg ML, et al. Preventing violence in developing countries: a framework for action. Int J Inj Contr Saf Promot 2008;15(4): 197–208.
25. García-Moreno C, Jansen H, Ellsberg M, et al. WHO multi-country study on women's health and domestic violence against women. Geneva (Switzerland): World Health Organization; 2005.
26. Philpart M, Goshu M, Gelaye B, et al. Prevalence and risk factors of gender-based violence committed by male college students in Awassa, Ethiopia. Violence Vict 2009;24(1):122–36.
27. Salaudeen AG, Akande TM, Musa OI, et al. Assessment of violence against women in Kano metropolis, Nigeria. Niger Postgrad Med J 2010;17(3):218–22.
28. Ardabily HE, Moghadam ZB, Salsali M, et al. Prevalence and risk factors for domestic violence against infertile women in an Iranian setting. Int J Gynaecol Obstet 2011;112(1):15–7.
29. Romero-Gutierrez G, Cruz-Arvizu VH, Regalado-Cedillo CA, et al. Prevalence of violence against pregnant women and associated maternal and neonatal complications in Leon, Mexico. Midwifery 2010. [Epub ahead of print].
30. Cooper C, Selwood A, Livingston G. The prevalence of elder abuse and neglect: a systematic review. Age Ageing 2008;37(2):151–60.
31. Fulmer T. Barriers to neglect and self-neglect research. J Am Geriatr Soc 2008; 56(Suppl 2):S241–3.
32. Haddon W. A logical framework for categorizing highway safety phenomenon and activity. J Trauma 1972;12:193–207.
33. Mock C, Peck M, Peden M, et al. A WHO plan for burn prevention and care. Geneva (Switzerland): World Health Organization; 2008.
34. Dissanaike S, Rahimi M. Epidemiology of burn injuries: highlighting cultural and socio-demographic aspects. Int Rev Psychiatry 2009;21(6):505–11.
35. Petrass LA, Finch CF, Blitvich JD. Methodological approaches used to assess the relationship between parental supervision and child injury risk. Inj Prev 2009; 15(2):132–8.
36. Van Niekerk A, Menckel E, Laflamme L. Barriers and enablers to the use of measures to prevent pediatric scalding in Cape Town, South Africa. Public Health Nurs 2010;27(3):203–20.
37. Mashreky SR, Rahman A, Khan TF, et al. Determinants of childhood burns in rural Bangladesh: a nested case-control study. Health Policy 2010;96(3):226–30.

38. Hyder AA, Borse NN, Blum L, et al. Childhood drowning in low- and middle-income countries: urgent need for intervention trials. J Paediatr Child Health 2008;44(4):221–7.

39. Guillemont J, Girard D, Arwidson P, et al. Alcohol as a risk factor for injury: lessons from French data. Int J Inj Contr Saf Promot 2009;16(2):81–7.

40. Driscoll TR, Harrison JE, Steenkamp M. Alcohol and drowning in Australia. Inj Control Saf Promot 2004;11(3):175–81.

41. Laflamme L, Hasselberg M, Burrows S. 20 years of research on socioeconomic inequality and children'—unintentional injuries understanding the cause-specific evidence at hand. Int J Pediatr 2010;2010:819687.

42. Giashuddin SM, Rahman A, Rahman F, et al. Socioeconomic inequality in child injury in Bangladesh—implication for developing countries. Int J Equity Health 2009;8:7.

43. Kim MH, Subramanian SV, Kawachi I, et al. Association between childhood fatal injuries and socioeconomic position at individual and area levels: a multilevel study. J Epidemiol Community Health 2007;61(2):135–40.

44. Cho HJ, Khang YH, Yang S, et al. Socioeconomic differentials in cause-specific mortality among South Korean adolescents. Int J Epidemiol 2007;36(1):50–7.

45. Wilkerson R, Northington L, Fisher W. Ingestion of toxic substances by infants and children: what we don't know can hurt. Crit Care Nurse 2005;25(4):35–44.

46. Koueta F, Dao L, Ye D, et al. Acute accidental poisoning in children: aspects of their epidemiology, aetiology, and outcome at the Charles de Gaulle paediatric hospital in Ouagadougou (Burkina Faso). Sante 2009;19(2):55–9.

47. Manzar N, Saad SM, Manzar B, et al. The study of etiological and demographic characteristics of acute household accidental poisoning in children–a consecutive case series study from Pakistan. BMC Pediatr 2010;10:28.

48. Oguche S, Bukbuk DN, Watila IM. Pattern of hospital admissions of children with poisoning in the Sudano-Sahelian North Eastern Nigeria. Niger J Clin Pract 2007; 10(2):111–5.

49. Pillai GK, Boland K, Jagdeo S, et al. Acute poisoning in children: cases hospitalized during a three-year period in Trinidad. West Indian Med J 2004;53(1):50–4.

50. Heila H, Isometsa ET, Henriksson MM, et al. Suicide and schizophrenia: a nationwide psychological autopsy study on age- and sex-specific clinical characteristics of 92 suicide victims with schizophrenia. Am J Psychiatry 1997;154(9):1235–42.

51. Voracek M, Loibl LM. Genetics of suicide: a systematic review of twin studies. Wien Klin Wochenschr 2007;119(15–16):463–75.

52. Milner A, McClure R, De Leo D. Socio-economic determinants of suicide: an ecological analysis of 35 countries. Soc Psychiatry Psychiatr Epidemiol 2010. [Epub ahead of print].

53. Uthman OA, Lawoko S, Moradi T. The role of individual, community and societal gender inequality in forming women's attitudes toward intimate-partner violence against women: a multilevel analysis. World Health Popul 2010;12(2):5–17.

54. Gass JD, Stein DJ, Williams DR, et al. Gender differences in risk for intimate partner violence among South African adults. J Interpers Violence 2010. [Epub ahead of print].

55. Norman R, Schneider M, Bradshaw D, et al. Interpersonal violence: an important risk factor for disease and injury in South Africa. Popul Health Metr 2010;8:32.

56. Wang JJ, Lin MF, Tseng HF, et al. Caregiver factors contributing to psychological elder abuse behavior in long-term care facilities: a structural equation model approach. Int Psychogeriatr 2009;21(2):314–20.

57. Macneil G, Kosberg JI, Durkin DW, et al. Caregiver mental health and potentially harmful caregiving behavior: the central role of caregiver anger. Gerontologist 2010;50(1):76–86.

58. Dong XQ, Simon MA, Beck TT, et al. Elder abuse and mortality: the role of psychological and social wellbeing. Gerontology 2010. [Epub ahead of print].
59. Carnegie Commission on Preventing Deadly Conflict. Carnegie commission on preventing deadly conflict series. Washington, DC: Carnegie Corporation of New York; 1997.
60. Pedersen D. Political violence, ethnic conflict, and contemporary wars: broad implications for health and social well-being. Soc Sci Med 2002;55(2):175–90.
61. Wang SJ, Modvig J, Montgomery E. Household exposure to violence and human rights violations in western Bangladesh: prevalence, risk factors and consequences. BMC Int Health Hum Rights 2009;9:29.
62. Gillespie LD, Robertson MC, Gillespie WJ, et al. Interventions for preventing falls in older people living in the community. Cochrane Database Syst Rev 2009;2: CD007146.
63. Ytterstad B, Sogaard AJ. The Harstad injury prevention study: prevention of burns in small children by a community-based intervention. Burns 1995;21(4):259–66.
64. Turner C, Spinks A, McClure R, et al. Community-based interventions for the prevention of burns and scalds in children. Cochrane Database Syst Rev 2004; 3:CD004335.
65. Thompson DC, Rivara FP. Pool fencing for preventing drowning in children. Cochrane Database Syst Rev 2000;2:CD001047.
66. Callaghan JA, Hyder AA, Khan R, et al. Child supervision practices for drowning prevention in rural Bangladesh: a pilot study of supervision tools. J Epidemiol Community Health 2010;64(7):645–7.
67. Nixon J, Spinks A, Turner C, et al. Community based programs to prevent poisoning in children 0-15 years. Inj Prev 2004;10(1):43–6.
68. Kendrick D, Smith S, Sutton A, et al. Effect of education and safety equipment on poisoning-prevention practices and poisoning: systematic review, meta-analysis and meta-regression. Arch Dis Child 2008;93(7):599–608.
69. Chandran A, Puvanachandra P, Hyder AA. Prevention of violence against children: a framework for progress in low- and middle-income countries. J Public Health Policy 2011;32(1):121–34.
70. Mock C, Kobusingye O, Joshipura M, et al. Strengthening trauma and critical care globally. Curr Opin Crit Care 2005;11(6):568–75.
71. Mock C, Nguyen S, Quansah R, et al. Evaluation of trauma care capabilities in four countries using the WHO-IATSIC guidelines for essential trauma care. World J Surg 2006;30(6):946–56.
72. Mock C, Arreola-Risa C, Quansah R. Strengthening care for injured persons in less developed countries: a case study of Ghana and Mexico. Inj Control Saf Promot 2003;10(1–2):45–51.
73. Aboutanos MB, Mora F, Rodas E, et al. Ratification of IATSIC/WHO's guidelines for essential trauma care assessment in the South American region. World J Surg 2010;34(11):2735–44.
74. Juillard CJ, Mock C, Goosen J, et al. Establishing the evidence base for trauma quality improvement: a collaborative WHO-IATSIC review. World J Surg 2009; 33(5):1075–86.
75. WHO. World report on road traffic injury prevention. Available at: http://whqlibdoc.who.int/publications/2004/9241562609.pdf. Accessed July 4, 2011.
76. WHO. World report on child injury prevention. Available at: http://whqlibdoc.who.int/publications/2008/9789241563574_eng.pdf. Accessed July 4, 2011.
77. WHO. Violence prevention, the evidence. Available at: http://whqlibdoc.who.int/publications/2002/9241545615_eng.pdf. Accessed July 4, 2011.

Basic Science Research and Education: A Priority for Training and Capacity Building in Developing Countries

Richard J. Deckelbaum, MD[a,b,]*, James M. Ntambi, PhD[c],
Debra J. Wolgemuth, PhD[a,d]

KEYWORDS

- Basic science research • Basic science education
- Global health • Developing countries

Does science education in developing countries really count?[1] The overall goal of this article is to provide evidence that basic science education and research are key priorities for global health training, capacity building, and practice. While an increasing number of scholars attest to the need of building basic science capabilities into education in developing countries, this is still largely a neglected area. To paraphrase from a 1964 article by J. Ronald Gass "The notion that science education should be considered as an investment is somewhat unheard of in the economic planning of many countries".[2] In this same article, he suggested "the great potentiality of science as a dynamic force in cultural change in the underdeveloped world." Dr Gass then continued to show the major lack of teachers, facilities, and even interest in developing basic science education that existed in the 1950s and 1960s—a situation which

---

Financial disclosure and conflict of interest obligations: None of the authors have any conflicts of interest or financial support relating to this manuscript.

[a] Institute of Human Nutrition, College of Physicians and Surgeons, Columbia University, 630 West 168th Street, PH1512, New York, NY 10032, USA

[b] Department of Pediatrics, Columbia University Medical Center, New York, NY, USA

[c] Departments of Biochemistry and Nutritional Sciences, 415B, 433 Babcock Drive, Madison, WI 53706-1544, USA

[d] Departments of Genetics & Development and Obstetrics & Gynecology, Columbia University Medical Center, Russ Berrie Pavilion, Room 608, 1150 Saint Nicholas Avenue, New York, NY 10032, USA

* Corresponding author. Institute of Human Nutrition, College of Physicians and Surgeons, Columbia University, 630 West 168th Street, PH1512, New York, NY 10032.
E-mail address: rjd20@columbia.edu

Infect Dis Clin N Am 25 (2011) 669–676
doi:10.1016/j.idc.2011.05.009
0891-5520/11/$ – see front matter © 2011 Elsevier Inc. All rights reserved.

id.theclinics.com

continues to the present day and is still underappreciated and most often not addressed.

More recently, the International Council for Science (ICSU), in its report "Science Education and Capacity Building for Sustainable Development,"[3] stressed that "science capacity-building encompasses a multiplicity of resources, actors, and of organizational and institutional components (of which the education and training of scientists is only one central and necessary component) interacting in a long-term systemic process".[3]

While this report makes a number of recommendations towards strengthening science education and capacity building, with a few exceptions, basic science research and education appear as low priorities in many developing as compared to developed countries (ie, the global South as compared with the global North). Expanding basic science capabilities will not only enhance the capacity of institutions in the South to enhance teaching and learning environments, but will more rapidly bring these institutions and their students and faculty into equal relationships with the currently dominant North. Importantly, it could have major impact upon halting or diminishing the massive brain drain of scientific researchers from the developing areas.

Traditionally, research in public health aspects of infectious diseases has been the major focus in developing areas and subsequently has consumed a significant portion of the available human and financial resources.[4] In terms of capacity building at the local level in the South, infectious disease research has been a major building block in establishing basic science research in order to train individuals in the South to serve initiatives that combat human immunodeficiency virus (HIV), malaria, parasitic diseases, and other infections. However, with the increasing recognition that noncommunicable diseases such as type 2 diabetes,[5] cardiovascular disease,[6,7] and cancer[8] are rapidly emerging as a significant burden in developing countries, similar to what has occurred in the developed countries, there is a major need for building laboratories and training personnel who can help manage these emergent problems locally in the South. There is a need to produce a cohort of researchers who possess the requisite competencies to address the priority challenges of the South relating to improving health, nutrition, food security, and rural livelihoods. Improvement in research in basic science in universities of the South will help guarantee sustainable development by strengthening local physical and human resources.[3]

Too often, researchers in the South have looked upon the North for handling biochemical analyses required for local population studies rather than developing the requisite capabilities. This needs to be discouraged. In a recent example, in the study of micronutrient status of children in the West Bank of the Jordan, local laboratory facilities were strengthened, and quality assurance was ensured by receiving blinded samples from the US Centers for Disease Control. Results obtained will likely lead to changes in fortification policy in Palestinian populations (Massad S, Deckelbaum RJ, Khammash U, unpublished data). The ability of basic scientists and public health scientists to provide a scientific and mechanistic basis to recommendations and policy will greatly enhance their ability to influence policy makers.[9]

WHAT IS THE CURRENT STATUS OF BASIC SCIENCE TRAINING IN GLOBAL HEALTH?

Even in North America and Europe, review of university curricula offered in global health tracks reveals that little emphasis is placed on basic science training. As an example, in an ad-hoc review by the authors of over 50 courses offered by two northeastern US universities for global health concentrations, only a single course with any molecular aspects was included, and this was a course in parasitology. Thus, even in the developed world, global health relates much more to public health, which is indeed very important, but without the accompanying basic science backup. Basic science training for students from the South often occurs in laboratories in the North where human resources and laboratory infrastructure and finances are strong. Well-trained students then return to faculty positions in their home countries with little physical infrastructure, low salaries, little research financing, and very large teaching burdens. Facing this situation, many choose either not to return to their countries of origin, or emigrate soon after their return to developed countries.

The ICSU report[3] writes that "...North America, Europe, Japan, and Asian newly-industrialized countries produce 60% of the world's gross national product, and are responsible for 85% of world expenditure in science and technology, even though they represent less than 25% of the world's population. In contrast, China, Latin America, and India account for a further 10% of the world's spending on research and development, and sub-Saharan Africa only 0.5%".[3] Of interest, the total budget projected for the US National Institutes of Health (NIH) for 2012 is approximately $32 billion, of which the Fogarty Institute, which stresses basic science training in developing countries, has a budget of only about $75 million. It is sobering to note that the total Kenyan national budget for 2010 of $12 billion is only slightly more than one-third of the total NIH budget spent for research and research infrastructure in the United States.

HOW CAN THE PROBLEMS OF LACK OF FINANCIAL AND HUMAN RESOURCES, PHYSICAL INFRASTRUCTURE, AND POOR RECOGNITION OF THE NEED FOR LOCAL BASIC SCIENCE RELATED TO INDIGENOUS HEALTH ISSUES BE ADDRESSED?

In building basic science research relating to health outcomes, clearly the major emphasis in training and research output should be tied to local problems. Thus, for example, women's health, reproductive health, and science relating to decreasing the burden of noncommunicable diseases should be a high priority in developing areas. Local social and environmental goals also need to be recognized in research priorities. Utilization of local resources and expertise needs to be encouraged much more in the framework of sustainable development.

A primary target must be convincing policy and decision makers in developing areas that investing in basic science, for example in fields with direct impact of human nutrition, will not only improve local health outcomes but also result in economic benefits in terms of increasing human productivity. The costs of doing nothing must be presented to political leaders and policy makers by demonstrating that the current human and economic burdens of carrying populations with not only high levels of infectious diseases, but also poor nutritional status, leads to low intellectual capacities and low productivity.[6,10]

It is increasingly obvious that the developing world is facing the health disparities associated with the double burden, both under- and overnutrition. Even with the long-standing emphasis on undernutrition in the developing world, few laboratories exist to even analyze the basics required for proper nutrition surveys in the South. For example, levels of micronutrients including vitamins A, and D, as well as folates and other micronutrients that need to be in order to assess nutritional status are commonly sent to laboratories in the North for analyses.

Overnutrition is associated with the substantial health care costs of type 2 diabetes and cardiovascular diseases.[6] In terms of overnutrition, Africa, as an example, is expected to see the largest proportional increase in obesity and associated diabetes over the next 20 years, a disease that markedly increases health care costs over many years due to the disease itself as well as its complications.[8] Moreover, some countries from the South already are losing men and women during their productive years (35–64 years) from cardiovascular disease rates 1.3 to 7 times higher for men and 1.8 to 2.4 higher for women compared with the United States.[6] The burden of losses of working people at younger ages is much higher in the South than in the North (**Table 1**). Genomic, pathophysiologic, and biochemical factors associated with noncommunicable diseases in the South share some commonalities, but likely also have major differences from populations in the North. These need to be defined by institutions in the South.

HOW WILL STRENGTHENING BASIC SCIENCE RESEARCH IN DEVELOPING COUNTRIES BE ACHIEVED?

Given the current status that few institutions, or no institutions in many areas, have the capability for providing laboratory infrastructure and human resources for graduate training, multi-institutional, cooperative research training facilities and consortia should be established. A very successful example of such a multi-institutional facility exists in the field of economics, where the African Economic Research Consortium (AERC) provides an infrastructure to "strengthen local capacity for conducting independent, rigorous inquiry into problems pertinent to the management of economies in sub-Saharan Africa".[11] This is achieved through a network ownership of multiple institutions in AERC's research and training agendas, which coordinate training needs for multiple institutions in Africa. Examples of some integrative efforts and consortia in sub-Saharan Africa are presented in **Table 2**.[10–14] Similar consortia can be established for training in biological sciences, whereby no single institution needs to provide all needed human and physical infrastructure for the training. Multiple institutions can share curricular development, teaching, and faculty and also use available information technology resources for training students at multiple sites. Regional core laboratories can be set up for specific needs to be used by students from multiple institutions. Regional and national coordinating bodies for facilitating working environments, setting priorities, and allocating resources need to be established.[3]

Quoting from a recent editorial in *Nature Genetics*[15] that reported on growing genetic and genomic capacity in developing countries, "Understanding human genome function and variation will require genetics capacity in population-rich as well as resource-rich regions of the globe".[15] Also, "Medicine based in genetics provides a route for developing countries to improve health care, from primary care, via prevention of genetic diseases to opportunities for new research…In attracting international collaborators, a developing region needs to put its own and its immediate

---

Table 1
Deaths from cardiovascular disease between the ages of 35–64 years (per 100,000 population in year 2000)

	Males	Females
United States	56	28
Brazil	71	49
India	81	56
South Africa	97	68

Data from Leeder S, Greenberg HM, Raymond S. A race against time: the challenge of cardiovascular disease in developing economies. Available at: www.earth.columbia.edu/news/2004/images/raceagainsttime_FINAL_051104.pdf.

Table 2		
Examples of African multi-institution consortia for promoting education and research in different disciplines		
Organization	**Discipline**	**Mission**
African Institute for Mathematical Science (AIMS–the Next Einstein Initiative)[11]	Mathematics	Training in mathematical thinking to address complex challenges in agriculture health and other areas of development
African Population and Health Research Center (APHRC)[12]	Public Health	Coordinating education and training to promote the well-being of Africans through policy relevant research on population, health, and education
African Economic Research Consortium (AERC)[10]	Economics	Strengthening local capacity for conducting rigorous inquiry and education related to the management of economies in sub-Saharan Africa
Training Health Researchers Into Vocational Excellence (THRiVE)[13]	Human health and disease	Empowering African institutions to develop human and laboratory infrastructures and administrative capacity "to support and lead in world class research programs"

neighbors' priorities first. So international collaborators must commit, so far as they can, to return benefits, training, and information to the developing region as the price of collaboration. Ideally, DNA should be genotyped and sequenced locally and not languish in a forgotten freezer overseas".[15]

It is not only the training in science that is required in developing areas, but also management of research and training. Currently a very large fraction of scientific research and training funds in developing countries derives from training relationships with institutions in the North. While institutions in the North often have grants and contract offices, these are relatively sparse, or nonexistent, in many institutions in the South. Researchers in the South need to be informed and supported to apply directly for funding through international sources. Fiscal reporting and responsibility must be part of these research and training offices in the South, much like they are in the North. Instruction is needed in data analysis, statistical approaches, and other skills that are integral parts of laboratory research. Often neglected, both in the developed and developing world institutions, is training in scientific writing and presentations. This is important not only writing research papers, but also in obtaining grants and presenting credible data to international audiences.

Another hindrance to overcome is the relatively low salary that academics receive in institutions in the South. This not only results in the aforementioned brain drain to the North, but also the departure of many local academics, or a large expenditure of their time, in pursuit of private sector opportunities. To decrease brain drain from the South, it is important to consider shortening the training periods of trainees from the South coming to the North. Training in a Northern institution for 3 to 6 years needs to be discouraged; rather periods of 6 to 12 months need to be considered, with the bulk of training to be provided at Southern institutions with South–South coordination and support. To discourage brain drain and enhance retention of young scientists, start-up research funds should be provided to Northern institutions to their graduates and trainees who return to the South. Such a practice is now being increasingly instituted by some institutions and organizations in the North.

While a number of alliances have emerged from the South from training relationships with institutions in the North, South–South cooperation in basic training is still at relatively low levels. A number of recommendations can be considered for enhancing South–South cooperation in education and training as suggested originally by the ICSU[3]:

> Develop South-South institutional networks to share innovative experiences and address critical economical, environmental, public health, and social problems
> Increase support for undergraduate, graduate, and postgraduate South–South fellowship programs devoted to quality education and science, and technology
> There should be mobilization of expatriate scientists living and working in the North to not only evaluate critical problems in the South, but also assist in local capacity and training in scientific institutions in the South
> Ensure that South–South research as well as North–South research is in the context of local policy development, equity, and relief of poverty.

From a global perspective, it is important to note that strengthening research capabilities received little specific attention in a recent report: Education of Health Professionals for the 21st Century.[16] Research training and education both in basic science and public health also need to be stressed more as part of developing professionals for an increasingly globalized world.

Are there indications that appreciation for basic research and training is increasing in developing countries? In a recent news interview in *Nature*, Dr Romain Murenzi, former science minister of Rwanda and current director of TWAS, the Italy-based Academy of Science for the Developing World provides a positive outlook on this. He states, "When the United Nations Millennium Development Goals were adopted in 2000, it was clear that most could not be achieved without science. Eradicating extreme poverty, improving access to water, securing the food supply; you need science for all those. As a result, the realization that science matters for economic growth has taken hold in developing countries."[17] Another *Nature* news article reported on the African Science, Technology ,and Innovation Endowment Fund, and suggested that African science ministers have agreed that the next decade would show increases in research budgets and that science and technology would have integrated roles in driving development.[18] Hopefully, with these increasing commitments to science as an integral part of capacity building, the large gaps between the North and South in science education and training will markedly diminish and contribute to the needed steps for capacity building and in improving human development.

In summarizing the great challenges facing the underdeveloped areas in the development of scientific and technical education, Dr Gass wrote in 1964 "For such expansion of higher education, cannot proceed without parallel expansion of science teaching at the secondary school level nor for reasons of social or political necessity, to the complete exclusion of introducing quantitative and scientific notations at the primary level…when the number of students required for rapid economic growth of developing countries is taken into account, it may be expected that the major bottleneck will be in the supply of teachers. Impressive teacher training programs will be needed to cope with this problem. Thus, what is needed is a radically new approach in teaching systems in which the teacher, the technology, and the curriculum are defined in relation to one another, bearing in mind the feasible teaching objective, the available resources, and the particular learning characteristics of the children. Such systems should, of course, be based on the current attempts, both in the United States and Europe, to filtrate the curricula so as to eliminate unnecessary material. They should also be based on the assessment of the possibilities and relative cost of film, television, radio, tape, and records as a teaching media."[2] While some of these suggestions regarding teaching media can be replaced with current information technology, clearly these recommendations written almost 50 years ago are meaningful and as yet unmet in many developing countries. Thus, one does not need to invent new wheels to move forward in terms of basic science education and training; the principles and guidelines are available. The will and monetary, physical and human resources to implement them are needed.

REFERENCES

1. Tyokumber ET. Does science education in developing countries really count? Bull Ecol Soc Am 2010;91:432–7.
2. Gass RJ. Science and science education in developing countries. Int Rev Educ 1964;10:77–84.
3. Series on science for sustainable development No. 5. Science education and capacity building for sustainable development. Paris (France): International Council for Science, ICSU; 2002.
4. Gotch F, Gilmour J. Science, medicine, and research in the developing world: a perspective. Nat Immunol 2007;8:1273–6.
5. Shaw JE, Sicree RA, Zimmer PZ. Global estimates of prevalence of diabetes for 2010 and 2030. Diabetes Res Clin Pract 2010;87:4–14.
6. Leeder S, Greenberg HM, Raymond S. A race against time: the challenge of cardiovascular disease in developing economies. Available at: www.earth.columbia.edu/news/2004/images/raceagainsttime_FINAL_051104.pdf. Accessed May 31, 2011.
7. Promoting cardiovascular health in the developing world: a critical challenge to achieve global health. Washington, DC: Institute of Medicine of the National Academies; 2010.
8. The global burden of disease: 2004 update. ISBN 978 92 4 1563710. Geneva (Switzerland): World Health Organization; 2008.
9. Deckelbaum RJ, Kennedy E, Akabas SR. Nutrition policy: strengthening the roles of science and research. In: Kennedy E, Deckelbaum R, editors. The nation's nutrition. Washington, DC: International Life Sciences Institute Press; 2007. p. 287–92.
10. Bendich A, Deckelbaum RJ. Health economics of preventive nutrition. In: Bendich A, Deckelbaum RJ, editors. Preventive nutrition: the comprehensive guide for health professionals. 4th edition. New York: Humana Press/Springer Science; 2010. p. 23–49.
11. Available at: http://www.aercafrica.org/. Accessed February 28, 2011.
12. Available at: http://www.nexteinstein.org/. Accessed February 28, 2011.
13. Available at: http://www.aphrc.org/. Accessed February 28, 2011.
14. Available at: http://www.thrive.or.ug/. Accessed February 28, 2011.

15. Developing genetics for developing countries. Nat Genet 2007;39:1287.
16. Frenk J, Chen L, Bhutta ZA, et al. Health professionals for a new century: trans-forming education to strengthen health systems in an interdependent world. Lancet 2010;376:1923–58.
17. Murenzi R. Giving the new generation a chance: Nature News. Nature 2011;474: 543.
18. Nordling L. African nations vow to support science. Nature 2010;465:994–5.

Global Laboratory Systems Development: Needs and Approaches

Robert Martin, MPH, DrPH[a],*, Scott Barnhart, MD, MPH[b]

KEYWORDS

- Laboratory quality • Laboratory strengthening
- International laboratory practice
- U.S. President's Emergency Plan for AIDS Relief
- Laboratory history

The development of functional laboratory systems is being increasingly recognized as a key component of country health care systems,[1–6] and development of laboratory systems has been addressed in several recent publications.[7–12] A laboratory system is defined as an entity whose components (physical facilities, human resources, procurement systems, quality-assurance activities, and so forth) and output (data) contribute to the goals of the broader health system to assure appropriate patient care and to assure availability of data to public health and related programs for the purpose of surveillance and monitoring of disease. A country's health laboratory system includes laboratories addressing both animal and human health at the national level, at the state/provincial/regional level, and at the district and local levels. The system supports interdependent partnerships of public health, clinical, environmental, agricultural, and veterinary laboratories through public-private collaboration. Laboratories addressing human health are clinical and public health laboratories. Clinical laboratories are those laboratories whose primary purpose is supporting the provision of patient care. Clinical laboratories may also perform tests the results of which are reported through disease surveillance and monitoring systems of the country's public health system. Public health laboratory functions have been well described[13,14] and include assurances of timely detection of public health threats, providing data and analysis to inform those who require information for action, and establishment of systems to assure collection and testing of specimens required for surveillance. These

The authors have nothing to disclose.

[a] Laboratory Systems Development, Department of Global Health, International Training and Education Center for Health, University of Washington, 901 Boren Avenue, Suite 1100, Seattle, WA 98104, USA

[b] Division of Health Systems, Department of Global Health and Medicine, International Training and Education Center for Health, University of Washington, 901 Boren Avenue, Suite 1100, Seattle, WA 98104, USA

* Corresponding author.

E-mail address: RMartin1@u.washington.edu

Infect Dis Clin N Am 25 (2011) 677–691

doi:10.1016/j.idc.2011.05.001

0891-5520/11/$ – see front matter © 2011 Elsevier Inc. All rights reserved.

id.theclinics.com

core functions of public health laboratories involve examining specimens from individual patients and may have an impact on treatment or diagnosis, but the primary purpose of public health testing is to assure community health.

In developed countries, medical care is often described as evidence based. That is, clinical decisions are made not only on the clinical acumen of the health care provider, but are most often combined with evidence that supports clinical diagnosis. However, in resource-limited countries, diagnosis is most often based on clinical judgment because clinicians either have no access to laboratories or the quality of testing is poor because of inadequate laboratory facilities, inability to procure quality reagents in a timely manner, and lack of quality-assurance practices. This limitation engenders a devaluation of laboratory practice that is often translated into lack of support (**Fig. 1**) for development of laboratory capacity.

Until recently, in resource-limited countries, laboratory strengthening activities have most often been linked to disease-specific initiatives that often resulted in the introduction of physical facilities and laboratory methods and procedures that could usually not be properly maintained. Although laboratory systems and networks were sometimes noted as critical components of effective programs to address specific diseases such as diabetes,[15] tuberculosis (TB)[16] and polio, there were few attempts to integrate activities that were common to all programs. Major health initiatives including the Global Fund and the President's Emergency Program for AIDS Relief (PEPFAR) have been, for the most part, vertical disease programs. In these programs, investment in laboratories has, until recently, been focused on physical infrastructure, purchasing of equipment and supplies (most often outside the country's own procurement system), and bench-level training.[17] The PEPFAR laboratory program area has historically addressed support for human immunodeficiency virus (HIV) testing and treatment, assuring quality of HIV testing, improving diagnosis of TB and opportunistic infections, infant diagnosis of HIV infection, viral load testing, and monitoring for drug resistance. These efforts have successfully introduced improved quality and capacity of testing in resource-limited countries but they also uncovered broader issues that have not commonly been addressed by disease-specific initiatives. These broader issues include the lack management and leadership skills. Also absent are more fundamental needs such as the lack of referral and transport systems and lack of a focus on areas such as quality assurance that have resulted in delays in implementing common quality practices for which training has been given.

Among the global health initiatives (GHIs), HIV/acquired immune deficiency syndrome (AIDS) funding has driven a previously unmatched response by governments and donor organizations to address both short-term (emergency) responses

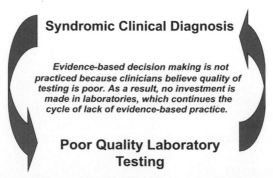

Fig. 1. The cycle that contributes to syndromic versus evidence-based diagnosis.

and, more recently, a shift to longer term approaches to assure country ownership and sustainability of health systems. In the last 10 years, the PEPFAR has provided billions of dollars to support program activities addressing HIV/AIDS detection, treatment, and care. The PEPFAR targets for the years 2010 to 2014 still include prevention, care and support, and treatment but now also highlight sustainability and country ownership as key issues. In addition to PEPFAR, other major drivers for the development of health systems include Millennium Development Goals and International Health Regulations, both of which require health systems (including laboratory services) capable of supporting activities to meet the goals of these internationally developed efforts.[18–21] Recently, the South-East Asia and Western Pacific Region (SEARO) of the World Health Organization (WHO) published a 5-year plan calling for strengthening of laboratory services in the region and calling for a view of laboratory services "not as a small component of a vertical health program but as a critical cross-cutting support service that needs to become an integral component of the health system at all levels."[6] This role for laboratories was also recognized and addressed in WHO/Centers for Disease Control (CDC) meetings on laboratory quality in which WHO and CDC have highlighted the advocacy roles of WHO, laboratory professionals, and ministries of health.[22,23]

Important issues that must be addressed include (1) law/regulation/policy specifying functions of laboratories; (2) educational programs for laboratory science (diploma, bachelor degree, and graduate degree); (3) procurement systems and a knowledge base that allows for the procurement of quality equipment reagents; (4) transportation systems for specimen referral; (5) quality-assurance measures at the national level with oversight/training responsibility for the laboratory system; (6) laboratory information systems (paper or electronic) that enable the accurate capture of date for patient treatment and for program evaluation; (7) biosafety office at the national level with oversight/training responsibility for the laboratory system.

In addition, a clear understanding of the technical aspects of internationally accepted laboratory practice, as well as an understanding of the critical role of leadership and management, is essential. It will be incumbent on donors who seek to support laboratory strengthening to address systems development with the same sense of passion and need as those who address disease-specific initiatives.

DEVELOPMENT OF HEALTH LABORATORIES

To better understand the complexities and challenges facing resource-limited systems in developing countries, it is important to understand the history of laboratory systems development in developed countries.

The history of development of laboratories as a standard component of the health care environment in the United States and western Europe dates to the early part of the twentieth century. Before that, physicians relied on signs and symptoms for diagnosis. Although some measurements were being used in the mid-1800s (eg, stethoscope, laryngoscope), to ascertain evidence of illness, it was not until the turn of the century that bacteriology, hematology, urinalysis, and coagulation were introduced and, by 1923, an American Medical Association survey showed that 48% of US hospitals had clinical laboratories.[24–27]

Accompanying the development of laboratories was the notion of laboratory science as a profession, and with that came development of various professional organizations representing professionals working in laboratory science. Laboratory practice as a discipline has evolved over the years and is now an accepted and recognized component of evidence-based practice. Several professional organizations represent either specific disciplines (eg, the American Society for Microbiology, established in 1899) or are member organizations representing those who work in laboratory medicine (eg, American Society for Clinical Pathology [ASCP]). The ASCP was founded in 1922 followed by a Board of Registry examination that required a college degree for certification. Since the turn of the century, more than 21 professional organizations representing laboratory science have been established. Along with these developments came the notion of quality in hospitals and in laboratories.

The development of national policy, law, and subsequent regulation of laboratory medicine in the United States is recent. It was not until 1967, because of fraud and abuse of Medicare, that the federal government developed the Clinical Laboratory Improvement Amendments (CLIA). In 1988, again in response to abuse that resulted in missed cases of cervical carcinoma, amendments to CLIA were developed.

In a recent editorial in Public Health Reports[28] the investigators point out that only in the past 10 years has the United States focused attention on the notion of a public health laboratory system that engages both clinical and public health laboratories. In 2001, the CDC and the Association of Public Health Laboratories (APHL) published the *Eleven Core Functions and Capabilities of State Public Health Laboratories*.[13] The introduction of the concept of a national laboratory system in the United States by the CDC in 2000 stimulated discussion of the need for such a system to better serve regional and national needs.[29,30] Those discussions took place in the historical context of laboratory development in the previous 100 years.

Resource-limited countries are only now going through a similar period of development of health laboratories (public health or clinical) and largely driven by outside interests. The lack of historical context and the lack of professional organizations are major barriers to rapid development of functional laboratory systems in these settings and are factors that must be considered by donor programs interested in development of quality health laboratories.

HISTORY OF DEVELOPMENT OF HEALTH LABORATORIES IN RESOURCE-CONSTRAINED COUNTRIES

While health laboratories were developing in the West, many resource-limited countries were occupied by colonial interests. Country development in all respects (including health) was not a priority and, as a result, minimal economic development occurred, and concurrent lack of development of human capital (eg, education) continued to weaken the economies of resource-limited countries.[31–33]

In the area of laboratory science, organizations such as the Pasteur Institute expanded in several resource-limited settings but were most often addressing research questions as opposed to development of country infrastructure. Overall, although laboratories were coming into their own as a presence in the health care environment in the West, there was little development of health care in resource-limited countries other than what was provided by benevolent organizations.

More recently in resource-limited countries, much of the attention to health has been from vertical programs focused on specific diseases (eg, the PEPFAR, Global Health Initiative [HIV/AIDS, TB, and malaria], polio eradication, Gates Foundation funding). However, this vertical approach has never sufficiently addressed broader health care issues and, as is the case with the polio eradication project, the question has become how to use the infrastructure more broadly.

In a Lancet editorial entitled, *Who runs global health?*[19] the commitment of GHIs is recognized, but several adverse effects on health systems are noted, among them "reduced quality of services to meet targets, decreases in domestic spending on health, misalignment between GHIs and country health needs, distraction of government officials from their overall responsibilities for health, and the creation of expensive parallel bureaucracies to manage GHIs in countries."

A compilation of data and commissioned reports[20] provides recommendations for how the disease-specific work of GHIs can be maximized if adjustments are made between the GHIs and country health systems.

Recommendations of the WHO Maximizing Positive Synergies Collaborative Group

Recommendation 1: Infuse the health system's strengthening agenda with the sense of ambition and speed that has characterized the GHIs.

Recommendation 2: Extend the targets of GHIs and agree to indicators for health systems strengthening.

Recommendation 3: Improve alignment of planning processes and resource allocations among GHIs, and between GHIs and country health systems.

Recommendation 4: Generate more realizable data for the costs and benefits of strengthening health systems, and evidence to inform additional and complimentary investments to those of GHIs.

Recommendation 5: Ensure an increase in national and global health financing, and in more predictable financing, to support the sustainable and equitable growth of health systems.

These recommendations addressing financing, quality, procurement, workforce, management systems, and coordination among and between donors apply directly to the development of laboratory systems as a component of an overall health system.

Easterly[34] describes the cycling between horizontal and vertical programs and marginal versus transformational approaches that have been going on for some years and cites this as an example "of an inability to learn transformational approaches in foreign aid to Africa." Advocates of both approaches tend to overpromise potential outcomes largely because of the impact of unknown variables. As could be predicted, there has been a recent attempt to move away from a disease-specific focus to a more horizontal approach. However, accompanying the desire to address health issues in a horizontal manner is an admonition to assure country ownership and sustainability. Easterly states that:

It would be worth testing and exploring more the hypothesis that most successful development is homegrown. And if so, research should concentrate more on homegrown determinants of development rather than spend so much time on outsider's actions. Perhaps then we might find that the ones most likely to "save Africa" are Africans themselves.

This statement is true not only for development of economic and educational programs but also of the development of country health care systems and their components including national laboratory systems. With an increased focus on country ownership, there may be an opportunity for even greater success in development of stronger health care systems, including laboratory systems.

NEEDS FOR DEVELOPMENT OF INTEGRATED LABORATORY SYSTEMS

To develop a functioning national laboratory system requires an understanding of the role of health laboratories and the complexity of the systems that support them. Health laboratories (public, clinical-government, and nongovernment) are a critical component for evidence-based clinical care and for disease detection, prevention, and control. In the WHO Integrated Framework Model for Health System, the laboratory is considered a component of Medical Products, Vaccines, and Technologies. As noted earlier, the quality and availability of laboratory services is often taken for granted in developed countries but, in most resource-limited countries, laboratory testing services are of poor quality and the test offerings are minimal other than in some donor-supported laboratories that are often more focused on research activities.

Given the history of efforts in the past 10 years, it has become increasingly clear that there are multiple and challenging elements all of which must be addressed to develop country ownership and sustainability of laboratory systems. Most efforts supported by donors and government programs to develop laboratories in countries have not focused on these elements but have focused on implementation of laboratory methods and training on how to perform those methods properly. Because of the lack of a compelling vision for a laboratory system within countries, there has been a lack of response on the part of donors and government programs to invest in the elements critical to country ownership and sustainability (**Table 1**).

Law and Regulation

Although building laboratories and introducing new tests, and the requisite training to perform tests, continues to be important, it is now clear that development of a laboratory system requires an underpinning of law and regulation that some have characterized as political will. Most resource-limited countries do not have laws (or they are weak and/or unenforced) requiring demonstration of adherence to standards (eg, personnel, safety, quality measures).

Laboratory Leadership and Management

Leadership and management skills must be strengthened among laboratory directors and managers. Because laboratories have often been marginalized in resource-limited settings, there is little understanding of why management and leadership are important characteristics to ensure development of a robust system. Several programs have been developed to provide laboratory management training (University of Washington, APHL/George Washington University, Royal Tropical Institute/KIT Biomedical Research). The lack of such skills is exemplified by lack of laboratory leadership engagement in discussions of national planning efforts, in addressing human resource issues (eg, retention, professional development), and in financial/procurement issues affecting laboratory practice. For example, procurement of equipment and reagents is a problem because those responsible for procurement have not been trained to write quality specifications, and because those with responsibility for purchasing within the procurement system have little or no understanding of the need for quality. Therefore, the decision point becomes only cost of the equipment/product. Although countries have been encouraged to develop a tiered approach to enable referral of tests, that system often exists on paper but the absence of management skills has often resulted in lack of referral because transportation systems are not available.

Quality

In the working definition of the word system provided earlier, laboratory systems or networks are more than the physical facilities that house laboratory equipment and laboratory scientists. The importance of a systems approach to quality, even for facilities with few services, is being increasingly recognized. Recently, the WHO, the CDC, and the Clinical Laboratory Standards Institute (CLSI) collaborated on the development of a management training package that addresses 12 Quality System Essentials. These 12 essential components (organization, facilities, equipment, purchasing and inventory, process control (sample management, quality control), assessment/audits [external quality assessment], personnel, customer service, error management, process improvement, document and records, laboratory information systems) are dependent on other systems within government infrastructure (eg, procurement, human resources) that must be responsive and supportive of laboratory requirements. In addition, laboratories exist to provide benefit to patient care and to public health programs; regular interaction between laboratory leadership and program leadership is essential. A functional laboratory system must be defined as not only a hierarchal referral arrangement of laboratory services (test results) but must include those components mentioned earlier that are essential to the functioning of a laboratory and contribute to high-quality testing and provision of interpretable data. Within laboratories, there has been little attention to development of internationally accepted standards. Even with training of laboratory management to better understand the importance of quality standards, without national policies/regulation there is little incentive to implement standards.

Education

Although these short programs contribute to the development of individuals currently working in laboratories, there is also a need for undergraduate and graduate educational programs that have taken into account internationally accepted accreditation standards. In the past, a common practice to develop a cadre of well-educated scientists was to send individuals to universities in developed countries. However, that practice often contributed to brain drain because these graduates often found more promising work in the countries in which they were educated or with donor organizations. These individuals comprised the diaspora that some believed would ultimately become the nexus for addressing the weaknesses of existing systems. However, these individuals were most often ill suited to return and engage in local science and technology systems because of the lack of development of those systems.[35] Although educating individuals in settings outside their own country may be a part of the solution, attention must be given to simultaneously developing educational programs in-country.

Another factor that has held back development of country systems is the lack of coordination among donors. Countries often do not have the capacity to coordinate various donor funding sources and, because of the lack of national plans for laboratory systems development, there is often no roadmap for coordinating donors who are driven by their own needs and agendas. Recently, within the US government, attention has been given to a whole-of-government approach that encourages US government agencies to collaborate in countries where they are working together.

CURRENT EFFORTS ADDRESSING LABORATORY SYSTEMS DEVELOPMENT

Developing better strategies for improving laboratory systems in resource-limited countries is being addressed by WHO and by major donor organizations including US government agencies and their programs.

WHO/SEARO in their Asia Pacific Strategy for Strengthening Health Laboratory Services (2010–2015)[6] has articulated a broad strategy for strengthening laboratory services including:

> ... a tiered laboratory network with each level having appropriate physical infrastructure, human resources, procurement and supply management, referral networks and information system. It promotes quality, biosafety, occupational health, and rational use of laboratory services and operational research to assure the use of appropriate technology.

Table 1
Elements critical for country ownership and sustainability

	Description	Benefit	Comments
Law and regulation and policy development	Laws permitting the establishment of appropriate regulation controlling performance of laboratory testing. National policies addressing the core principles of a national laboratory system	Establishes country ownership and helps assure sustainability Assures scarce resources are used to provide reliable data Data from all laboratories will meet a minimum standard of quality Test kits will have met requirements established by the country or by the international community (eg, WHO validation of HIV test kits) Safety of workers and the community in which the laboratory is located can be assured National policies guide both the public and private sector in creation of services	Introduction of the underpinning of law and regulation helps assure a sustainable presence In the absence of regulatory authority, the quality and validity of data are unknown and will contribute little to either patient care or to public health programs Regulation addressing importation of test kits and reagents (FDA role in United States) is essential to provide for care and for program information Regulation can clearly define roles and responsibilities in health emergencies
Leadership and management	Leadership and management skills to assure best use of resources required for quality laboratory results	Leadership and management skills help assure: that the responsible individuals have the capabilities to develop appropriate policy an owner-driven agenda and country-appropriate direction of donor funding development of strategic plans for the laboratory network development of system-oriented approaches to assuring availability of testing (eg, establishment of referral systems) responsiveness to health emergencies provision of working environments (eg, career paths) that limit brain drain to donor programs or to jobs outside the country integration of disease-specific initiatives	Possessing appropriate leadership and management skills helps assure laboratory leadership participation in development of programs addressing national or international initiatives (eg, International Health Regulations) Management of a country's network of laboratories (public and private) requires modern management skills Laboratory leadership is required to help address broader issues such as examination of future workforce needs at various levels in the health care system

National quality program	National quality programs that provide for periodic auditing, delivery of proficiency testing, and establishment of courier systems help provide consistency of national data that allows country-wide evaluation when addressing national health issues	Provides assurances to the public and to health programs about the accuracy and reliability of test results (information) Can lead to international accredition (eg, WHO/AFRO)	Most resource-limited countries have no quality programs and clinicians and public health programs cannot rely on the accuracy of information produced by laboratories A national approach helps assure broad availability of external quality assessment (eg, proficiency testing from other countries)
Educational programs	MoH leadership in development national preservice and in-service educational and training activities is essential to develop and maintain skills of laboratory scientists	Assures an adequately educated and trained entry-level workforce (provides for ongoing education and training of existing workers) Addresses a national standard curriculum that includes current best practices	Implementation of new technologies is delayed or is not possible in the absence of timely training

Abbreviations: FDA, US Food and Drug Administration; MoH, Ministry of Health; WHO/AFRO, World Health Organization Regional Office for Africa.

Although the laboratory tests performed within the system may vary by country, the *Asia Pacific Strategy for Strengthening Health Laboratory Services*[6] and the *Technical and Operational Recommendations for Clinical Laboratory Testing Harmonization and Standardization* provide[36] examples of the types of testing that may be offered at each level. The issues addressed in the plan are not unique to the Asia-Pacific region. The description of major issues and a framework for laboratory services provide essential information and guidance for countries hoping to strengthen their laboratory networks. The complete table of recommended tests at various levels of service can be found at this WHO Web site: (http://www.who.int/hiv/amds/WHOLabRecommendationByLevelFinal.pdf). However, it is critical to consider a variety of issues when implementing a tiered approach, including resource allocation, procurement and supply chain, instrument service, technology selection, quality, and training.[5]

Guidance such as this is important when engaging donors in discussion of need and where funds should be spent. There have been major accomplishments by various donor programs to move countries toward development of country-owned sustainable models addressing many of the issues described in this plan.

For example, the World Health Organization Regional Office for Africa; (WHO/AFRO) and the PEPFAR program have implemented a regional laboratory accreditation program[37] in Africa. A 5-step accreditation program has been implemented that will prepare limited-resource countries to develop a process enabling them to move toward accreditation in a manner suitable for the resources available in those countries. Rather than relying on a pass-fail system, this process enables laboratories to be recognized for progress toward the ultimate goal of accreditation. The process does not replace international accreditation schemes (eg, ISO15189) but provides a pathway for resource-limited laboratories to better prepare laboratories to enroll.

PEPFAR has made major contributions to the development of laboratory capacity and capability in resource-limited countries. From 2004 to 2009, PEPFAR supported more than 2000 laboratories and approximately 20,000 HIV testing sites in 15 focus countries in sub-Saharan Africa. This support has included testing for monitoring of disease for prevention programs, and for care and treatment of individuals infected with HIV. Quality of testing has been addressed by assuring availability of high-quality test kits, implementing the use of standardized methods for testing and standardization of accessioning and reporting documents, and development of simple procedures to enable appropriate quality control at the local level.[38]

In addition to addressing HIV-specific needs, the PEPFAR program has supported improvement of laboratory methods for diagnosis of TB and other opportunistic infections, support for development of supply chain management within countries, and support for development of laboratory information systems using established guidelines.[39]

For example, in Tanzania, PEFAR has supported harmonization of testing and standardization of laboratory equipment that led to reduced procurement costs for equipment, reagents, and service contracts.[40] Accomplishment required strong support from the Ministry of Health and Social Welfare. In Nigeria, PEPFAR supported development of infrastructure to support infant diagnosis of HIV (polymerase chain reaction suites that can be used for other molecular assays).[41] In Zimbabwe, PEPAR is supporting the strengthening of the TB program (renovation of facilities and mentoring in implementation of methods and in managing the laboratory). In Ethiopia, PEPFAR supported the Ethiopian Health and Nutrition Research Institute (EHNRI) to implement a coordinating task force led by the director of EHNRI and whose members include implementing partners. This group meets regularly to address issues related to work being performed in the various regions of Ethiopia and to coordinate activities from EHNRI in Addis Ababa. Implementing partners, including the University of Washington/University of California San Francisco's International Training and Educational Center for Health, participate in this process and are guided by EHNRI and by regional health bureaus in various laboratory strengthening activities including building renovations, management training, and implementation of new methods.

The PEPFAR program is also supporting the development on the African Society for Laboratory Medicine (ASLM). An inaugural meeting is being held in Addis Ababa, Ethiopia, in March 2011. For many countries, and certainly for most African laboratory scientists, this is likely their first opportunity to participate in a professional organization addressing the concerns of their profession.

These examples of PEPFAR activities that address strengthening laboratories beyond the disease-specific interests around HIV make clear the recognized need for a broader approach to building country ownership and sustainability.

The Laboratory Systems Development Branch of the Center for Emerging and Zoonotic Infectious Diseases at the CDC, working with the State Department (Biosecurity Engagement Program [BEP]) and the Department of Defense (Defense Threat Reduction Agency [DTRA] program) specifically addresses "training in infectious disease surveillance and molecular diagnostics, and laboratory capacity building activities" and is participating in a whole-of-government approach to laboratory systems strengthening in a number countries in central Asia and the southern Caucuses. In Pakistan, these agencies are collaborating to provide assistance in the development of an integrated disease surveillance system that includes strengthening of both laboratory and epidemiology capacity and capability. In Georgia, Kazakhstan, and Azerbaijan, laboratory capacity has been developed including central reference laboratories and often regional laboratories. This infrastructure serves as a basis for further development of national systems in these countries.

An extensive overview of laboratory strengthening activities was undertaken by the RAND (Research and Development) corporation[42] by reviewing published reports, interviews of major donor organizations, and case studies of laboratory systems in 3 countries (Thailand, Kenya, and Ethiopia). Major findings included the following:

- Laboratory systems: countries are developing multitiered systems, but infrastructure declines rapidly at each successive level.
- Coordination: a disease-specific focus by funding agencies and their programs continues to be a barrier to integration.
- Quality systems: although countries and donors are aware of the issues of quality, there has been little progress toward developing the notion of a quality systems approach.

SUMMARY

A country-owned and sustainable laboratory system is recognized as an essential component of the health system infrastructure, and many US government agencies and their partners have been providing support to resource-limited countries to develop laboratory infrastructure that will support the countries' health system needs (eg, accurate burden of disease information) as well as supporting the countries' international responsibilities (eg, International Health Regulations and Millennium Development Goals). Because donor funding is not likely to increase in the current global economic climate, addressing factors that will lead to country ownership becomes even more critical. Although disease-specific programs have provided much in the way of physical laboratory infrastructure and implementation of laboratory methods, several additional factors must be considered to assure progress toward country-owned sustainability.

To assure future contributions of vertical programs, donor program leadership must address the complexity of laboratory systems, the need for integration, and the scale of effort required to establish such systems in resource-constrained settings. That can only be accomplished through assurance that future grants/contracts/cooperative agreements contain language that requires recipients to address systems development.

Attempting to develop a system of interconnected laboratories in countries where the laboratories have only existed as independent entities presents major difficulties beyond learning how to implement new methods and perform procedures. Even when implementing disease-specific initiatives, political will and commitment, providing leadership and management training (development of strategic plans, understanding the interconnectedness of financial systems, human resource systems, and the regulatory/policy areas), addressing educational needs, assuring a national focus on quality, and assuring coordination among donors are critical to success.[16] A major barrier for systems development is the lack of awareness or understanding of how a system will improve the ability to address health issues. Although providing training around laboratory management is important, if participants in that training do not have a vision for how the system in their country might function to support health programs, it will be difficult to implement sustainable management practices. Study tours or assessments by a country's leadership should be supported to provide experience of how such a system works in developed countries, or in neighboring countries where there has been advancement, and to talk with colleagues who work in the system.

Building the evidence to inform the development of laboratory systems is a difficult undertaking. Using concepts introduced by implementation science may be an important consideration. Because disease-specific strategies have proved too focused and limited for sustainability, broadening the understanding of the many factors involved in developing a laboratory system would be an important contribution. The Fogarty International Center has designated implementation science as one of its 5 priority areas for research and research training in global health, and a March 2010 report of the Implementation Science Working Group[43] outlined the types of implementation science research and their importance for improvement of global health programs and policies. Implementation research examines both health and nonhealth determinants of successful public health programs. For laboratory systems development, the science base (laboratory methods) is critically important, but the elements required for a successful laboratory system go far beyond the laboratory; a successful system requires those building blocks (discussed earlier) of organizational structure (are laboratories located in the right place in the organizational structure?), leadership (are there the skills and abilities to form critical partnerships and to provide advocacy?), management (are laboratories managed in ways that lead to international accreditation, and are financial systems in place that enable rapid procurement of appropriate supplies, equipment, and so forth?), national approaches to quality, educational systems that provide sustainable human resources, and information technology infrastructure (accurate accessioning of specimens, rapid reporting of results, and ability to analyze data).

These are key elements for consideration as donors consider the implementation of functional laboratory systems in resource-limited countries.

Continuing the prevailing strategy of focusing on single diseases and the interventions associated with those diseases is too limited and does not contribute to the development of sustainable, country-owned programs. An immediate focus of resources on the components required for a functioning system, combined with continued technical support, will provide a strong base that will enable countries to assume responsibility for their country-specific needs as well as improving their capability to address international responsibilities.

REFERENCES

1. Martin R, Hearn TL, Ridderhof JC, et al. Implementation of a quality systems approach for laboratory practice in resource-constrained countries. AIDS 2005; 19(Suppl 2):S59–65.
2. Nkengasong JN. Strengthening laboratory services and systems in resource-poor countries. Am J Clin Pathol 2009;131(6):774.
3. Birx D, de Souza M, Nkengasong JN. Laboratory challenges in the scaling up of HIV, TB, and malaria programs: the interaction of health and laboratory systems, clinical research, and service delivery. Am J Clin Pathol 2009;131(6): 849–51.
4. Justman JE, Koblavi-Deme S, Tanuri A, et al. Developing laboratory systems and infrastructure for HIV scale-up: a tool for health systems strengthening in resource-limited settings. J Acquir Immune Defic Syndr 2009;52(Suppl 1):S30–3.
5. Peter TF, Shimada Y, Freeman RR, et al. The need for standardization in laboratory networks. Am J Clin Pathol 2009;131(6):867–74.
6. WHO. Asia Pacific Strategy for Strengthening Health Laboratory Services (2010–2015). 2009. Manilla (Phillipines): South-East Asia Region: World Health Organization; 2010.
7. Petti CA, Polage CR, Quinn TC, et al. Laboratory medicine in Africa: a barrier to effective health care. Clin Infect Dis 2006;42(3):377–82.
8. Berkelman R, Cassell G, Specter S, et al. The "Achilles heel" of global efforts to combat infectious diseases. Clin Infect Dis 2006;42(10):1503–4.
9. Bates I, Maitland K. Are laboratory services coming of age in sub-Saharan Africa? Clin Infect Dis 2006;42(3):383–4.
10. Muula AS, Maseko FC. Medical laboratory services in Africa deserve more. Clin Infect Dis 2006;42(10):1503.
11. Okeke IN. Diagnostic insufficiency in Africa. Clin Infect Dis 2006;42(10):1501–3.
12. Frieden TR, Henning KJ. Public health requirements for rapid progress in global health. Glob Public Health 2009;4(4):323–37.
13. Witt-Kushner J, Astles JR, Ridderhof JC, et al. Core functions and capabilities of state public health laboratories: a report of the Association of Public Health Laboratories. MMWR Recomm Rep 2002;51(RR-14):1–8.
14. Inhorn SL, Astles JR, Gradus S, et al. The state public health laboratory system. Public Health Rep 2010;125(Suppl 2):4–17.
15. Windus DW, Ladenson JH, Merrins CK, et al. Impact of a multidisciplinary intervention for diabetes in Eritrea. Clin Chem 2007;53(11):1954–9.
16. Paramasivan CN, Lee E, Kao K, et al. Experience establishing tuberculosis laboratory capacity in a developing country setting. Int J Tuberc Lung Dis 2010;14(1): 59–64.
17. Ridderhof JC, van Deun A, Kam KM, et al. Roles of laboratories and laboratory systems in effective tuberculosis programmes. Bull World Health Organ 2007; 85(5):354–9.
18. Alva S, Kleinau E, Pomeroy A, et al. Measuring the impact of health systems strengthening (USAID). Geneva (Switzerland): World Health Organization; 2009.

19. Who runs global health? Lancet 2009;373(9681):2083.
20. Samb B, Evans T, Dybul M, et al. An assessment of interactions between global health initiatives and country health systems. Lancet 2009;373(9681): 2137–69.
21. Taboy CH, Chapman W, Albetwkova A, et al. Integrated disease investigations and surveillance planning: a systems approach to strengthening national surveillance and detection of events of public health importance in support of the International Health Regulations. BMC Public Health 2010;10(Suppl 1):S6.
22. WHO. Joint WHO-CDC Conference on Health Laboratory Quality Systems. Weekly epidemiological record. WHO; 2008. p. 285–92.
23. WHO/AFRO. Maputo-declaration. WHO/AFRO; 2008. Available at: www.who.int/diagnostics.laboratory/Maputo.Declaration.2008.pdf. Accessed May 24, 2011.
24. Berger D. A brief history of medical diagnosis and the birth of the clinical laboratory. Part 4–Fraud and abuse, managed-care, and lab consolidation. MLO Med Lab Obs 1999;31(12):38–42.
25. Berger D. A brief history of medical diagnosis and the birth of the clinical laboratory. Part 3–Medicare, government regulation, and competency certification. MLO Med Lab Obs 1999;31(10):40–2. p. 44.
26. Berger D. A brief history of medical diagnosis and the birth of the clinical laboratory. Part 2–Laboratory science and professional certification in the 20th century. MLO Med Lab Obs 1999;31(8):32–4. p. 36, 38.
27. Berger D. A brief history of medical diagnosis and the birth of the clinical laboratory. Part 1–Ancient times through the 19th century. MLO Med Lab Obs 1999; 31(7):28–30. p. 32, 34–40.
28. Downes FP, Ridderhof JC. The evolving Public Health Laboratory System. Public Health Rep 2010;125(Suppl 2):1–3.
29. Astles JR, White VA, Williams LO. Origins and development of the national laboratory system for public health testing. Public Health Rep 2010;125(Suppl 2): 18–30.
30. Martin R, Astles JR, Kushner JW. Are we ready for a national laboratory system? A call for stronger working relationships among the medical care community, hospital/independent laboratories, and public health laboratories. Journal of the Clinical Laboratory Management Association Vantage Point 2001;5(12/13):1–4.
31. Fieldhouse DK. The West and the third world: trade, colonialism, dependence, and development. Oxford (United Kingdom); Malden (MA): Blackwell Publishers; 1999.
32. Snodgrass DR. Inequality and economic development in Malaysia. Kuala Lumpur (Malaysia). New York: Oxford University Press; 1980.
33. Hill CB. World development report 1990 – poverty - world-bank. Econ Dev Cult Change 1993;41(2):427–30.
34. Easterly W. Can the West Save Africa? J Econ Lit 2009;47(2):373–447.
35. Gaillard J. Gaillard AM. Can the scientific diaspora save African science? 2003. Available at: www.scidev.net/en/opinions/can_the_african_diaspora_save_African_science.html. Accessed May 24, 2011.
36. WHO. Consultation on technical and operational recommendations for clinical laboratory testing harmonization and standardization. Maputo (Mozambique): WHO; 2008.
37. Gershy-Damet GM, Rotz P, Cross D, et al. The World Health Organization African region laboratory accreditation process: improving the quality of laboratory systems in the African region. Am J Clin Pathol 2010;134(3):393–400.
38. Parekh BS, Anyanwu J, Patel H, et al. Dried tube specimens: a simple and cost-effective method for preparation of HIV proficiency testing panels and quality

control materials for use in resource-limited settings. J Virol Methods 2010;163(2): 295–300.

39. Kakkar R, Maryogo-Robinson L, Morgan M, et al. Guidebook for implementation of laboratory information systems in resource-poor settings. Silver Spring (MD): Association of Public Health Laboratories; 2005.

40. Massambu C, Mwangi C. The Tanzania experience: clinical laboratory testing harmonization and equipment standardization at different levels of a tiered health laboratory system. Am J Clin Pathol 2009;131(6):861–6.

41. Abimiku AG. Building laboratory infrastructure to support scale-up of HIV/AIDS treatment, care, and prevention: in-country experience. Am J Clin Pathol 2009; 131(6):875–86.

42. Olmsted SS, Moore M, Meili RC, et al. Strengthening laboratory systems in resource-limited settings. Am J Clin Pathol 2010;134(3):374–80.

43. Fogarty. Implementation science and global health meeting report. Bethesda (MD): Fogarty International Center; 2010.

Drugs and Diagnostic Innovations to Improve Global Health

Rosanna W. Peeling, PhD[a],*, Solomon Nwaka, PhD[b]

KEYWORDS

- Drugs - Diagnostics - Innovation

Infectious diseases continue to cause millions of deaths every year, disproportionately affecting the poor and young children in developing countries.[1] Strategies for reducing the burden of disease due to infectious causes include vaccination programs, health education, vector control, provision of clean water and sanitation, and treatments including mass drug administration for some neglected tropical diseases. However, for most infected patients, access to diagnostic tests and appropriate treatment remains an urgent priority. In the last 30 years, only 1% of the drugs that have come to the market were developed for infectious tropical diseases.[2] Existing drugs for these diseases are often toxic and are becoming less and less effective because of the development of resistance. Highly accurate diagnostic tests and effective therapies are available for patients with infectious disease in the developed world but they are neither affordable nor accessible for patients in the developing world.[3]

For diseases with a specific clinical presentation, management decisions can be made without the use of a diagnostic laboratory. For example, UNICEF and the World Health organization (WHO) have developed guidelines for the Integrated Management of Childhood Illness (IMCI), under which children with fever, cough, and rapid breathing are treated with an antibiotic that covers the common causes of bacterial pneumonia.[4] Patients presenting with symptoms of sexually transmitted infection, such as urethral discharge or genital ulcers, are treated for the common causes of those syndromes.[5] Syndromic management can be highly effective, but inevitably leads to overtreatment, resulting in wasted resources and increased risk of development of antimicrobial resistance. For infectious diseases where patients are asymptomatic or where clinical

The authors have nothing to disclose.
a Department of Clinical Research, Faculty of Infectious and Tropical Diseases, London School of Hygiene and Tropical Medicine, Keppel Street, London WC1E 7HT, UK
b UNICEF/UNDP/World Bank/World Health Organization Special Programme for Research and Training in Tropical Diseases, Avenue Appia, Geneva 27, Switzerland
* Corresponding author.
E-mail address: rosanna.peeling@lshtm.ac.uk

Infect Dis Clin N Am 25 (2011) 693–705
doi:10.1016/j.idc.2011.06.002
0891-5520/11/$ – see front matter © 2011 Elsevier Inc. All rights reserved.

id.theclinics.com

features are nonspecific but the consequences of infection are serious such as human immunodeficiency virus (HIV) or syphilis, diagnostic tests are needed for early detection to guide treatment, reduce the risk of development of long-term complications, and prevent onward transmission. Ideally, the diagnosis should be made at the point-of-care (POC), so that treatment can be started without delay, and should not depend on the availability of a laboratory or highly trained staff.[6,7]

Accurate diagnostics for surveillance, outbreak investigations, monitoring the effectiveness of interventions, detecting and monitoring drug resistance, and certifying disease elimination are critical for effective disease control. However, these are often overlooked because of lack of resources and sustainable systems in most developing countries to support these. The performance and operational characteristics of these diagnostics are often different from those required for patient management. The development of these tools for diseases of public health importance in the developing world is an urgent priority. Strengthening the development and access of these diagnostics tools along with the required treatments in developing countries will support both disease control and elimination programs.

This article examines the landscape of drugs and diagnostics in the developing world and highlights major barriers to access to existing drugs and diagnostics. New research developments and innovative funding schemes to drive drugs and diagnostics innovations in the developing world to fulfill the promise of delivering affordable drugs and diagnostics in a faster timeframe are also reviewed. Concomitant developments on the demand side such as harmonized regulatory standards, technology assessment, and capacity building for quality assurance and health systems management are needed to ensure efficient uptake and sustainable adoption of products of drugs and diagnostics innovations.

DRUGS AND DIAGNOSTICS IN THE DEVELOPING WORLD
Lack of Investment in Drug Development for Diseases Prevalent in the Developing World

The costs of research and development (R&D), and the time from target discovery to bringing diagnostics, drugs, or vaccines to market vary. Each R&D investment has its opportunity costs. It is estimated by the pharmaceutical industry that the cost of bringing a new drug to market ranges from US$500 million to about US$1 billion including the cost of failures and can take up to 15 years.[8–10] Recent experience from public-private partnerships show that the cost of developing a new drug for treating infectious tropical diseases ranges from $100–200 million. However, it is not clear whether this estimate includes discovery and development of products or just clinical development alone.

The dearth of new antibacterial drug candidates in the R&D pipeline is an urgent concern. Compared with many therapeutic classes, antiinfectives are considered a relatively small commercial market compared with lifestyle drugs or drugs for chronic diseases. The antibacterial drug pipeline is almost empty. In the past 3 decades, only 2 novel classes of antiinfectives have been marketed: the oxazolidinones and cyclic lipopeptides, both of which are for the treatment of gram-positive bacterial infections, and resistance has already been documented for both compounds.[11] Currently, only 5 (1.6%) of drugs in the R&D pipelines of the top 15 drug companies are antibacterials.

The Long Road to Product Development

In addition to the lack of investment, the pathway from target discovery to clinical trials is slow with significant attrition.[12] There is an enormous valley of death as many promising leads have fallen by the wayside, making the process inefficient (**Fig. 1**). Traditionally, the success rate of pharmaceutical companies is only around 6% to 7% in producing lead compounds. For example, only 5 leads were delivered from 70 high-throughput screening campaigns conducted by GlaxoSmithKline between 1995 and 2001.[11] In addition, discovery research and innovation in public health are often complicated by the unclear role of intellectual property in access to medicines for the poor.[13]

Two case studies are presented to demonstrate the lengthy process from development to licensing and production. These examples are drawn from products that have originated from the developing world.

1. NIPRISAN The National Institute for Pharmaceutical Research and Development (NIPRD), based in Abuja, Nigeria, developed a therapy from plant extracts for sickle-cell disease, a genetic disease affecting millions of people in Africa; for example, in Nigeria about 4 million people in Nigeria's population of 150 million are affected. With the help of the United Nations Development Program (UNDP) and others, NIPRD and the traditional health practitioner patented the drug and conducted further R&D in 1993 but the clinical trial result was published in 2001.[8] Niprisan was licensed to the Nigerian subsidiary of US chemical company Xechem International in 2002. But last year, the company closed its factory. The next step for the production of the drug is unclear. NIPRD also has encouraging results for phytocompounds to treat malaria and tuberculosis (TB) but research on all these projects has almost ground to a halt recently because of lack of funding (Nature.com, published online 18 November 2010, doi:10.1038/news.2010.602).

2. Qinghaosu was isolated by Chinese chemists in 1971 from the leaves of the plant, *Artemisia annua* but it was not until 1991 that Novartis (then Ciba-Geigy) began collaborating with Kunming Pharmaceuticals on Coartem production. Marketing approval was obtained in 1998 and Novartis partnered with the WHO in 2001 to make Coartem available in malaria-endemic countries on a not-for-profit basis.

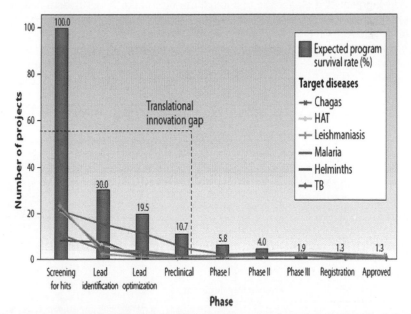

Fig. 1. Attrition rates (the valley of death) in the drug development pipeline for infectious diseases. (*Courtesy of* S. Nwaka, PhD, Geneva, Switzerland.)

Access to Affordable and Efficacious Drugs

In the developing world, access to medicines varies across countries, depending on income levels, coverage and quality of health system infrastructure, political commitment, and the resources allocated to health care. The problem is acute for HIV, TB, malaria, and diarrheal diseases that cause high mortality, for example, 5 million people were on HIV/AIDS treatment in developing countries in 2010, but another 10 million are in urgent need and will die within the next few years without it. Even when political commitment to adopt new medicines is made, rollout of more effective medicines is too slow in developing countries and often plagued by shortage of health workers, supply chain issues, and other health infrastructure barriers.

In 1999, Médecins Sans Frontières (MSF) set up an Access Campaign to improve access to existing health care tools including medicines, diagnostics, and vaccines, and to stimulate the development of improved health care tools for people in countries where MSF works. WHO, national governments, nongovernmental organizations, multilateral organizations, academic institutions, and the pharmaceutical industry have responded to this effort. We are now witnessing increasing access to medicines and support for the building of health care infrastructure to facilitate universal access to basic health care, including medicines. In 2001, the Doha declaration on trade-related aspects of intellectual property rights and public health and the use of flexibilities in trade agreements by countries such as India, Thailand, or Brazil has helped to improve access for some HIV drugs.

The WHO estimates that 1.8 million people die from TB each year. As a consequence of the slow progress of drug R&D taking more than 10 years to come to market and then another 2 to 5 years to roll out, how many people will die while waiting for the next new drug to come to those who need them?

Lack of Investment in Diagnostic R&D and in Diagnostic Services

The development of a diagnostic test is estimated to take 2 to 10 years with investment ranging from $2 million to $100 million.[14] For products with a viable commercial market, the development pathway is driven, funded, and managed largely by the private sector (**Fig. 2**). For diagnostics needed in the developing world, there has

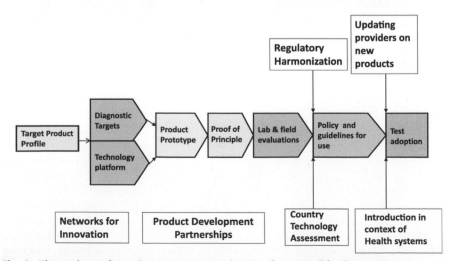

Fig. 2. The pathway from discovery to test adoption for accessible diagnostics.

been little private sector interest in investing in diagnostic product R&D, because of a perceived lack of return for investment.

Diagnostics services are often undervalued. The Lewin report on the value of diagnostics noted that although diagnostics comprise less than 5% of hospital costs and about 1.6% of all USA Medicare costs, their findings influence 60% to 70% of health care decision making.[15] In the developing world, expenditure on diagnostics is often a negligible proportion of health care spending. A WHO report showed that only 6% of health expenditure at a district hospital in Malawi is on diagnosis.[16]

Patients in rural areas may have to walk for hours to reach a clinic where laboratory services are available. If they are asked to come back for their results the following day or week, many will fail to do so. The result is that most patients in developing countries are treated presumptively at health facilities that do not have laboratory facilities. The 2004 World Development Report cites lack of accessibility as one of the major reasons why health services fail.[17]

Variable Quality of Laboratory Services

Laboratory diagnosis improves patient care most efficiently within well-managed health care systems. Such a system requires technical competence, access to good quality reagents and a quality assurance program, and a timely communication system between the laboratory and the health care provider. In addition, health care providers need to value and should be able to interpret laboratory results to guide clinical management. In the developing world, the quality of laboratory services are often compromised because of lack of resources, supply logistics, and trained personnel. These problems lead to physicians not trusting laboratory results, which in turn lead to further neglect of laboratory services.[18]

Lack of International and National Regulatory Standards for Approval of Diagnostics

National regulatory processes for drugs provide safeguards for the safety and effectiveness of drugs used in a country. Most countries have a process for reviewing the evidence from drug trials to support the introduction of new drugs, and this has done much to improve the quality of drugs used in developing countries. That said, there is the strong need to strengthen drug regulatory capacity in developing countries especially Africa. Unfortunately, apart from tests used for blood banking, regulatory standards are often lacking for diagnostic tests; especially those targeting diseases that are uncommon in industrialized countries.[19] As a result, diagnostic tests are often sold in most of the developing world without any formal evaluation of their performance and effectiveness.

THE WAY FORWARD

2008 marked the 30th anniversary of the declaration of Alma-Ata at the International Conference of Primary Health Care, at which United Nations member states committed to strengthen primary health care for the attainment of health to permit people to lead socially and economically productive lives.[20] At the dawn of the new millennium, United Nations member states committed to the attainment of 8 Millennium Development Goals (MDGs), of which 3 are health related (**Fig. 3**).

Based on current trends, goals set for reducing maternal and childhood mortality (MDG 4 and 5) are the least likely to be met in most of the developing world. Although progress is being made in the control of malaria and TB, problems of drug resistance continue to be urgent priorities. Unmet needs for universal access for care and treatment of HIV infections remains unacceptably high. The availability of diagnostics and

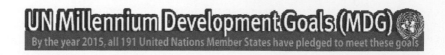

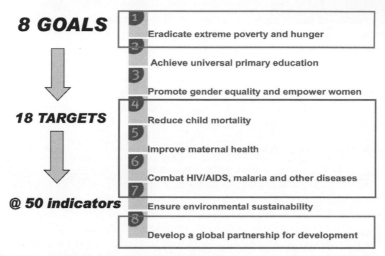

Fig. 3. The UN Millennium Development Goals.

drugs that are affordable, relevant to the needs of the population, and appropriately used is an urgent priority. But the current models of development of new drugs and diagnostics are too slow to keep up with the rapid emergence and spread of infectious diseases around the world and too costly in these days of financial constraints. Attainment of the health-related MDGs requires global commitment on multiple fronts and a new paradigm for innovation.

A New Paradigm in the Making

A new R&D paradigm and business models are urgently needed to accelerate progress along the path from discovery to product adoption and implementation (see **Fig. 2**). Although funding for R&D is critical, an accompanying increase in investment to build capacity for drug and diagnostic R&D, access, and robust health care infrastructure are critical if the full impact of these innovative approaches is to be realized.

A new paradigm is emerging from a convergence of several key insights and developments:

- Simiyu and colleagues[21] examined technology development in Kenya, Uganda, Rwanda, Ghana, and Tanzania and concluded that 3 important needs emerged: proof-of-concept funds, networks linking scientists and entrepreneurs, and physical centers providing shared research infrastructure.
- Health technology innovation needs to be played out on a global stage.[22]
- WHO's Global Strategy and Plan of Action developed by the Inter-Governmental Working Group on Innovation, Intellectual Property and Public Health promotes innovation as a way to improve R&D, access, and build sustainable capacity in developing countries for a range of affordable interventions for diseases that disproportionately affect developing countries.[13]

- The African Network for Drugs and diagnostics Innovation (ANDI) has been established to help build a sustainable platform for R&D innovation in Africa.[23,24] This landmark initiative is already establishing pan-African Centers of Excellence to support product R&D and access in Africa, the first of its kind in Africa. Projects are also being identified for funding through a competitive call for proposals (www.andi-africa.org).
- Several pharmaceutical companies are also establishing R&D facilities in developing countries to support R&D into neglected diseases.[23] Examples include the Novartis Institute in Singapore and AstraZeneka in Bangalore, India. Recently, NovoNordisk donated its compound library to the National Center for Drug Screening in Shanghai to support drug discovery for neglected diseases in collaboration with TDR (WHO Special Program for Research and Training in Tropical Diseases).
- The launch of the African Society for Laboratory Medicine in March 2011 signals a new commitment to improving diagnostic quality and capacity for the continent.

Although the new paradigm is still evolving, steady progress has been made in the following areas.

Drive for Innovation in the Developing World

The product pipeline of drugs and diagnostics for infectious diseases of public health importance in the developing world is meager as traditionally the private sector has shown little interest and companies in the developing world generally do not have sufficient research funding or expertise. In 2008, WHO convened an Inter-Governmental Working Group on Innovation, Intellectual Property and Public Health to examine barriers for innovation in public health such as lack of R&D capacity, intellectual property, and political will. A Global Strategy and Plan of Action (GSPOA) was developed as a result of these discussions and will change the way R&D is prioritized and supported.

In response to the GSPOA, WHO through TDR and several African institutions, initiated the African Network for Drugs and Diagnostics Innovation (ANDI), aimed at promoting and building R&D capacity for target discovery and product development in Africa.[23,24] ANDI is now hosted by United Nations Economic Community for Africa (UNECA) in Addis Ababa Ethiopia and supported by the WHO including TDR, WHO Regional Office for Africa (AFRO) and East Mediterranean region (EMRO), UNECA, the African Development Bank, the European Union, and governments in the region. ANDI is seen as a promising mechanism to support sustainability of product R&D and access to health products in Africa. It is also promoting local ownership and leadership research agenda. ANDI was formally established after a meeting in Abuja, Nigeria in 2008, and a task force was charged with developing the strategic and business plan for ANDI in Geneva, Switzerland, in February 2009. Mapping of the landscape for R&D and manufacturing in Africa was conducted to inform the development of strategic and business plans for ANDI.[13] The mapping revealed that substantial capacity for R&D, clinical trials, and manufacturing of vaccines and generic drugs exists, but available capacity needs to be synergized and harnessed systematically because of a lack of a sustainable mechanism to support translation of research and innovation. Several African institutions have outstanding success stories and they should provide the foci around which concrete actions can be undertaken to strengthen R&D capacity across the continent. The rapid implementation of the ANDI business plan, shared broadly with stakeholders at the 2010 ANDI meeting in Nairobi, Kenya, has now started with the goal to increase African-led capacity for product research and innovation through the discovery, development, manufacturing, and delivery of affordable tools to diagnose and treat diseases that are prevalent on the continent. ANDI could also catalyze local innovation through south-south, north-south, and public-private collaborations, not only for health products and other interventions. Mentorship in quality management is also an important component of ANDI. Calls for project proposals and centers of excellence have resulted in a substantial number of projects now being reviewed by the Scientific and Technical Committee of ANDI and will soon be selected for funding to support ANDI's plan of action.

Similar networks have been initiated in China, India, and Association of Southeast Asian Nations (ASEAN) countries for Asia. The first meeting of the China NDI was held in Shanghai in October 2009 with 149 participants from 48 institutions in 12 provinces, including representatives from Ministries of Science and Technology, Ministry of Health, the Shanghai Municipal Government, and Chinese pharmaceutical, diagnostic, and vaccine companies. A working group of national experts was set up and a home page of the ChinaNDI was launched at www.asiandi.org/china and, to date, several hundred scientists from 20 provinces have registered with the Web site. India had its first meeting in April 2010 at which initial mapping results were discussed. The ASEAN countries have completed an R&D mapping exercise and a business plan is now being developed. It is anticipated that a broad meeting of the Asian networks will be convened in due course. An Americas network has also been implemented in collaboration with the Pan American Health Organization.

Novel Funding Schemes to Accelerate Technological Advances

The human genome and genomes of major infectious disease pathogens have been sequenced, making it possible to identify novel drug targets, microbial diagnostic targets and biomarkers as a signature of infection. Rapid progress in microbial genetics and proteomics, together with breakthroughs in innovative technologies are currently creating opportunities for the field to move drug and diagnostic target discovery rapidly forward. The European Union, in collaboration with several large pharmaceutical companies, is now funding an Innovative Medicines Initiative (IMI) to develop POC diagnostics that can rapidly and accurately identify infections and antimicrobial resistance in patients (http://www.imi.europa.eu/). Although IMI is aimed at reducing the cost of drug trials, the POC technologies would potentially be of tremendous benefit to patients in the developing world.

There are now more funding and players in the field of diagnostics R&D. Donors and funders, notably the Bill & Melinda Gates Foundation, the US National Institutes of Health, the Wellcome Trust, The UK Department of International Development (DFID), and the European Commission have increasingly invested in the development of improved or novel diagnostics for the developing world. In particular, Grand Challenges Canada and the US National Institutes of Health have posted calls specifically targeted at developing country diagnostic developers. It is hoped that this increase in funding will result in a robust pipeline of candidates and products along the diagnostic developmental pathway. But advocacy for diagnostic leadership in developing countries to create or strengthen the health infrastructure for better use of existing and improved diagnostics is still needed.

Funding for the development of POC diagnostics has also been made available from the Bill & Melinda Gates Foundation and Grand Challenges Canada using a novel funding strategy. Separate grants were given for developing novel platforms to improve specimen processing, amplify diagnostic targets, improve signal transduction, develop enabling technologies such as mobile phones, and for developing models to enable rapid and sustainable adoption. The grantees are given 3 years to conduct their R&D, at the end of which, the best-in-class in each category will be asked to collaborate in a convergence of these novel technology platforms to deliver promising POC technologies on integrated platforms that will require little user input other than loading the specimen. The test result can be displayed in hand-held devices or, if necessary, built-in communications modules will allow data transmission for communicating patient results or for surveillance purposes.

Leveraging Investments in Global Health to Strengthen Health Systems

Global health initiatives such as the Global Fund for AIDS, TB, and malaria, the President's Emergency Program for AIDS Relief (PEPFAR), and the President's Malaria Initiative (PMI), in addition to funding improved care and treatment, have the potential to strengthen health systems. However, in a fragile health system, there is the potential to weaken the health system by attracting the best trained health workers to leave their posts in rural settings to work for these global programs as they tend to offer better pay and opportunities for advancement. A WHO initiative to find synergies between global health initiatives and health system strengthening has identified successes and best practice to maximize opportunities to improve the health system in developing countries and offer quality care and treatment.[25]

Educating and Updating Health Care Providers

Health providers need to be educated on how to use and interpret POC technologies correctly and to prescribe appropriate drugs based on the results. Medical and nursing school curricula should be continuously updated through continuing medical education seminars provided to doctors and other health providers on diagnostics, similar to those for drugs, often provided by the pharmaceutical industry.

SPECIAL CONSIDERATIONS FOR DIAGNOSTICS
Advocacy for Appropriate Diagnostics and Diagnostics R&D

There has been increasing realization that the lack of diagnostics is a bottleneck for improving global health but more effort is needed to draw attention to the importance of improved diagnostics. The Bill & Melinda Gates Foundation organized a Global Health Diagnostics Forum, and published a supplement with the Nature Publishing Group on the use of mathematical models to estimate the potential impact of improved diagnostics for the developing world.[26-30] Advocacy should be aimed at donors, at policy makers in developing countries, and at the diagnostic and pharmaceutical industry.

Product Development Partnerships

Diagnostic product development partnerships such as the Foundation for Innovative New Diagnostics (FIND), the Program for Appropriate Technology in Health (PATH), the Infectious Diseases Research Institute (IDRI) and the US National Institutes of Health consortia for Point of Care Diagnostics are working with diagnostic companies to develop POC technologies for TB, malaria, sexually transmitted infections, and neglected tropical diseases. These partnerships create opportunities for researchers in both public and private sectors with disease expertise and knowledge of diagnostic targets to work with those in science and engineering.

An innovation that is urgently needed is the establishment of a network of diagnostic optimization and evaluation centers. Traditionally, most diagnostic products are developed in industrial countries and then sold to developing countries for use in settings that are drastically different from those where the products were designed, engineered, and optimized. Often, the performance and operational characteristics of these products are adversely affected by conditions such as heat, humidity, dust, vibrations, and electrical surges. As a result, these products often require extensive reoptimization and reassembly to work properly, or, as is often the case, they simply break down and are never used again. The establishment of these optimization and evaluation centers will accelerate the development of appropriate diagnostics and has the potential to allow scientists from developing countries to be exposed to cutting edge technologies and perhaps collaborate in product development and validation.

Development of Harmonized Regulatory Standards

The lack of regulatory standards in developing countries has resulted in POC technologies of low quality being sold and used in many developing countries.[31] Companies with high-quality tests cannot compete in markets flooded with cheap low-quality tests. There is an urgent need for countries to adopt quality standards in the approval of diagnostic tests. As most companies do not have funds to conduct trials in every country, securing agreements among countries to reduce regulatory bureaucracy by adopting harmonized regulatory standards with an international or regional platform would reduce the cost for companies seeking to register their products in multiple countries. Those savings can be passed onto the customers, while ensuring purchasing options and competition to maximize choice of proven diagnostic technologies.

Formation of an International Diagnostics Association

Although there are diagnostic manufacturers' associations in Europe, United States, Japan, China, and India, the establishment of an international federation of diagnostic manufacturers' associations would give the diagnostics industry a single voice and an enhanced ability to negotiate with governments and international agencies. Using the International Federation of Pharmaceutical Manufacturers' Association (IFPMA) as a model, this international federation should set quality standards and develop a code of conduct for its members so that the industry has credibility and can work with governments to deal with counterfeit products entering the health system. Creative solutions are also needed to regulate Internet services that promote and sell unproven diagnostic tests.

Technology Assessment to Bridge the Gap Between Research and Policy

Even when diagnostic products are available, many governments do not have clearly defined processes to perform a technology assessment to determine if a new or improved diagnostic tool addresses the country's public health needs. In the last 5 years, the STOP TB Partnership in the WHO has approved the use of several new diagnostic tests to detect pulmonary TB and TB drug resistance. These new tests use different technologies and are not appropriate for all settings. A TB control program in each country needs to develop a framework and a process to assess the test performance, reproducibility, heat stability, whether they are cost-effective for their setting, and whether laboratories in the country have the capacity to use these tests to improve patient care. Data from the technology assessment would form the basis for informed policy decisions and guidelines for the sustainable adoption of new tests. An important component of the assessment is to define criteria for the selection and procurement of new diagnostics. However, the evaluation of test performance and other operational characteristics often suffers from a lack of rigor, such as insufficient sample size or inappropriate study population. To address the lack of quality standards in diagnostic evaluations, WHO/TDR has assembled a Diagnostics Evaluation Expert Panel to provide advice on the design and conduct of diagnostic evaluations. In collaboration with the Nature Publishing Group, supplements on evaluating diagnostics have been published for malaria, sexually transmitted infections, and visceral leishmaniasis, and most recently on CD4 tests.[32]

Capacity Building for Uptake and Delivery of POC Technologies

Technological advancement is only one side of the coin.[33] Even when a test with acceptable performance is available, there are considerable challenges and difficulties in introducing new tests in developing countries. Test introduction and sustainable adoption depend on a robust health care system and many other factors, including adequate human resources, supply chain management, to avoid frequent stock outs of diagnostics and/or drugs. Screening of pregnant women for syphilis is recommended policy in most countries, yet it is estimated that 500,000 babies die each year of congenital syphilis in sub-Saharan Africa because of lack of access to antenatal screening.[34] Although several rapid syphilis tests have been found to have acceptable performance characteristics and to be cost-effective, few countries have taken advantage of these new tools.[35] The Bill & Melinda Gates Foundation is funding a multicountry project on the feasibility and cost-effectiveness of using rapid syphilis tests for screening prenatal women and high-risk populations. By engaging policy makers, national program managers, and stakeholders in the design and implementation of these projects, the investigators managed to bring about policy change to adopt the rapid tests in a timely manner, strengthen health systems, and save lives.

Quality Assurance (QA)

QA is often considered a luxury in developing countries and, as a result, diagnostic testing is performed without QA. Health providers have little confidence in the results of diagnostic tests and in turn, do not order laboratory tests even where they are available. POC tests are often read by eye and the quality of the results are dependent on the quality of the training and the quality of tests procured and stored for long periods at ambient temperatures in rural clinics. It is important to make proficiency panels widely available to ensure that the tests are still valid and that they are correctly used.[36,37] The recent launch of the African Society for Laboratory Medicine is a welcome development that will support quality management of laboratories and build much needed laboratory infrastructure for drug and diagnostic R&D and diagnostic services, especially to perform antimicrobial susceptibility testing to yield data for the development of strategies to combat drug resistance.

SUMMARY

Infectious diseases remain the major causes of morbidity and mortality in the developing world. Affordable effective drugs and diagnostics are critical for patient management and disease control but the development of new drugs and diagnostics is too slow to keep up with the rapid emergence and spread of infectious diseases and drug resistance around the world. A drive for innovative approaches to funding product development has forged new partnerships that will share resources, risks, and hopefully rewards. New R&D paradigms and business models are evolving and will potentially accelerate progress along the path from discovery to product adoption and implementation. This should be accompanied by an increased investment in capacity building for product R&D in the developing world if the full impact of these innovative approaches and investments is to be realized.

REFERENCES

1. Bryce J, Boschi-Pinto C, Shibuya K, et al. WHO estimates of the causes of death in children. Lancet 2005;365:1147–52.
2. African Network for Drugs and Diagnostics Innovation (ANDI) (2008) Part I: Health product R&D landscape in Africa, and Part 2: Collection of meeting, abstract. Founding meeting in Abuja (Nigeria). Available at: http://apps.who.int/tdr/news-events/news/pdf/ANDI-rd-landscape-abstracts.pdf. Accessed July 7, 2011.
3. Mabey D, Peeling RW, Ustianowski A, et al. Diagnostics for the developing world. Nat Rev Microbiol 2004;2:231–40.
4. World Health Organization. Guidelines on the integrated management of childhood illness. Geneva (Switzerland): WHO; 2004.
5. World Health Organization. Guidelines on the management of sexually transmitted infections. Geneva (Switzerland): WHO; 2003.
6. Peeling RW, Mabey D. Point-of-care tests for diagnosing infections in the developing world. Clin Microbiol Infect 2010;16:1062–9.
7. Yager P, Domingo GJ, Gerdes J. Point of care diagnostics for global health. Annu Rev Biomed Eng 2008;10:107–44.
8. Nwaka S, Ridley R. Virtual drug discovery and development for neglected diseases through public-private partnership. Nat Rev Drug Discov 2003;2:919–28.
9. DiMasi JA, Hansen RW, Grabowski HG. The price of innovation: new estimates of drug development. J Health Econ 2003;22(2):151–85.
10. Moran M, Strub-Wourgaft N, Guzman J, et al. Registering new drugs for low-income countries: the African challenge. PLoS Med 2011;8:e1000411.
11. World Health Organization. Antimicrobial resistance: no action today, no cure tomorrow. Geneva (Switzerland): World Health Organization; 2011. Available at: http://www.who.int/world-health-day/2011/world-health-day2011-brochure.pdf. Accessed July 7, 2011.
12. Nwaka S, Hudson A. Innovative lead discovery strategy for tropical diseases. Nat Rev Drug Discov 2006;1:941–55.
13. The strategic and business plan for the African Network for Drugs and Diagnostics Innovation (ANDI) Creating a sustainable platform for R&D innovation in Africa; 2009. Available at: http://apps.who.int/tdr/svc/publications/tdr-research-publications/sbp-andi. Accessed July 7, 2011.
14. Kettler H, White K, Hawkes S. Mapping the landscape of diagnostics for sexually transmitted infections. Geneva (Switzerland): WHO/TDR publication; 2004.
15. The Lewin Group. The value of diagnostics: innovation, adoption and diffusion into health care. Geneva (Switzerland): The Lewin Group; 2005. Available at: http://www.socalbio.org/pdfs/thevalueofdiagnostics.pdf. Accessed July 7, 2011.
16. WHO Task Force on Health Economics. Cost containment and cost analysis of TB control programmes: the case of Malawi. Geneva (Switzerland): World Health Organization; 2003.
17. World Bank. World development report 2004: making services work for poor people. New York: Oxford University Press for the World Bank; 2004.
18. Petti CA, Polage CR, Quinn TC, et al. Laboratory medicine in Africa: a barrier to effective health care. Clin Infect Dis 2006;42:377–82.
19. WHO/TDR Tuberculosis Diagnostics Economic Working Group. Regulation of in vitro diagnostics: a global perspective Diagnostics for tuberculosis: global demand and market potential. The Special Programme for Research and Training in Tropical

Diseases. Geneva (Switzerland): WHO/TDR publication; 2006. p. 194–203. Available at: http://apps.who.int/tdr/svc/publications/tdr-research-publications/diagnostics-tuberculosis-global-demand. Accessed June 1, 2011.

20. Haines A, Horton R, Bhutta Z. Primary health care comes of age. Looking forward to the 30th anniversary of Alma-Ata. Lancet 2007;370:911–3.

21. Simiyu K, Daar AS, Singer PA. Stagnant health technologies in Africa. Science 2010;330:1483–4.

22. Thorsteinsdóttir H, Ray M, Kapoor A, et al. Health biotechnology innovation on a global stage. Nat Rev Microbiol 2011;9:137–43.

23. Mboya-Okeyo T, Ridley RG, Nwaka S. The African network for drugs and diagnostics innovation. Lancet 2009;373:1507–8.

24. Nwaka S, Ilunga T, Da Silva J, et al. Developing ANDI: a novel approach to health product R&D in Africa. PLoS Med 2010;7(6):e1000293.

25. Samb B, Evans T, Dybul M, et al. World Health Organization Maximizing Positive Synergies Collaborative Group. An assessment of interactions between global health initiatives and country health systems. Lancet 2009;373:2137–69.

26. Hay Burgess DC, Wasserman J, Dahl CA. Global health diagnostics. Nature 2006;444(Suppl 1):S1–2.

27. Urdea M, Penny LA, Olmsted SS, et al. Requirements for high impact diagnostics in the developing world. Nature supplement: determining the global health impact of improved diagnostic technologies for the developing world. Nature 2006;444(Suppl 1):73–9.

28. Lim YW, Steinhoff M, Girosi F, et al. Reducing the global burden of acute lower respiratory infections in children: the contribution of new diagnostics. Nature 2006;444(Suppl 1):9–18.

29. Aledort JE, Ronald A, Rafael M, et al. Reducing the burden of sexually transmitted infections in resource-limited settings: the role of improved diagnostics. Nature 2006;444(Suppl 1):59–72.

30. Aledort JE, Ronald A, Le Blanq SM, et al. Reducing the burden of HIV/AIDS in infants: the contribution of improved diagnostics. Nature 2006;444(Suppl 1): 19–28.

31. Peeling RW, Smith PG, Bossuyt PM. A guide for diagnostic evaluations. Nat Rev Microbiol 2006;4(Suppl):S2–6.

32. Nature supplements: evaluating diagnostics are accessible at. Available at: http://apps.who.int/tdr/svc/publications/journal-supplements/mal-guide; http://apps.who.int/tdr/svc/publications/journal-supplements/sti-guide; http://apps.who.int/tdr/svc/publications/journal-supplements/vl-guide. Accessed July 7, 2011.

33. Pang T, Peeling RW. Diagnostic tests for infectious diseases in the developing world: two sides of the coin. Trans R Soc Trop Med Hyg 2007;101:856–7.

34. Schmid G. Economic and programmatic aspects of congenital syphilis prevention. Bull World Health Organ 2004;82:402–9.

35. Senior K. The complex art of making diagnostics simple. Lancet Infect Dis 2009;9:467.

36. Plate DK, on behalf of the Rapid HIV Test Evaluation Working Group. Evaluation and implementation of rapid HIV tests: the experience in 11 African countries. AIDS Res Hum Retroviruses 2007;23:1491–8.

37. Martin R, Hearn TL, Ridderhof JC, et al. Implementation of a quality systems approach for laboratory practice in resource-constrained countries. AIDS 2005; 19(Suppl 2):S59–65.

Index

Note: Page numbers of article titles are in **boldface** type.

A

Accident(s)
   global health–related, 627–629
African Science Academy Development Initiative, 493–494
AITRP, 519
Altruism
   in global health, 540
APACPH. *See* Asia Pacific Academic Consortium for Public Health (APACPH)
Asia Pacific Academic Consortium for Public Health (APACPH), **537–554**
   in N-S partnerships
      case study of, 546–547
   S-S-N collaborative model of
      development of
         catalysts in, 547–549
   in vulnerable populations, 549–550
Association of Schools of Public Health (ASPH) Competency Initiatives
   in global health
      current status of, 579–583
Association of Schools of Public Health (ASPH) Global Health Competencies
   Model Development Project, 583–586

B

Bangladesh
   childhood injuries in, 627
BASIC, 487
Basic science research and education, **669–676**
   described, 669–670
   in global health
      in developing countries, **669–676**
         current status of, 670–671
         methods for strengthening of, 672–675
         problems related to, 671–672
BHP. *See* Botswana-Harvard AIDS Institute Partnership (BHP)
Botswana-Harvard AIDS Institute Partnership (BHP), 519
BRIC, 487

C

Capacity building
   as empowerment

Infect Dis Clin N Am 25 (2011) 707–717
doi:10.1016/S0891-5520(11)00070-5
0891-5520/11/$ – see front matter © 2011 Elsevier Inc. All rights reserved.
id.theclinics.com

Moving?

Make sure your subscription moves with you!

To notify us of your new address, find your **Clinics Account Number** (located on your mailing label above your name), and contact customer service at:

Email: journalscustomerservice-usa@elsevier.com

800-654-2452 (subscribers in the U.S. & Canada)
314-447-8871 (subscribers outside of the U.S. & Canada)

Fax number: 314-447-8029

Elsevier Health Sciences Division
Subscription Customer Service
3251 Riverport Lane
Maryland Heights, MO 63043

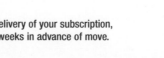

ELSEVIER

Printed and bound by CPI Group (UK) Ltd, Croydon, CR0 4YY

14/10/2024

01773693-0001